DIAGNOSTIC IMAGING FOR
REPRODUCTIVE FAILURE

Dedication

This book is dedicated to those caring for couples with reproductive failure, and to the continued quest for successful and minimally invasive diagnostic and therapeutic imaging modalities for these patients.

Lisa Barrie Schwartz

DIAGNOSTIC IMAGING FOR
REPRODUCTIVE
FAILURE

EDITED BY

Lisa B. Schwartz MD
Assistant Professor, New York University Medical College

David L. Olive MD
Professor and Chief, Reproductive Endocrinology and Infertility
Yale University School of Medicine

Shirley McCarthy MD
Professor, Yale University School of Medicine

WITH AN INTRODUCTION BY

Alan H. DeCherney MD
Professor and Chairman, Department of Obstetrics and Gynecology
UCLA School of Medicine

The Parthenon Publishing Group
International Publishers in Medicine, Science & Technology

NEW YORK   LONDON

Library of Congress Cataloging-in-Publication Data
Diagnostic imaging for reproductive failure / edited by
Lisa B. Schwartz, David L. Olive, Shirley McCarthy
    p. cm.
Includes bibliographical references and index.
ISBN 1-85070-561-5
   1. Infertility – Diagnosis.   2. Generative
organs – Imaging.   3. Infertility – Imaging
  I.   Schwartz, Lisa B.   II.   Olive, David L.
  III. McCarthy, Shirley
[DNLM: 1. Infertility – diagnosis.   2. Diagnostic
Imaging – methods. WP 570 D536 1997]
RC889.D54   1997
616.6'920754-dc21
DNLM/DLC
for Library of Congress   97-12274
                      CIP

British Library Cataloguing in Publication Data
Diagnostic imaging for reproductive failure
   1. Infertility – Imaging.   2. Reproductive organs –
Imaging.   I. Schwartz, Lisa B. II. Olive, David L.
III. McCarthy, Shirley
616.6'92'0754

ISBN 1-85070-561-5

Published in North America by
The Parthenon Publishing Group Inc.
One Blue Hill Plaza
Pearl River
New York 10965, USA

Published in the UK and Europe by
The Parthenon Publishing Group Limited
Casterton Hall, Carnforth
Lancs. LA6 2LA, UK

Copyright © 1998 Parthenon Publishing Group Ltd

First published 1998

Composition by Speedlith, Manchester, UK

Printed and bound by TG Hostench S.A., Spain

Contents

List of principal contributors

Janis M. Brown
Department of Diagnostic Radiology
Yale University School of Medicine
333 Cedar Street
New Haven, CT 06510, USA

Alan H. DeCherney
Department of Obstetrics and Gynecology
UCLA School of Medicine
10833 Le Cont Avenue,
Los Angeles, CA 90095-1740, USA

Morton G. Glickman
Department of Diagnostic Radiology
Yale University School of Medicine
333 Cedar Street
New Haven, CT 06510, USA

Stanton C. Honig
Department of Urology
Yale University School of Medicine
333 Cedar Street
New Haven, CT 06510, USA

Andrew W. Litt
MRI Department of Radiology
HCC Basement
New York University School of Medicine
550 First Avenue
New York, NY 10016, USA

Shirley McCarthy
Department of Diagnostic Radiology
Yale University School of Medicine
333 Cedar Street
New Haven, CT 06510, USA

Margaret J. Nachtigall
Department of Obstetrics and Gynecology
Division of Reproductive Endocrinology and
    Infertility
New York University Medical Center
550 First Avenue
New York, NY 10016, USA

David L. Olive
Department of Obstetrics and Gynecology
Division of Reproductive Endocrinology and
    Infertility
Yale University School of Medicine
333 Cedar Street
New Haven, CT 06510, USA

John A. Rizzo
Institute for Social and Policy Studies
Yale University School of Medicine
10076 Armory Street
Handem, CT 06517, USA

Lisa Barrie Schwartz
Department of Obstetrics and Gynecology
Division of Reproductive Endocrinology
New York University Medical Center
550 First Avenue
New York, NY 10016, USA

Robert C. Smith
Department of Diagnostic Radiology
Yale University School of Medicine
333 Cedar Street
New Haven, CT 06510, USA

Robert N. Troiano
Department of Diagnostic Radiology
Yale University School of Medicine
333 Cedar Street
New Haven, CT 06510, USA

Marlene Zawin
Department of Diagnostic Radiology
Yale University School of Medicine
333 Cedar Street
New Haven, CT 06510, USA

LEGENDS TO COLOR PLATES

Color plate A Normal uterus. Transverse color Doppler scan demonstrates the peripheral arcuate vessels (curved arrow) located between the echogenic endometrial stripe (clear arrow) and the myometrium (short arrow)

Color plate B Laparoscopic view of the anterior peritoneum showing the left obliterated umbilical and epigastric vessels. The inferior ports are inserted lateral to the epigastric arteries

Color plate C Laparoscopic view of the uterus and left ovary

Color plate D Laparoscopic chromopertubation documents tubal patency by allowing visualization of the free flow of blue dye from the fimbriated end of the Fallopian tube

Color plate E Hysteroscopic view of the normal ostia

Color plate F The many laparoscopic appearances of endometriosis. (i) Traditional blue-black lesion. (ii) Traditional lesions, white plaques, and clear vesicles. (iii) Red lesion surrounded by white, fibrotic lesions. (iv) Multiple small reddish-blue cystic lesions. (v) Small red and clear vesicles, white fibrotic plaques, and punctate red lesions

Color plate G The presence of prominent peripheral vascularity on color flow imaging (i) and low-impedance flow on spectral Doppler (ii) are typical and aid in identification.

Color plate H Purely cystic masses in the ovary are common and virtually always physiological, non-neoplastic lesions, although they may be large and occasionally produce symptoms. This figure shows corpus luteal cysts which are similar in appearance to follicular cysts but show typical peripheral vascularity

Color plate I A corpus luteum cyst typically shows prominent peripheral vascularity on color flow imaging. Neoplastic lesions may also be quite vascular and the appearance is often non-specific. In premenopausal patients, the study should be repeated early in a subsequent cycle, when there should be no luteal flow

Color plate J Although lesions with soft tissue components, thick or vascular septations and low-impedance flow are more likely to be malignant, there is considerable overlap in both appearance and vascularity. This figure shows a primarily cystic mass with mural nodularity and high-velocity, low-impedance flow which was resected and diagnosed as an ovarian cancer

Color plate K Normal testis: color flow Doppler ultrasound scan. Straight arrows (CA) to red show normal capsular (circumferential) arteries; curved arrows to blue show centripetal arteries. From reference 50, with permission

Color plate L Varicocele: color flow Doppler scans. (i) Note dilated tubular structure with minimal flow at rest, accentuated with Valsalva maneuver. (ii) Flow in veins at rest and increased flow (yellow hue) with the Valsalva maneuver. From reference 50, with permission

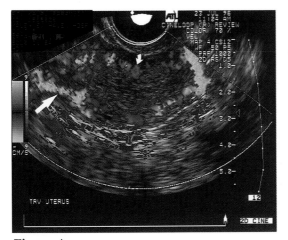

Figure A

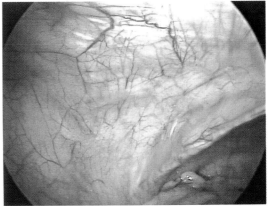

Figure B

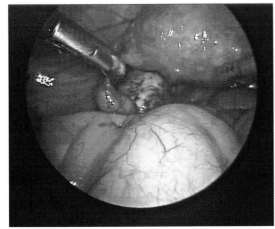

Figure C

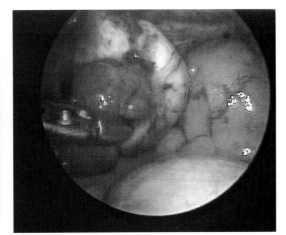

Figure D

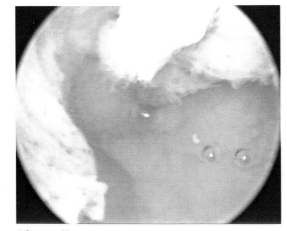

Figure E

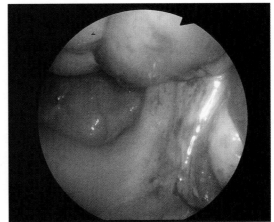

Figure F (i)

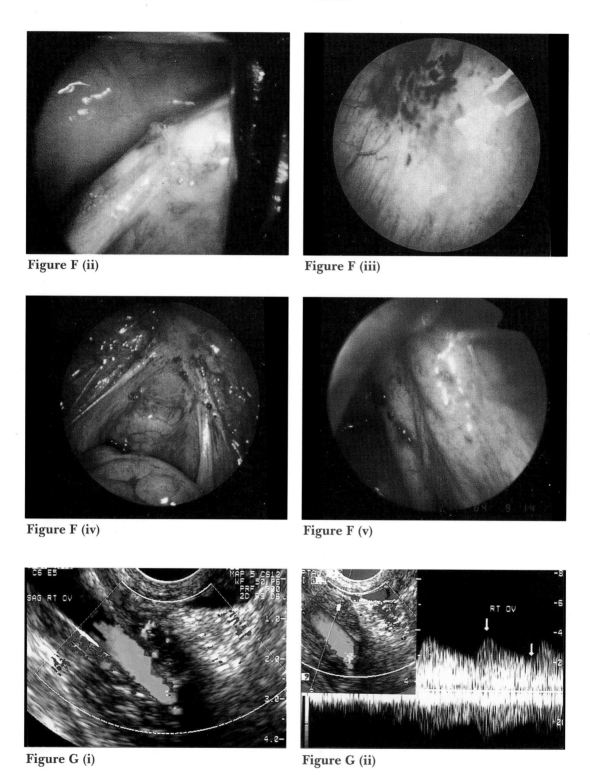

Figure F (ii)

Figure F (iii)

Figure F (iv)

Figure F (v)

Figure G (i)

Figure G (ii)

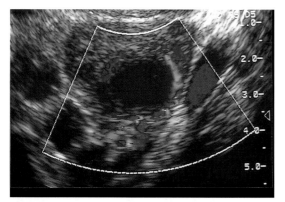

Figure H

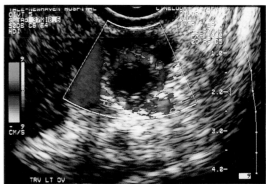

Figure I

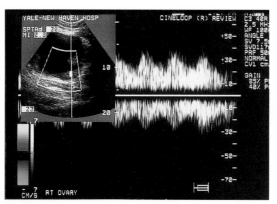

Figure J

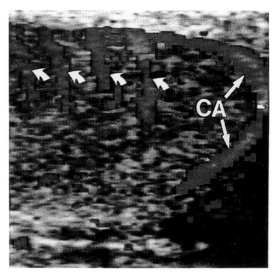

Figure K

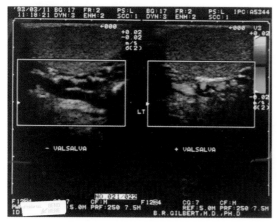

Figure L (i)

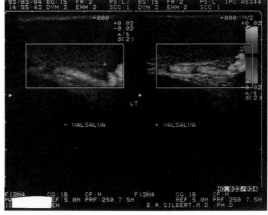

Figure L (ii)

Foreword

Today imaging techniques have become an integral and indispensable part of the practice of obstetrics and gynecology. The application of imaging modalities has provided minimally invasive diagnostic and therapeutic options that were previously unavailable for the couple with reproductive failure.

After an insightful introduction by Dr DeCherney, this book begins with a unique, in-depth review of the basic physics underlying the technique of magnetic resonance imaging, and also reviews the principles of ultrasonography, transvaginal Doppler flow ultrasound and computerized tomography scanning. The choice of distension media for hysteroscopic procedures is reviewed so that the practitioner can be familiar with the advantages and disadvantages of each. Throughout the book, emphasis is placed on imaging techniques and procedures available for the diagnosis and treatment of both female and male causes of reproductive failure. Another unique aspect of this book is that, in addition to pelvic imaging modalities, it also addresses neuroradiology and imaging of the adrenal glands as related to reproductive failure. Both normal and abnormal anatomy is described. The ways in which ultrasonography has shaped the new field of assisted reproductive technologies is discussed. Illustrations, including color images, are provided liberally, and can be used as a guide for practitioners. Current, relevant literature has been referenced in a critical fashion.

The contents of this book can also assist the practitioner in choosing the appropriate diagnostic tests during the investigation of the couple with reproductive failure. Furthermore, a chapter is dedicated to assisting the practitioner with the interpretation of results of diagnostic tests. Especially relevant in this era of cost containment and managed care, the issue of cost-effectiveness is addressed in a separate chapter.

We are grateful for the participation and contributions of experts in the fields of both reproductive endocrinology and radiology, as well as urology. By combining the input of these specialties, the breadth and depth of the information presented in this book is more expansive than if it had been written by members of only one of these groups in isolation. This book will therefore be useful for radiologists, gynecologists, urologists and health care workers in all these fields. These experts have provided us not only with state-of-the-art clinical information, but also with glimpses into the future.

Lisa Barrie Schwartz

Introduction

A. H. DeCherney

THE INTEGRATION OF TECHNOLOGY AND CLINICAL MEDICINE

When I was a medical student some 30 years ago, I remember the professor who taught Physical Diagnosis telling us that our clinical acumen had reached such a high level of perfection that autopsies were no longer necessary to define and confirm clinical diagnoses. Perhaps this was provocation on his part. But nevertheless, three decades later, with exploding technological advances in medicine, this is probably true. Nowhere is this more apparent than in imaging techniques.

The use of diagnostic imaging in cases of reproductive failure illustrates this concept in a profound way. Most clinicians are already aware of the profound impact that advancements in imaging techniques have had on neurological diagnosis. After completing a perusal of this text, I know you will agree with me that the marriage between imaging techniques and reproductive medicine is equally exciting. The menu of available techniques is impressive. Our diagnostic capabilities have been greatly enhanced by the advent of ultrasound and hysterosalpingography, but now Doppler, transcervical tuboplasty, CT scanning and pelvic MRI have dramatically impacted on our practice. Who could imagine practicing today without the use of an office ultrasound machine to make and confirm diagnoses?

In my opinion, it is gratifying to understand the technology associated with the various imaging techniques available to us today; in fact, such an understanding is often of use in arriving at an accurate and thorough interpretation of diagnostic images. This text defines and presents the requisite physical principles and their application to imaging technology in a clear and comprehensive manner.

The authors have selected topics in reproductive medicine on the basis of anatomy and pathology. They begin with a description of normal female pelvic anatomy as visualized with various imaging techniques. Subsequently, diseases of the peritoneum (adhesions), the ovary (ovarian cysts), the tube (salpingitis) and the uterus (adenomyosis) are discussed in an encyclopedic fashion.

If, 30 years ago, someone had proposed that in the future we would be able to write an all-inclusive textbook of gynecology and reproductive endocrinology based on imaging techniques alone, we would have considered it an impossibility. Recall that at that time, all we had at our disposal in the way of imaging options were the hysterosalpingogram, flatplates of the abdomen and pelvic pneumograms (although I have no personal experience of these). It is truly amazing to contemplate how far we have come in expanding on these techniques. A favorite interest of mine is uterine anomalies. In my opinion, all uterine anomalies can be diagnosed through the use of appropriate imaging methods, making it no longer necessary for imaginative mental pictures to be produced from physical findings.

A 14-year-old girl presents with amenorrhea and severe abdominal pain. Her anatomical lesion can now easily be diagnosed and treated appropriately, demonstrating in an albeit simplistic fashion how technology and clinical medicine can be combined to make a difficult diagnosis easy.

Any textbook that addresses reproductive failure must also look at male factor infertility.

A chapter on normal male pelvic anatomy is included, and the authors describe specific tests for examining the prostate, seminal vesicles, vas deferens and testes. These are important and timely inclusions, and constitute an enlightening complement to the approach to the female genital/reproductive tract.

The authors deserve a great deal of credit for including images of the brain in this text. We are all aware of several regulatory mechanisms that are mediated by the brain, such as the effect of prolactinomas on fertility, yet I would never have thought to include this in a text on imaging. This addition is insightful and well-placed, because it is an area of some ignorance in the practice of reproductive endocrinology. In the American Board Examination for Reproductive Endocrinology, a magnetic resonance image of the skull is usually presented to the examinee. I daresay this is one of the most frequently missed kodachromes on the test.

If one had to choose an area of technology that is most important in the explosive interest in reproductive failure, it would have to be assisted reproductive technology (ART). Ultrasound techniques have been, and continue to be, extremely important in the ongoing development of ART, not only for monitoring follicles but also for oocyte retrieval. Ultrasound-guided retrieval has revolutionized ART, removing it from the laparoscopic operating room and converting it to an office procedure. This is addressed in a comprehensive, intelligent manner, even for the person with no experience in the advanced techniques.

I will end on an outcome-oriented note. Evaluation of cost-effectiveness and risk–benefit modalities is extremely appropriate. All agree that these techniques have added a great deal to what we do – how we diagnose clinical conditions and how we treat them. But the issue of cost now must be considered, and this coda to the text explains the relevance of this kind of testing.

This compilation is a wonderful example of the integration of technology and clinical medicine. The old saw of Osler, that if you knew syphilis you knew medicine, I daresay could be altered to 'if you know diagnostic imaging you know reproductive endocrinology and reproductive failure'.

Imaging of the female pelvis: technical considerations

1

R. C. Smith

INTRODUCTION

In order to perform and interpret imaging studies of the female pelvis, one must be familiar with the imaging appearance of normal structures as well as the disease entities which may be encountered. However, it is also important to be familiar with and understand the basic physical principles of the available imaging techniques. This discussion is intended to describe the physical principles of the available imaging techniques used in the evaluation of the female pelvis.

GYNECOLOGICAL ENDOSCOPY

For many of the female pelvic disorders that may lead to reproductive failure, definitive diagnoses are derived from histological interpretation of pathology specimens. However, many pelvic diseases can also be adequately diagnosed by visualization through the laparoscope or hysteroscope. The explosive development of technological advances in gynecological endoscopy has resulted in revolutionary changes in the area of reproductive failure. With the availability of new and improved instrumentation and equipment, laparoscopy and hysteroscopy have recently changed from diagnostic to therapeutic procedures.

LAPAROSCOPY

Laparoscopy has become widely used not only as a diagnostic tool, but also as a means to operate within the abdominal and pelvic cavities. Instruments have been developed which enable a wide range of surgery to be performed through the laparoscope. This includes minor procedures such as lysis of adhesions, to more involved procedures including tubal surgery (fimbrioplasty, neo-salpingostomy, salpingo-ovariolysis, chromo-pertubation), excision of ectopic pregnancies and treatment of severe endometriosis, ovarian cystectomies and myomectomies.

The essential equipment for performing laparoscopy includes: pneumoperitoneum apparatus and insufflating needles, laparoscope, light source, trocars, coagulation apparatus, laser equipment, suction (aspirator) and irrigation cannulas, and forceps and scissors[1]. Modern advances in the technology include the development of: automated pneumoflaters for safe abdominal distension; fiberoptic cables for light transmission; telescopes with rod lens systems which provide clear undistorted views; electro-coagulation, hemostatic clips and ligatures for better hemostatic control and improved safety; atraumatic forceps for gentle tissue handling; dissecting instruments including hydrodissectors for precise tissue dissection; and disposable trocars, which promote sterility and also avoid the problem of becoming blunt with use[1].

The introduction of the video camera is perhaps the most crucial advance that has enabled laparoscopy to move from the role of diagnostics into the realm of therapeutics. The camera not only allows the surgeon to operate more comfortably, but more importantly, allows better understanding, involvement and co-operation from the operating room staff, including the assistants, nurses and anesthesiologists. Before the addition of the video system, only the surgeon was able to view the operative field, rendering the surgical assistant unable to participate in the surgery at full potential. Video laparoscopy allows more than one surgeon to work while watching the image on the screen instead of through-the-lens viewing.

Producing a pneumoperitoneum, with intra-abdominal pressure and the volume of gas – carbon dioxide (CO_2) – within safe limits, is the first requirement for laparoscopy. The gas is introduced into the abdomen using a spring-loaded needle (Veress) inserted through the 'tented-up' umbilicus. The 7-cm needle is commonly used, but longer ones up to 15 cm are available for obese patients or for introducing the pneumoperitoneum through the posterior vaginal fornix[1]. The primary trocar and cannula is inserted blindly after production of the pneumoperitoneum, and has a port to maintain CO_2 flow. The secondary trocars and cannulae are then introduced under direct visualization. A 5-mm laparoscope may be satisfactory for diagnostic laparoscopy, but the 1–11-mm telescope is preferred for video laparoscopy and operative procedures. The standard light source with a power of 150 W is used for diagnostic laparoscopy, but a cold light fountain with a 250-W halogen lamp is necessary for performing operative laparoscopy or using closed-circuit color television[1].

Initially, diagnostic laparoscopy was used primarily to investigate infertility. However, before proceding to a laparoscopy, the infertile couple should first receive a complete 'work-up', including a detailed history and physical examination, hormonal testing, documentation of ovulation, semen analysis and hysterosalpingogram. Other indications have since developed, including: acute or chronic pelvic pain, suspected endometriosis, suspected ectopic pregnancy, pelvic inflammatory disease, suspected adnexal torsion, uterine anomalies and myomas and anticipation of tubal reanastomosis[1]. Once inspection of the upper abdomen is complete, there should be systematic, detailed examination of the pelvic organs, including the uterus,

anterior and posterior cul-de-sacs, both fallopian tubes in their entirety from cornua to fimbriae and both ovaries. Visible signs of endometriosis should carefully be assessed while each pelvic structure is inspected. Fallopian tube abnormalities that can be diagnosed include salpingitis isthmica nodosa (appearing as oval thickenings in the proximal isthmus), adhesive disease and hydrosalpinx. Chromopertubation is performed by injecting dilute methylene blue transcervically to assess tubal patency. Dye will spill at the fimbrial opening if the tubes are open. Dye will not be seen in the tubes if there is proximal blockage, and instead may be seen in the uterine veins due to intravasation of fluid under pressure. Dye will be located inside distended tubes in the case of distal blockage, but will not spill. Normal ovarian activity can be diagnosed by the presence of a follicular cyst, the stigma following ovulation, or the corpus luteum. Other conditions such as polycystic ovaries, streak ovaries, ovotestis, endometriomas and dermoid cysts can be diagnosed.

Operative laparoscopy was initially confined to tubal sterilization. Infertility surgery such as periadnexal adhesiolysis and neosalpingostomy was among the initial laparoscopic procedures to be performed. Operative laparoscopy requires cutting instruments, electrosurgical instruments, probes, grasping instruments and irrigation and suction cannulae. The patient should be placed in a modified lithotomy position, legs abducted and flexed to 5°[1]. Procedures that are of proven value in improving fertility include adhesiolysis, salpingo-ovariolysis, fimbrioplasty and neosalpingostomy[1-3]. Fallopian tube diameter, wall thickness, ampullary mucosal integrity and extent and severity of adhesions all determine the outcome[1]. Patients whose tubal status predicts poor prognosis may benefit more by referral for *in vitro* fertilization and embryo transfer (IVF-ET). Other more recently developed laparoscopic treatments for pelvic diseases related to reproductive failure include myomectomies, ovarian drilling for recalcitrant polycystic ovaries, excisions of endometriomas and dermoid cysts and treatment of severe endometriosis.

Absolute contraindications to laparoscopy include mechanical and paralytic ileus, large abdominal or pelvic masses, hypovolemic shock, cardiac or respiratory failure, severe obstructive airway disease, recent myocardial infarction and irreducible external hernia[1]. Relative contraindications include multiple abdominal incisions, abdominal wall infections, gross obesity, blood dyscrasias and coagulopathy and hiatus hernias[1]. Most laparoscopic complications are avoidable. However, there is a small but significant risk of complications which include extraperitoneal gas insufflation, pneumo-omentum, penetration of a hollow viscus, blood vessel injury, gas embolism, organ perforation, thermal injury, incisional hernias, infections, anesthesia complications and injuries from the operating table[1].

HYSTEROSCOPY

Hysteroscopy is used for diagnosis and treatment of endometrial diseases. A diagnostic hysteroscope consists of a 3.5-mm telescope and a 4-mm sheath, and can be used in the operating room or the office. The Hopkins rod lens system is the optical system in most rigid telescopes, and gives a bright and undistorted image. A flexible hysteroscope does not provide as clear a view, but may provide more ease in visualizing the cornual orifices and is advantageous for visualizing the anomalous uterine canal such as the complete bicornuate uterus. Before a hysteroscopy can be performed, the uterine cavity must be distended either with CO_2 gas or with fluid (e.g. saline, Hyskon, 1.5% glycine). For a diagnostic hysteroscopy using CO_2 gas, the intrauterine pressure should not exceed 40–50 mmHg and the flow rate should not exceed 60 ml/min[1]. Cameras and video systems are available from various manufacturers. Most resectoscopes are modifications of cystoscopes. The sheaths are 7 mm in diameter. The electrosurgical generators have a basic frequency of 475–750 kHz[1], and can deliver cutting and coagulating currents.

Hysteroscopy is useful in the diagnosis and management of uterine lesions, which contribute to approximately 4% of infertility cases[1]. Furthermore, hysteroscopy is important as a component of the evaluation of patients with recurrent miscarriages, affecting 1% of the population, with uterine lesions responsible for 15–25% of cases[1]. Diagnostic hysteroscopy enables directed biopsy of the endometrial lesion rather than a blind curettage. Visible pathological findings may include endometrial polyps, submucosal myomas, intrauterine adhesions, congenital malformations (such as a septum) and retained products of conception; all of these can also be treated with the operative hysteroscope. The hysteroscope can also be used to catheterize the cornual orifice of the fallopian tube to treat proximal occlusions. Endometritis is an absolute contraindication to hysteroscopy. The major potential complication of hysteroscopy is uterine perforation. This can be avoided by using the proper technique, including inserting the telescope through the cervical canal under direct vision without force and operating under laparoscopic guidance for complex procedures.

MAGNETIC RESONANCE IMAGING

Basic physics

Protons contained within the nuclei of hydrogen atoms in both water and fat molecules are the origin of the magnetic resonance signal. When protons are placed within a strong external magnetic field, their behavior is similar to that of a spinning top placed within the gravitational field of the earth. When a conventional top is set spinning, it initially spins undisturbed about its own axis. The axis of the top is initially in perfect alignment with the gravitational field of the earth. As the top slows, its axis begins to tip away from the gravitational field of the earth, and the top then precesses (i.e. the spinning top itself rotates) around the axis of the earth's gravitational field. Eventually, the top stops spinning around its own axis and falls over.

Protons are charged particles that possess 'spin'. The property of spin is a quantum mechanical phenomenon. The proton (and other elementary particles) can be crudely thought of as a small charged particle that rotates around its own axis, similar to a spinning top. The rotational motion gives rise to a small 'intrinsic' magnetic field, since any moving charge (such as a current in a wire) gives rise to a magnetic field.

When protons are placed in a strong external magnetic field (the field denoted as B_0), they behave like tiny magnetic tops. However, the rate of their intrinsic spinning motion is fixed (i.e. they do not 'slow down') and, therefore, the strength of the intrinsic magnetic field is fixed and constant for all protons. Analogous to a conventional spinning top, as long as the intrinsic magnetic field of an individual proton remains aligned with B_0, the proton will rotate around its own axis but will not precess. However, if the intrinsic field of a proton is not aligned along B_0, the proton will not only rotate around its own axis but will also precess around B_0. The rate of precession is directly proportional to the strength of B_0. At 1.5 T, this precessional frequency will be 63.87 MHz.

When protons are placed within an external magnetic field (B_0), the axis of their intrinsic magnetic field can only assume one of two possible orientations: one orientation somewhat along B_0 and one orientation somewhat against B_0 (Figure 1). This is a quantum mechanical effect. Neither of these orientations are directly along B_0. Therefore, all of the protons will be spinning around their own axis and will also precess around the axis of B_0. Since there are only two possible orientations, there will be two populations of protons (Figure 2).

Suppose a large sample of protons (e.g. a patient) is placed in a strong magnetic field (B_0). Due to the presence of B_0, it is energetically more favorable to be aligned somewhat along B_0. However, the energy difference between

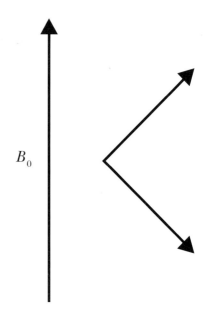

Figure 1 *In the presence of an external magnetic field* B_0, *there are two allowable orientations for an individual proton: one orientation somewhat along and one orientation somewhat against the external field direction*

the two alignment states is very small. At body temperature, the energy of thermal motion greatly exceeds this energy difference, so that individual protons are constantly changing between the two alignment states. Over time, an equilibrium will be reached at which there will be a small net excess of protons in the alignment state along the external field direction, since this is energetically more favorable. This is analogous to a chemical equilibrium.

When equilibrium is achieved, the small net excess of protons aligned along the B_0 direction causes the sample to obtain a net magnetization in the direction of B_0. The precessional motion of the protons in the two alignment states causes the individual protons to be randomly distributed around the axis of the external field as they precess. This random distribution results in zero net magnetization along the plane perpendicular to B_0. Therefore, at equilibrium, the net magnetization of the entire sample of protons will point precisely along B_0.

By convention, magnetization along the external field direction (B_0) is referred to as

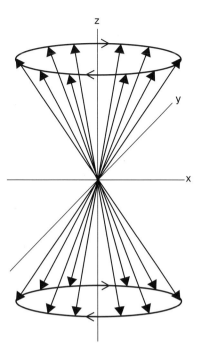

Figure 2 *A group of protons is placed in an external field which is oriented along the z axis of a Cartesian coordinate system. The magnetic field of each individual proton is represented by an arrow. The individual protons rotate (around the z axis) and are randomly distributed (around the z axis) as they rotate. This random distribution results in zero net magnetization in the xy plane. There are two populations of protons: one oriented somewhat along the positive z axis and one oriented somewhat along the negative z axis*

'longitudinal magnetization'. Magnetization in the plane perpendicular to the external field direction is referred to as 'transverse magnetization'. Also by convention, when using a Cartesian coordinate system, the direction of B_0 is defined as the z axis and the transverse plane as the plane formed by the x and y axes.

It suffices to specify the net magnetization when describing an entire sample of protons. Any disturbance of the sample can then be described in terms of its effect on the net magnetization. The individual protons within the sample possess 'spin'. Likewise, the net magnetization can be treated as an object that also has the property of 'spin'. At equilibrium, the net magnetization points exactly along B_0

and will therefore not precess around B_0. However, if any disturbance causes the net magnetization to be no longer aligned with B_0, the net magnetization will precess just like the individual protons.

It can be shown mathematically that the energy difference between the two alignment states is equal to the energy of a photon of frequency equal to the precessional frequency of the individual protons. Therefore, at 1.5 T, this energy difference is equal to the energy of a photon at a frequency of 63.87 MHz. This is a photon in the FM radio frequency (RF) range. Magnetic resonance imaging (MRI) is performed by exposing a sample of protons to external RF radiation (usually referred to as an RF pulse) in the presence of a strong external magnetic field. The RF radiation will serve to disturb the equilibrium state. If the frequency of the RF radiation exactly matches the precessional frequency of the protons, then it will be absorbed and will cause transitions between the two alignment states.

Two independent phenomena will occur when a sample of protons is placed in a strong external magnetic field (B_0) and is exposed to an RF pulse. First, the equilibrium distribution of the individual protons within the two alignment states will be disturbed. The photons of the RF radiation will induce transitions between alignment states. This will cause some protons aligned with B_0 to become aligned against B_0. As more RF energy is applied, the number of protons in the two alignment states will become equal. At this point, the net longitudinal magnetization within the sample will become zero. If additional RF energy is applied, the sample will acquire a net longitudinal magnetization opposite the direction of the external field.

The second effect of an RF pulse is an alteration of the relationship of the individual protons as they precess around the axis of the B_0 field. Recall that at equilibrium, the individual protons precess in a random distribution around the axis of the B_0 field such that there is no net transverse magnetization. An RF pulse not only alters the distribution of protons with respect to the alignment states, it also alters the distribution of protons as they precess. It causes the protons to be no longer randomly distributed but to precess in phase. This results in the development of net transverse magnetization (Figure 3). Since the individual protons precess around the axis of B_0, the net transverse magnetization will also precess around the axis of B_0. This is the origin of the magnetic resonance signal.

To summarize, an RF pulse will have two independent effects:

(1) It will induce transitions between the two alignment states of the individual protons. This will change the net longitudinal magnetization of the sample.

(2) It will cause the individual protons to precess in phase around the axis of the external field. This will create net transverse magnetization.

Once the RF pulse is turned off, the system will return to equilibrium:

(1) Protons will undergo transitions between the two alignment states until the net longitudinal magnetization equals the equilibrium distribution. This is usually referred to as T_1 relaxation. That is, T_1 relaxation is the rate at which the longitudinal magnetization recovers following an RF pulse.

(2) The net transverse magnetization will decay as the individual protons again become randomly distributed around the axis of the external field instead of precessing in phase. This is usually referred to as T_2 relaxation. That is, T_2 relaxation is the rate at which the transverse magnetization decays following an RF pulse.

The greater the T_1 relaxation rate, the more quickly longitudinal magnetization recovers following an RF pulse. The reciprocal of the T_1 relaxation rate is the T_1 relaxation time. Therefore, the greater the T_1 relaxation time, the longer it takes to recover longitudinal magnetization. The greater the T_2 relaxation rate, the more quickly transverse magnetiza-

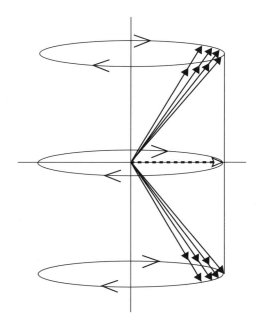

Figure 3 *Following a 90° radio frequency pulse, the protons in the two populations are no longer randomly distributed around the z axis. They begin to precess in phase and rotate as a group. This results in net transverse magnetization within the xy plane (represented by the dashed arrow with the open arrowhead). This net transverse magnetization itself rotates around the z axis and generates the magnetic resonance signal*

tion decays following an RF pulse. The reciprocal of the T_2 relaxation rate is the T_2 relaxation time. Therefore, the greater the T_2 relaxation time, the longer transverse magnetization persists following an RF pulse.

For most structures, T_2 relaxation times are much shorter than T_1 relaxation times. This means that, for most structures, transverse magnetization will decay much more quickly than longitudinal magnetization will recover following an RF pulse.

Instead of looking at the effect of the RF pulse on the individual protons, we can look at its effect on the net magnetization of the sample as a whole. When viewed as a wave phenomenon, RF radiation consists of alternating electric and magnetic fields. The magnetic field of an RF pulse is usually denoted as B_1. Suppose the RF pulse is applied such that the direction of B_1 is perpendicular to the net magnetization of the sample (i.e. within the transverse plane). Since the net magnetization does not lie along the direction of B_1, the net magnetization will precess around the direction of B_1 (since the net magnetization possesses the property of 'spin'). This will cause the net magnetization to rotate toward the transverse plane. The rate of rotation of the net magnetization around B_1 is much smaller than the precessional frequency of the individual protons around B_0, since B_1 is substantially smaller than B_0. Since the RF pulse is of short duration, the B_1 field is present for only a very short time.

Once the net magnetization is no longer oriented along the direction of the B_0 field, it will start to precess around the axis of B_0 (since the net magnetization possesses the property of 'spin'). As the net magnetization rotates around B_0, it induces a current in a receiver coil. This is the origin of the magnetic resonance signal. The frequency of the signal induced in the receiver coil will equal the frequency of rotation of the net transverse magnetization. Recall that this frequency of rotation is determined by the strength of the applied field. As a result of T_2 relaxation, the magnetic resonance signal quickly decays following an RF pulse.

Each RF pulse is usually specified in terms of the degree of rotation of the net longitudinal magnetization toward the transverse plane. For example, a 90° RF pulse would cause all of the longitudinal magnetization to be converted into transverse magnetization. A 180° RF pulse would completely invert the longitudinal magnetization and create no transverse magnetization.

The above discussion shows how a signal can be generated from a sample of protons placed within an external magnetic field and exposed to an RF pulse. In order to generate a useful image, however, the signal emitted must be spatially encoded. Spatial encoding is accomplished in several independent steps. If only the B_0 field is applied, then all portions of a sample will experience the same field strength (assuming the field is perfectly homogeneous). Under this circumstance all

protons within the sample will precess at exactly the same frequency. For standard high field systems, the B_0 field has a strength of 1.5 T and the precessional frequency is equal to 63.87 MHz.

Small changes in the local magnetic field strength will result in small changes in the precessional frequency of the protons. The frequency of the signal emitted by protons following an RF pulse is equal to their precessional frequency. Therefore, if a group of protons all precess at the same frequency, they will all emit a signal at the same frequency following an RF pulse. Likewise, protons that precess at different frequencies will emit a signal at different frequencies.

As long as the local field strength remains constant throughout a sample of protons, all protons will precess at the same frequency. However, suppose we superimpose (on the B_0 magnetic field) an additional small magnetic field, which varies along a specified direction (usually referred to as a gradient field). The magnitude of the gradient field is very small compared with the B_0 field. The result of the gradient field is to cause the precessional frequency of the protons within a sample to vary in a known manner along a specified direction. For example, if a gradient field is applied along the z direction, then precessional frequencies will vary as a function of z. Since the gradient field is small, it will cause only a small variation in frequency. The gradients used in clinical MRI are such that the frequency change they induce is of the order of several kilohertz (kHz) per centimeter.

Suppose a small gradient is applied along the z direction, and induces a change in frequency of magnitude 2 kHz/cm. At the center of this section the field strength is 1.5 T. At one end of the section the field strength is slightly less than 1.5 T and at the other end of the section the field strength is slightly greater than 1.5 T. Protons within this section will precess in the frequency range from 63.87 MHz − 1 kHz to 63.87 MHz + 1 kHz. The difference between the highest and lowest frequencies is 2 kHz. Protons outside this section of tissue will precess at frequencies less than 63.87 MHz – 1 kHz or greater than 63.87 MHz + 1 kHz.

If an RF pulse is applied which contains frequencies between 63.87 MHz – 1 kHz and 63.87 MHz + 1 kHz, then it will excite only the 1-cm section of tissue that contains protons precessing in this frequency range. In this same manner, by applying a gradient along the x or y direction, sagittal or coronal sections of tissue can be selectively excited. The associated gradients are usually referred to as section (or slice) select gradients. This is how a section of tissue is selectively excited during MRI.

Once a section of tissue is selectively excited, there still remains the problem of spatially encoding the signal such that a useful image can be obtained. Suppose we excite an axial section of tissue by applying the section select gradiant along the z axis. We then have to spatially encode the signal along the x and y axes. Prior to measuring the signal, we can apply a small gradient along the y axis. While this gradient is on, the precessional frequency of protons within the sample will vary as a function of position along the y axis. Once the gradient is turned off, all the protons will again precess at the same frequency (63.87 MHz when the main magnetic field strength is 1.5 T). However, while the gradient was on, some protons will precess more rapidly than others (and vice versa). This will alter the phase relationships as a function of position along the y axis. This gradient is referred to as the phase encoding gradient.

Next, during the process of signal measurement, a third gradient can be applied along the x axis such that the precessional frequency of protons within the excited section of tissue will vary as a function of position along the x axis. This is referred to as the read gradient (or frequency encoding gradient). The measured signal will therefore consist of a superposition of signals at different frequencies. Each frequency component will itself consist of a superposition of signals with different phases. The strength of the read gradient determines the range of frequencies

present within the signal. For most clinical applications, the strength of the read gradient is such that the signal will contain frequencies in a range of ± 16 kHz above or below the center frequency of 63.87 MHz. Such a signal is said to have a 'bandwidth' of 16 kHz.

The received signal is an analog signal (which is a continuous function of time). The received signal is actually 'sampled' (i.e. measured) at multiple discrete points of time (typically a power of 2, such as 256 times) during the signal measurement process. In this manner, an analog signal is converted into a digital signal (which is a discrete function of time). The number of samples taken is equal to the size of the image matrix along the frequency direction.

It can be shown mathematically that a discrete Fourier transform can then be applied to convert the digital signal into multiple (typically 256) component frequencies. The Fourier transform converts a function of time (expressed as signal intensity at a given time) into a function of frequency (expressed as signal intensity at a given frequency). After a Fourier transform is performed on the received signal, the signal intensity of the 256 component frequencies is determined. But each of these 256 frequencies consists of multiple phase components. The number of phase components equals the size of the image matrix along the phase-encoding direction (typically 128 or 192).

The signal intensity of each phase component cannot be measured directly. Only the composite signal at each frequency can be determined. Therefore, an individual signal measurement yields 256 different signal intensities, each of which equals the sum of 128 unknown phase components. In order to determine these 128 unknown quantities, 128 different equations must be generated (recall that the solution for n unknowns requires n equations).

By repeating the signal measurement process 128 times, 128 equations are generated for each frequency component. The phase gradient is varied for each measurement in order to generate data that are not redundant. This process is equivalent to sampling the phase data just as we sampled the frequency data in order to be able to perform a Fourier transform. The interval of time between repeated measurements is denoted the TR (time of repetition).

The MRI process therefore consists of the following steps:

(1) A collection of protons (i.e. a patient) is placed within a strong external magnetic field of known strength (B_0).

(2) A small magnetic field gradient is applied along the x, y, or z axis. For illustrative purposes assume this gradient is applied along the z axis to generate an axial section.

(3) An RF pulse is applied in a specific frequency range to selectively excite a thin section of tissue at a specific location. For most applications, optimal excitation is achieved by using a 90° RF pulse. This creates net transverse magnetization within the section of interest.

(4) A small gradient is applied along the y axis to induce phase changes as a function of position along the y axis. This is done after the 90° pulse but prior to signal measurement.

(5) At a specified time (usually referred to as the echo time, TE) following the 90° pulse, a small gradient is applied along the x axis and the signal is measured in the presence of this gradient. A Fourier transform is then applied, to break up this signal into its component frequencies.

(6) This process is repeated as many times as there are phase-encoding steps. The time interval between the different excitation pulses (i.e. the TR interval) is typically much greater than TE. Once the signal is measured from one section, there is nothing left to do with that section until the TR interval has expired. This allows multiple different sections to be excited during the same TR interval. This is usually referred to as multiplanar imaging.

In addition, in order to improve the signal/noise ratio, not only is the process repeated 128 times for 128 phase-encoding steps, but it can be repeated many times for each phase-encoding step. The number of excitations per phase-encoding step is usually referred to as the number of signal averages (NSA) or number of excitations (NEX).

Therefore, the total imaging time for the MRI sequence as described above is given by:

$$\text{Total imaging time} = (\text{TR}) \times (\text{NSA}) \times (\text{number of phase encodings})$$

The imaging sequence described up to this point leaves out one important facet. Ideally, the main external magnetic field would be of equal magnitude at all points within the magnet. In reality, however, small imperfections always exist. These imperfections result in fixed heterogeneities in the main field. That is, due to imperfections, some places within the bore of the magnet will always be at slightly higher field strengths than others. These fixed heterogeneities cause local differences in precessional frequencies.

What is the effect on the magnetic resonance signal of local imperfections in the main magnetic field? Recall that the transverse magnetization created by an RF pulse precesses about the axis of the main magnetic field to generate the MR signal. The frequency of this precession (and hence the frequency of the signal) in any small region of a patient being imaged is dependent upon the local field strength.

The signal will be maximal in a small region if all the transverse magnetization within that region precesses at precisely the same frequency. Otherwise, if there is precession at multiple different frequencies, the individual signals in even very small regions will be out of phase and the overall signal will not be maximal. This type of signal loss is said to be due to dephasing.

Were it not compensated for, this dephasing would cause significant signal loss in clinical imaging. In order to compensate for fixed heterogeneities of the main external field, an additional RF pulse is incorporated into each imaging sequence. This additional pulse is actually a 180° pulse that is applied at time TE/2 after each 90° RF pulse. This compensates for the fixed heterogeneities in the following manner. When there is a fixed heterogeneity in the external field, one portion of the field has a slightly greater strength than does another portion. Transverse magnetization in the stronger area precesses slightly faster than in the weaker area of the field and therefore acquires a relative positive phase.

Following application of a 180° pulse, this phase relationship is reversed, such that transverse magnetization that had been precessing ahead gets behind. Since the transverse magnetization that is then behind is still in the stronger field (assuming that the heterogeneities are fixed) it will once again catch up. The time required for it to catch up will equal a second interval of time of length TE/2 following the 180° pulse.

By applying the 180° pulse at time TE/2, the decay in signal that would otherwise occur due to field heterogeneity is cancelled out at time TE when the signal is measured. In fact, the signal initially decays up to the time of the 180° RF pulse. The signal then transiently increases to a maximal value at time TE, at which time signal measurement is performed. The transient increase in signal caused by the 180° pulse is like an echo. It is due to the rotation (or spin) of the net magnetization by the 180° pulse. The term spin echo sequence is applied to those sequences that use a 180° RF pulse.

Image weighting

The meanings of the terms T_1-weighted, T_2-weighted and proton density (or intermediate)-weighted images are now reviewed. For conventional spin echo images, the signal intensity (S) is proportional to $N(h)(1 - e^{-TR/T_1})e^{-TE/T_2}$. That is, S is directly proportional to the density of protons (denoted by $N(h)$). All other factors being equal, the greater the density of protons the greater the signal. S is directly proportional to an exponential term in T_1. The greater the T_1 value the less the signal (for a given TR, $1 - e^{-TR/T_1}$ decreases as T_1 increases). S is directly proportional to an exponential term in T_2. The greater the T_2 value, the greater the signal (for a given TE, e^{-TE/T_2} increases as T_2 increases).

This is meant to show that all images, regardless of the parameters chosen, will have signal intensity dependent upon T_1, T_2 and proton density. However, depending upon the choice of TR and TE, one parameter can be made to dominate the signal intensity characteristics. Hence, the term weighting is used.

Recall that 90° pulses convert longitudinal magnetization into transverse magnetization. It is the transverse magnetization rotating around the axis of the external field that generates the magnetic resonance signal. In order to determine spatial position, the excitation process is repeated many times. The time interval between 90° pulses is the TR (or repetition time).

Following each 90° pulse the net longitudinal magnetization becomes zero. During the TR interval longitudinal magnetization will recover to a degree dependent upon the T_1 relaxation time. For tissues with a short T_1 (such as fat) there is near complete recovery during each TR interval. For tissues with a long T_1 (those with a high water content) there is not complete recovery of longitudinal magnetization when the TR interval is short. It is for this reason that, in order to generate 'T_1-weighted' images, short TR intervals are used. This allows differential recovery of longitudinal magnetization between different tissues, depending on their T_1 values.

When long TR intervals are used almost all tissues have enough time to undergo complete recovery of longitudinal magnetization ($1 - e^{-TR/T_1}$ approaches 1 as TR >> T_1 for all tissues). Therefore, to eliminate T_1 contrast, long TR intervals are used.

The other major factor that determines tissue contrast is echo time (TE). This is the time at which the signal is measured after the 90° pulse. Immediately after a 90° pulse the net transverse magnetization is at its maximum. It decays rather quickly as the precessing protons get out of phase. The rate at which this dephasing occurs is dependent on T_2. The greater the T_2 value, the longer the transverse magnetization persists. Therefore, in order to develop T_2 contrast, the echo time is chosen to be relatively long, so that some tissues will have lost a significant amount of transverse magnetization and others will have retained a significant amount.

In order to eliminate (or reduce) T_2 contrast, a relatively short echo time is used. That way, no tissue will undergo a significant loss of transverse magnetization during the TE interval (i.e. e^{-TE/T_2} approaches 1 for TE $<<$ T_2).

To summarize:

(1) To eliminate T_2 contrast we choose a short TE. To develop T_1 contrast we choose a short TR. Hence, a 'T_1-weighted' image uses a short TR and a short TE (e.g. TR = 400–600 ms, TE = 10–20 ms).

(2) To eliminate T_1 contrast we use a long TR. To develop T_2 contrast we use a long TE. Hence, a 'T_2-weighted' image uses a long TR and a long TE (e.g. TR = 2000–2500 ms, TE = 60–80 ms).

(3) By using a long TR to eliminate T_1 contrast and a short TE to eliminate T_2 contrast, a 'proton density-weighted' image is obtained (e.g. TR = 2000–2500 ms, TE = 10–20 ms).

Contrast characteristics in clinical imaging

Both T_1- and T_2-weighted sequences should be acquired when the female pelvis is imaged. T_1-weighted images provide a general overview of all the structures of the pelvis. They are useful for the detection of lesions which contain lipid and/or blood products, lymph nodes and bony abnormalities, and for the visualization of bowel. On T_1-weighted images, the normal uterus and ovaries have a homogeneous intermediate signal intensity. No internal architecture is usually discernible.

T_2-weighted images are essential to delineate the normal zonal anatomy of the uterus and to depict the internal architecture of the ovaries. In virtually all premenopausal patients, three distinct zones of signal intensity can be visualized in the uterine corpus[1]. An inner zone of high signal intensity corresponds to the endometrium. An adjacent zone of low signal intensity corresponds to the so-called junctional zone. The remainder of the myometrium has intermediate signal intensity.

The cervix also has a unique zonal anatomy on T_2-weighted images[1]. At least three distinct zones of signal intensity can always be seen. An inner zone of high signal intensity corresponds to the endocervical canal. An adjacent zone of very low signal intensity corresponds to the predominantly fibrous portion of the cervical stroma. An outer zone of intermediate signal intensity is continuous with and isointense to the outer myometrium. Sometimes a fourth zone of intermediate signal intensity can be seen between the endometrial canal and fibrous stroma. This most probably represents the mucosa of the endocervical canal.

In virtually all premenopausal patients, the ovaries are readily identified on T_2-weighted images. They appear as ovoid structures with a stroma of intermediate to low signal intensity, and this usually contains multiple round follicular cysts with very high signal intensity. In most postmenopausal patients, the ovaries are smaller in size and usually contain only a few tiny cysts within the stroma.

The normal vagina shows walls of low signal intensity and may contain some fluid or mucus of high signal intensity. The peri-vaginal venous plexus is usually visualized as curvilinear serpiginous high-signal structures surrounding the vaginal walls. The urethra is clearly visible on axial images as a round structure just anterior to the vagina below the bladder base.

Imaging sequences

Imaging sequences used when the female pelvis is evaluated include conventional spin echo (CSE), fast spin echo (FSE) and chemical selective sequences. Until recently, all T_2-weighted imaging of the pelvis was performed using CSE sequences. However, the FSE sequence can be used to provide improved image quality and resolution while also providing a reduction of imaging time. There are a number of different imaging parameters that must be chosen when FSE sequences are used. In addition, there are unique contrast characteristics of FSE T_2-weighted images as compared to CSE T_2-weighted images.

In order to facilitate determination of the appropriate imaging parameters and understanding of the contrast characteristics of the FSE sequence, the CSE technique and some of the physical concepts that form the basis of the FSE technique are reviewed.

Conventional spin echo

CSE pulse sequences acquire data as described previously. For each section, a section-selective 90° excitation pulse is followed by a 180° pulse at time TE/2 and an echo (or signal) is then measured at time TE. The phase-encoding gradient is usually applied between the 90° and 180° pulses. The term multiplanar (or multisection) imaging is used because multiple sections can be excited during each TR interval. This allows multiple different sections to be imaged in the same amount of time. The total number of sections that can be acquired is dependent upon the TR and TE times. The greater the TR, the greater the number of sections that can be acquired for a given TE. The greater the TE, the fewer the number of sections that can be acquired for a given TR.

In a similar manner, there is nothing to prevent the acquisition of multiple echoes following a 90° excitation pulse. This is achieved by applying multiple 180° pulses after each 90° pulse. This is referred to as multi-echo imaging. For example, a 180° pulse can be applied at time $TE_1/2$ after a 90° pulse. An echo can then be measured at time TE_1. A second 180° pulse can then be applied at time $(TE_1 + TE_2)/2$ and a second echo measured at time TE_2.

When a CSE sequence is used to generate T_1-weighted images, it is performed with a single echo in a multiplanar acquisition. By definition, the TE is usually chosen as short as possible in order to maximise T_1 weighting. When a CSE sequence is used to generate T_2-weighted images, a much longer TE is required. If only the long TE echo were measured, there would be significant 'dead' time in waiting to measure such a late echo. Therefore, it is customary to measure an earlier echo as well and generate a proton density-weighted (also called an intermediate-weighted) image. There is no additional time required to do this, as the earlier echo is measured while waiting for the late echo. Thus, most CSE T_2-weighted sequences are multi-echo and multiplanar.

When a multi-echo CSE sequence is performed, each echo measured following a given section-selective 90° excitation is acquired with the same phase-encoding gradient. By the time the next 90° pulse is applied (i.e. after the TR interval has elapsed), all of the transverse magnetization created by the prior 90° pulse will have decayed to zero. Therefore, all of the phase changes induced by the prior phase-encoding gradient will no longer be present. This means that, for CSE pulse sequences, each phase-encoding gradient affects the signal of only echoes measured during the same TR interval.

CSE sequences are very time efficient at generating T_1-weighted images. The TR is usually of the order of 400–600 ms and the minimum TE is usually chosen. The minimum TE value is usually between 10 and 20 ms. Even for a 192-phase matrix and NSA = 1 or 2, images of a large number of locations can be obtained in 2–4 min. However, CSE sequences are not very time efficient at generating T_2-weighted images. This results from the obligatory use of a much longer TR (usually at least 2000 ms) and a much longer TE. The longer TE results in a long 'dead' time waiting to measure late echoes.

Due to the inherently lower signal/noise ratio of T_2-weighted images, at least two signal averages are usually required. This means that even with a 128-phase matrix size, the imaging time of CSE T_2-weighted sequences is at least 8–9 min. This limits the attainable resolution and necessitates the use of additional imaging options to help reduce motion-related artifacts associated with the long imaging times.

Fast spin echo

The FSE technique is a variation of the CSE technique. One of the reasons that it takes so long to generate T_2-weighted images with CSE sequences is that a large value of TE must be used. This means that a large amount of imaging time is simply wasted waiting to measure a late echo. Is there a more efficient means of data collection?

Each signal measurement of a CSE sequence is made following the application of a different strength phase-encoding gradient. The number of different phase-encoding gradient strengths is equal to the size of the phase matrix. In general, the simplest scheme for applying the phase-encoding gradients is to go from the strongest negative gradient to the strongest positive gradient (or vice versa) in sequential fashion. If a 128-phase matrix size is used, then we can number the gradients as $-G_{64}, -G_{63}, \ldots, -G_1, +G_1, \ldots, +G_{63}, +G_{64}$. The subscript then corresponds to the strength of the gradient; the plus or minus signs correspond to the polarity.

The greater the strength of the phase-encoding gradient, the lower the signal of the echo. This makes intuitive sense, since the greater the phase-encoding gradient strength, the greater the amount of dephasing and signal loss. This effect is so pronounced that the vast majority of the magnetic resonance signal is actually determined by a small number of echoes acquired with the weakest phase-encoding gradients. An image with reasonable signal/noise ratio could be recon-

structed by acquiring only echoes with, say, the 16 or 32 weakest phase-encoding gradients. Unfortunately, such an image would appear very blurred.

Most of the signal and contrast characteristics of MRI are determined by echoes acquired with the weak phase-encoding gradients. These are usually referred to as low-order echoes. The stronger phase-encoding gradients (i.e. high-order echoes) provide mainly spatial resolution information. An image with reasonable resolution could be reconstructed by acquiring only echoes with the 16 or 32 strongest phase-encoding gradients. Unfortunately, such an image would appear very noisy.

By combining the data from the low-order and high-order echoes (as well as all echoes in between), an image with adequate signal/noise ratio and without blurring can be obtained. These concepts are important for the understanding of the fast spin echo sequence. To summarize: echoes acquired with weak phase-encoding gradients provide mainly signal and contrast. Echoes acquired with strong phase-encoding gradients provide mainly spatial resolution.

FSE sequences exploit the relationship of the strength of the phase-encoding gradient to the signal and spatial resolution of an image. To increase imaging speed, a different phase-encoding gradient can be used for each echo of a multi-echo train following a 90° RF pulse. This increases the amount of phase-encoded data acquired per section per TR interval.

The FSE sequence acquires a train of up to 32 spin echoes following each section-selective 90° pulse. This is achieved by applying multiple 180° pulses in rapid succession to generate multiple spin echoes. A different phase-encoding gradient is used for each echo. The number of 180° pulses applied is referred to as the echo train length (ETL) and the spacing between echoes is referred to as the echo spacing (ESP). Thus, the FSE sequence acquires up to 32 points of phase-encoded data in each section per TR interval before moving on to the next section. Therefore, for equal TR, phase matrix size and NSA, the FSE sequence can reduce imaging time (compared with CSE sequences) by a factor equal to the ETL. The pulse sequence diagram for a CSE sequence is shown in Figure 4. For comparison, the pulse sequence diagram for a FSE sequence is shown in Figure 5.

The method of data collection used for FSE sequences leads to unique imaging characteristics. Multiple echoes, each with a different TE and different phase-encoding gradient, are measured during each TR interval. The signals from all of these measurements are used to generate a single image. There is T_2 decay of the magnetic resonance signal between echoes of the multi-echo train. Therefore, the early echoes have the most signal and the late echoes have the least signal, owing to T_2 decay. The signal loss for later echoes will therefore be greatest for tissue components with a short T_2 value.

The greater the strength of the phase-encoding gradient, the greater the degree of phase-induced signal loss. Therefore, those echos acquired with the weak phase-encoding gradients will have the least phase-induced signal loss and those echoes acquired with the strong phase-encoding gradients will have the most phase-induced signal loss. Those echoes acquired with the low-order (i.e. weak) phase-encoding gradients determine the signal and contrast of an image, and those echoes acquired with the high-order (i.e. strong) phase-encoding gradients determine the spatial resolution and edge sharpness of an image.

What does all of this have to do with how contrast is determined for an FSE image? Suppose the low-order phase-encoding gradients are applied to the late echoes of the multi-echo train. This will cause the least amount of phase-induced signal loss for the late echoes. Since most of the signal and contrast of such an image will come from echoes with a long TE, the image will appear T_2-weighted. The signal from these late echoes will be relatively enhanced, since there is little phase gradient-induced signal loss compared with a CSE sequence with an equivalent TE.

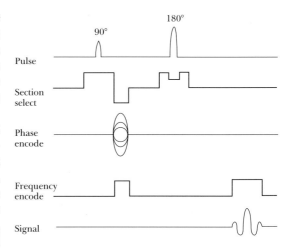

Figure 4 *Pulse sequence diagram for a conventional spin echo technique. This occurs for each section during each time of repetition interval. Note that the phase-encoding gradient is applied prior to the 180° pulse*

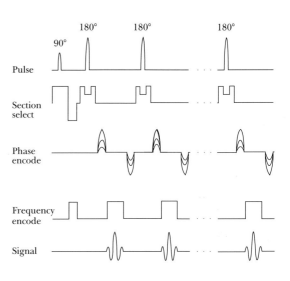

Figure 5 *Pulse sequence diagram for a fast spin echo technique. Multiple 180° pulses are applied following each 90° pulse. This also occurs for each section during each time of repetition interval. Each 180° pulse generates an echo (signal) which is measured in the presence of the frequency-encoding gradient. Note that the phase-encoding gradients are applied after each 180° pulse and then rebound prior to the next 180° pulse*

At the same time, the high-order (i.e. strong) phase-encoding gradients will be applied to the early echoes. Echoes acquired with the high-order phase-encoding gradients determine the spatial resolution and edge sharpness of the image. Since these are the earliest echoes, they will have the least amount of signal loss due to T_2 decay. Therefore, the signal of the echoes which determine spatial resolution and edge sharpness will be relatively enhanced compared with a CSE sequence with an equivalent TE.

Suppose the low-order phase-encoding gradients are applied to the early echoes of a multi-echo train. Since most of the signal and contrast of such an image will come from echoes with a short TE, the image will appear T_1-weighted or proton density-weighted, depending upon the TR. At the same time, the high-order phase-encoding gradients will be applied to the late echoes. The late echoes will therefore undergo significant signal loss, both due to T_2 decay and induced by the strong phase-encoding gradient. These echoes will therefore have little useful residual signal. Since these echoes are necessary for spatial resolution and edge sharpness, the images will appear blurred, with structures having unsharp edges.

The blurring effect will be most pronounced for structures with a short T_2, since these structures will have the greatest T_2 decay for the late echoes. This edge blurring will be along the phase-encoding direction, as a result of the method of phase-encoded data collection for FSE images. The frequency-encoded data for FSE images are collected in the same manner as the frequency-encoded data for CSE images. The edge blurring (and loss of spatial resolution) of T_1-weighted and proton density-weighted FSE images is most pronounced for small objects with a short T_2 and thin objects oriented perpendicular to the phase-encoding direction. The degree of image blurring can be dramatic (Figure 6).

The choice of ETL and ESP will clearly affect the amount of blurring for T_1-weighted and proton density-weighted FSE images. Blurring will be minimized for a shorter ETL

and shorter ESP. In most applications related to the pelvis, there is no need for proton density-weighted FSE images, so this is of little concern. T_1-weighted images are best acquired with CSE techniques. Some T_1-weighted images use the earliest possible echo, there is little advantage in using an FSE technique. The imaging time would be the same with both techniques in acquiring the same number of sections.

If the FSE technique is used to generate T_1-weighted or proton density-weighted images, an ETL no greater than 6 should be used to minimize image blurring. The minimum possible ESP should also be used. In addition, the use of a higher phase matrix will reduce blurring along the phase-encoding direction.

FSE images do not have a single TE time that can be specified. In general, when a TE (usually referred to as an effective TE) is chosen for an FSE sequence, the phase-encoding scheme is as follows: if the effective TE is chosen as $n \times ESP$, then the weakest phase-encoding gradients are applied to the nth echo of each multi-echo train ($n \leq ETL$). For example, suppose that ESP = 20 ms and ETL = 16. Echoes will be collected at 20 ms, 40 ms, 60 ms, ..., 320 ms for each 16 echo multi-echo train. If the phase matrix size is 192, then 12 multi-echo echo trains will be required (192/16 = 12). If an effective TE of 100 ms is chosen, then the 12 weakest phase-encoding gradients will be applied to the 5th echo (5×20 ms = 100 ms) of each multi-echo train.

What about the choice of TR for FSE sequences? For a given value of TR, phase matrix size and NSA, the imaging time is inversely proportional to the ETL. However, the number of section locations is also inversely proportional to the ETL. It is advantageous to use as long a TR as possible. The greater the TR value, the greater the degree of recovery of longitudinal magnetization between excitations and hence the greater the signal/noise ratio of the image. In addition, the greater the TR, the greater the elimination of T_1-weighting. Beyond a certain point, however, there is little if any significant

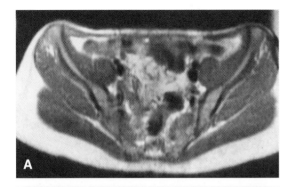

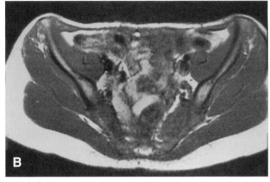

Figure 6 (A) *Conventional spin echo T_1-weighted image through the mid-pelvis (600/18, 256×192 matrix). (B) Fast spin echo T_1-weighted image through the same location (600/18, 256×192 matrix, echo train length = 16, echo spacing = 18). Note the severe blurring of the fast spin echo image*

additional recovery of longitudinal magnetization as the TR is increased further. For most tissues, including water, there is near complete recovery of longitudinal magnetization for a TR value of about 5000 ms or greater. Therefore, there is little advantage (with respect to improving the signal/noise ratio and degree of T_2-weighting) in using a TR of much greater than 5000 ms. An exception is the use of a higher TR in order to obtain a greater number of sections.

As the ETL is increased, echoes are acquired with later echo times. The later the echo time, the less the signal. This is most pronounced for tissues with a short T_2. These tissues will have virtually no signal left for very late echoes. This loss of signal for late echoes will be most pronounced when the high-order phase-encoding gradients are applied to the late echoes (e.g. for a T_1- or

proton density-weighted FSE image). This will increase the blurring of such images. This effect is much less pronounced for T_2-weighted FSE images, since for these images the high-order phase-encoding gradients are applied to the early echoes anyway.

When obtaining T_2-weighted images, a long effective TE must be chosen. The maximum value of the effective TE is directly proportional to the ETL (it is equal to the product of ETL and ESP). Therefore, the ETL must be chosen such that the desired effective TE can be attained. For example, suppose ESP = 20 ms and ETL = 4. Then the maximum achievable effective TE is 80 ms (4×20 ms = 80 ms). If an effective TE of 120 ms is desired, then an ETL of at least 6 would have to be used.

Ideally, then, assuming the ETL is long enough to attain the desired effective TE, the TR should be chosen to be between 5000 and 6000 ms, and the ETL then adjusted accordingly to obtain the desired number of section locations.

Contrast characteristics of FSE images

The contrast characteristics of T_2-weighted FSE images will be very similar to CSE T_2-weighted images. One important exception is the appearance of lipids (e.g. subcutaneous fat). Depending on the choice of parameters, the relative signal from lipids will be greater on FSE T_2-weighted images than on CSE T_2-weighted images.

Lipids within the human body contain long-chain fatty acids. Most of the protons within these molecules are contained in methyl ($-CH_3$), methylene ($-CH_2$) and methine ($-CH$) groups. In a high-resolution nuclear magnetic resonance (NMR) spectrum, the protons in each of these three groups have slightly different resonance frequencies when exposed to the same external magnetic field. This results from the fact that the local field experienced by each type of proton is slightly different owing to their different chemical nature. One might expect three different peaks within the NMR spectrum of long-chain fatty acids owing to protons in each of these three groups. However, the signal emitted by protons in each group is split into multiple closely spaced peaks. This splitting results from the interaction of protons on adjacent carbon atoms. For example, at the end of a long-chain fatty acid, a methyl group and a methylene group are adjacent to one another ($-CH_2$ $-CH_3$). Each of the two protons on the methylene group can assume one of two possible orientations with respect to the external field. Each of the two protons can be independently aligned with or against the external field. Hence, three distinct configurations of the two methylene protons are possible (both aligned with or both aligned against the field, or one aligned with and one aligned against the field). Each of these three configurations will result in a small distinct change in the local magnetic field experienced by the methyl protons. Therefore, the observed magnetic resonance signal from the methyl protons is split into three peaks. In an identical manner, the signal from the methylene protons will be split into four peaks by the three methyl protons. This results from the fact that there are four possible configurations of the three methyl protons with respect to the external field.

Protons on the same carbon atom do not cause splitting of each other's peaks. This results from the rapid rotation of the carbon atoms around the carbon–carbon bonds. Each proton on a given carbon atom experiences the same average local field from the protons bonded to the same carbon atom due to the rapid rotation.

Each peak in an NMR spectrum corresponds to a different resonance frequency. If the signal corresponding to the methyl protons is split into three peaks, this means that the methyl protons can precess at three closely spaced but different frequencies. At any instant of time, each individual proton precesses at a single frequency. However, over time, as the configuration of the protons on adjacent carbon atoms changes, the precessional frequency of an individual proton will change.

The protons on the interacting groups are said to be coupled. A coupling constant, usually denoted by J, is used as a measure of the splitting of the peak of one group of protons by another group to which they are coupled. Such J-couplings are expressed in hertz and, unlike chemical shift differences (e.g. between water and lipid protons) they do not vary with the external magnetic field strength. This results from the fact that the local field changes which give rise to the coupling effects are derived from the intrinsic magnetic field of the protons. This intrinsic field is of fixed magnitude.

The rate at which protons change their alignment with respect to the external field is by definition determined by their T_1 value. The T_1 value of lipid protons is relatively small. Therefore, lipid protons will rapidly change their alignment with respect to the external field over time.

Each time a proton changes its alignment, the field experienced by other protons to which it is coupled also changes. These local field changes result in dephasing of protons on adjacent carbon atoms. This is equivalent to T_2 decay. However, 180° pulses will compensate for fixed local field differences. 'Fixed' means that the field difference remains constant over the interval of application of the 180° pulse and subsequent signal measurement (i.e. over the interval TE).

When conventional spin echo T_2-weighted images are acquired, a long TE is used. As a result, coupled protons will undergo one or more local field changes during the interval TE. These field changes are therefore not fixed and are not compensated for by the 180° pulse. This lowers the T_2 value of lipid protons. If, however, the 180° pulses are very closely spaced, then the local field changes will essentially become fixed between 180° pulses. Under this circumstance, the local field changes caused by adjacent protons will not induce dephasing. The application of closely spaced 180° pulses decouples coupled protons and therefore prevents dephasing.

When FSE T_2-weighted images are acquired (with a long effective TE), multiple closely spaced 180° pulses are used. This results in decoupling of the lipid protons, causing their signal to be relatively increased. The closely spaced 180° pulses of an FSE sequence cause the T_2 value of lipid protons to increase. It is for this reason that the signal from fat is significantly greater on T_2-weighted FSE images compared to T_2-weighted CSE images, when the same effective TE is used.

This has important implications for clinical pelvic imaging. If a lesion is surrounded by fat, it may be less conspicuous (due to the higher fat signal) on a T_2-weighted FSE image than on a T_2-weighted CSE image. However, such lesions will be readily detected on T_1-weighted CSE images. Therefore, it is always important to use the CSE T_1-weighted images to complement the FSE T_2-weighted images.

Chemical selective sequences

Even when lipid and water protons are exposed to the same external magnetic field, they will precess at slightly different frequencies. This means that, following excitation, lipid and water protons will emit signals at slightly different frequencies. At a field strength of 1.5 T, this difference in frequency is approximately 220 Hz. This results from slight differences in the local environment of the lipid and water protons at the molecular level, causing the lipid protons to experience a slightly smaller local field strength than the water protons, even when placed in the same external field.

These differences in precessional frequency between lipid and water protons can be used selectively to suppress the signal from one of these two species. At 1.5 T, water protons precess at 63.87 MHz, and lipid protons precess at approximately 63.87 MHz – 220 Hz.

The selective suppression of lipid signal is achieved as follows. Suppose a multisection acquisition is being performed. A non-section-selective narrow bandwidth 90° excitation pulse centered at 63.87 MHz – 220 Hz is applied to the entire imaging volume. The bandwidth of this pulse is of the order of

± 100 Hz, so that the maximum frequency component is 63.87 MHz – 120 Hz and the minimum frequency component is 63.87 MHz – 320 Hz. The maximum frequency component is below the precessional frequency of water protons. Thus, only the lipid protons are excited.

Immediately following the lipid-selective 90° excitation, all of the longitudinal magnetization in lipid-containing tissue is converted into transverse magnetization. A strong gradient (spoiler gradient) is then applied, resulting in complete loss of this transverse magnetization. Therefore, following the selective excitation and the spoiler gradient, lipid-containing tissue has no net transverse or longitudinal magnetization. Immediately following the spoiler gradient the standard spin echo imaging sequence for a given section is performed. The lipid protons are unexcitable, as they possess zero longitudinal magnetization. They therefore emit no signal. The same process is repeated prior to the imaging of each section in the multisection acquisition.

The fact that the lipid-selective excitation pulse is non-section selective means that no gradients are applied during its application, so that a large volume is excited. All lipid protons in the homogeneous portion of the field (i.e. that portion of the field which is at 1.5 T) are therefore excited. If a gradient were applied to selectively excite lipid protons in a single section, then water protons in an adjacent section at the low end of the section-selected gradient would also be excited. This would interfere with imaging of this section. This technique is therefore effective for only those portions of a sample located near the isocenter in the homogeneous portion of the field.

In an identical manner, if the narrow bandwidth pulse is centered on the precessional frequency of water protons, the signal from water is selectively suppressed. This is referred to as water suppression.

Selectively suppressing the signal from water or lipid protons is probably the least technically demanding implementation of chemical selective imaging. It is the technique most commonly employed on commercially available imaging systems.

Chemical selective techniques should be used to distinguish between fat and blood. This most commonly arises in attempting to distinguish between a dermoid cyst and an endometrioma. Depending upon the components present, blood products can be isointense with fat on both T_1- and T_2-weighted images. Therefore, if any lesion is detected which is isointense with fat, an additional water and/or fat suppression sequence should be performed.

Motion artifact reduction techniques

Regardless of the imaging sequence, motion during the acquisition of the MRI data will result in image artifacts. Inadvertent patient movements as well as physiological motion will lead to artifacts. Physiological motion includes respiratory motion, vascular pulsation, blood flow and cardiac motion. The most troublesome is the ghost artifact.

In order to reconstruct a magnetic resonance image of a section of tissue, multiple excitations must be performed. A single phase-encoding gradient is applied following each excitation and prior to signal measurement (when CSE sequences are used). This changes the phase of the signal within each voxel as a function of position along the phase-encoding direction. The signal is then measured in the presence of the frequency-encoding gradient.

The signal is measured at discrete time points in the presence of the frequency-encoding gradient, in order to convert the analog signal into a digital signal. The number of frequency samples is equal to the size of the frequency matrix. When a 16-kHz bandwidth is used, all of the samples are obtained over an 8-ms interval. The time between frequency samples is very short and is $8/256 = 1/32$ ms. Therefore, there will not be significant physiological motion between frequency samples.

However, the signal at each component frequency consists of a superposition of signals, which differ in phase. Unlike frequency, the different phase components cannot be measured directly and can be determined only by performing multiple excitations, each excitation with a different phase-encoding gradient. Thus, although the frequency components of each individual signal measurement can be directly determined, the phase components cannot. The signal from each excitation contains all of the necessary information to determine position along the frequency-encoding direction. However, the signal measurements from all of the excitations are needed to determine position along the phase-encoding direction.

With CSE sequences, only a single phase sample is obtained for the signal following each excitation. The time between phase samples will then equal the TR interval (0.5 to several seconds). Therefore, there will be significant physiological motion between phase samples.

The magnetic resonance signal emitted by an object following an excitation is strictly determined by the amount of transverse magnetization present at the echo time TE. The transverse magnetization within each voxel at the time of signal measurement is determined by the T_1, T_2 and proton density of the tissue within each voxel. For a stationary object, the tissue within each voxel remains constant over time. If there is motion between signal measurements, the tissue within each voxel will change over time. (In this context, time refers to the time between signal samples.) The effect of motion then is to change the tissue content (and hence the emitted signal) of voxels through which structures move between signal samples. This results in image artifacts. The artifacts are different with respect to the frequency- and phase-encoding directions.

Each signal contains all of the information necessary to determine position along the frequency-encoding direction. Following each excitation, the signal emitted by each voxel will remain essentially constant during the frequency-sampling process. Therefore, the effect of motion along the frequency-encoding direction between excitations is to cause a slight offset of the position of the object along the frequency-encoding direction (for each excitation). This will appear as a loss of sharpness in the image.

The situation is very different with respect to the phase-encoding direction. The signal arising from a given voxel is uniquely determined by its frequency and phase. The frequency of the signal emitted by tissue within a given voxel is strictly determined by its position along the frequency-encoding direction. Since the read gradient strength is the same magnitude for all signal measurements, the frequency of the signal emitted by each voxel is always the same.

The strength of the phase-encoding gradient is incremented between phase-encoded signal measurements. The signal from voxels with the same spatial coordinate along the phase-encoding direction will undergo the same incremental phase change between one phase-encoding step and the next. Therefore, position along the phase-encoding direction is not determined by the absolute value of the phase of the signal but by the incremental phase change between one phase-encoding step and the next.

If the tissue content of a given voxel remains constant during each signal measurement (other than signal intensity changes caused by T_2 decay and by the read or phase-encoded gradients), the location of the signal arising from that voxel will be accurately determined. The Fourier transform process will assign a location based upon the unique frequency and unique phase increment of the signal. Any motion that occurs between signal samplings will change the tissue content of a voxel and therefore change the signal arising from the voxel.

It can be shown mathematically that, when the signal of a voxel changes in a periodic manner between signal samples, it is as if the signal arises from multiple voxels. When the signal from a voxel changes between phase samples, it is therefore equivalent to having the signal arise from multiple voxels along the phase-encoding direction. These additional (phantom or ghost) sources of signal are displayed in the image. Since this effect is seen only along the phase-encoding direction, it is referred to as phase ghosting.

The spacing between the phase ghosts is directly proportional to the frequency of the motion which gives rise to the ghost. The amplitude of the phase ghosts progressively decreases as they are further displaced from the true signal source. However, the absolute intensity of the ghosts is directly related to the signal intensity of the structure giving rise to the ghost and to the number of voxels traversed by the moving structure. The intensity of ghosts is inversely related to the NSA. Since the motion giving rise to ghosts is random (as is noise), the averaging of multiple signal measurements averages out the signal from the ghosts.

Since phase ghosts are usually superimposed on other tissue within the image, the net signal at the location of a ghost is the sum of the signal from the ghost and the signal from the underlying tissue. If these two signals are in phase, there will be an increase in signal intensity. If these two signals are out of phase, there will be a decrease in signal intensity. This accounts for the seemingly paradoxical areas of low signal that can occur from ghosts which arise from structures (such as vessels) with a very high signal. The phase of the ghost signal is determined by the phase of the motion. In turn, the phase of the motion is independent of the phase of tissue signals.

Since ghosts arise from periodic motion, if one can eliminate periodic motion, one can eliminate ghosts. The most troublesome ghosts arise from respiratory motion and vascular pulsation and flow variations. There are two techniques that are commonly used to reduce the ghosts which arise from these types of motion.

Respiratory ordered-phase encoding (ROPE) is commonly employed when imaging the abdomen and/or pelvis with CSE pulse sequences. This technique essentially converts periodic motion into non-periodic motion with respect to the phase-encoding process. To achieve this, a different phase-encoding gradient strength is used for each excitation of an MRI sequence. The number of different phase-encoding gradient strengths is equal to the size of the phase matrix. The difference in strength between successive phase-encoding gradients is a constant. For most imaging sequences, the phase-encoding gradients are applied in sequential fashion from the strongest negative gradient to the strongest positive gradient. Suppose the size of the phase matrix is 128. Denote the most negative gradient as $-G_{64}$, and denote the most positive gradient as $+G_{64}$.

As an example, suppose the respiratory rate is equal to one-half the TR. In addition, suppose the first excitation is begun at full inspiration. Then the second excitation will occur at full expiration. The third excitation will occur at full inspiration, and so on. If the phase-encoding gradients are applied in sequential fashion, this would result in a periodic variation of the signal intensity between successive phase-encoded signal measurements. There is a simple method to avoid this. Suppose the phase-encoding gradients are applied in the order $-G_{64}$, $+G_{64}$, $-G_{63}$, $+G_{63}$, etc. This means that successive negative phase-encoding gradients are all applied at full inspiration and successive positive phase-encoding gradients are all applied at full expiration. This is equivalent to applying the phase-encoding gradients in sequential fashion from the strongest negative gradient to the strongest positive gradient with only a single breath in between. Thus, by reordering the phase-encoding gradients with respect to the respiratory cycle, periodic motion between successive phase-encoding gradients has been eliminated.

ROPE is implemented by using a hollow tube closed at one end with the other end connected to a pressure transducer. The tube is wrapped around the patient's abdomen or pelvis. The average respiratory rate is determined and the order of application of the phase-encoding gradients is determined on the basis of the respiratory cycle, to reduce the effective periodic motion between successive phase-encoding gradients.

The reduction of phase ghost artifacts by using ROPE can be dramatic (Figure 7). ROPE should be routinely employed with all CSE pulse sequences when the abdomen and/or pelvis are imaged. Unfortunately, ROPE is not currently compatible with FSE sequences. This results from the fact that, when an FSE sequence is used, the order of the phase-encoding gradients is already constrained by the choice of effective TE. Further reordering would therefore require a more sophisticated algorithm. The inability to use ROPE with FSE sequences can result in significant image degradation and loss of contrast.

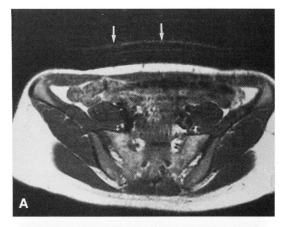

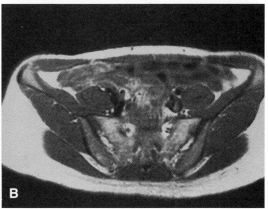

Figure 7 (A) *Conventional spin echo T_1-weighted image through the mid-pelvis obtained without respiratory ordered-phase encoding (ROPE). Note the prominent ghost artifact from the anterior subcutaneous fat (arrows). The phase direction in anteroposterior. (B) Otherwise identical parameters and section location as in (A) but with ROPE. Note the elimination of the phase ghost artifact*

These effects are usually minimal in the pelvis (where respiratory motion is usually minimal), but can be substantial within the abdomen.

Ghost artifacts affect the contrast of an image, because the object itself loses signal when it gives rise to image ghosts. This can result in significant loss of signal intensity within moving objects. A dramatic example is the loss of signal intensity within the gallbladder when the liver is imaged with FSE sequences (Figure 8). That this is due to respiratory motion is readily seen by using the

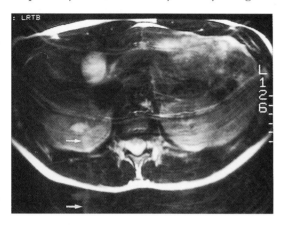

Figure 8 *Multicoil fast spin echo T_2-weighted image of the liver through the level of the gallbladder. Phase ghosts (arrows) are seen originating from the gallbladder and the gallbladder signal intensity is heterogeneous. There is marked degradation of the image due to respiratory motion artifact*

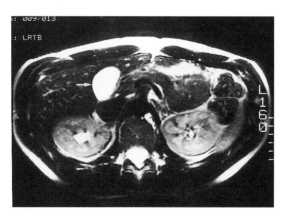

Figure 9 *Otherwise identical parameters to those in Figure 8, but with patient-controlled respiratory gating. The gallbladder (arrow) is of higher uniform signal intensity and the motion artifact is eliminated*

same FSE sequence with data acquisition triggered by the patient at the end of expiration during a short intermittent breath-hold (Figure 9). Fortunately, these effects are usually minimal within the pelvis.

What about ghost artifacts from blood vessels? Depending on flow velocity and direction, vessels will not always appear as a signal void on magnetic resonance images. When present, intravascular signal is problematic, because of the phase ghost artifact that results (Figure 10). This ghost artifact arises in two ways. The pulsatile motion of the blood vessels themselves causes ghost artifacts. As vessels expand and contract, they move through adjacent voxels. This expansion and contraction is periodic with the cardiac cycle. As with respiratory motion, this causes a periodic amplitude modulation of the signal in voxels located adjacent to the vessel. This gives rise to phase ghosts. These ghosts are usually manifest as circular rings, since they arise only from voxels through which the periphery of a vessel moves. The voxels within the center of a vessel remain within the vessel throughout the motion of the vessel wall.

In addition to the motion of the vessel wall, flow velocity in a vessel varies with the cardiac cycle. Unless an acquisition is gated to the

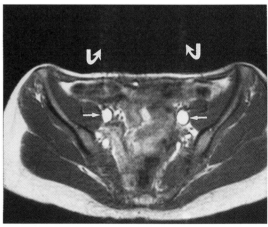

Figure 10 *Conventional spin echo T_1-weighted image through the mid-pelvis obtained without saturation pulses. Note the high intravascular signal in the iliac arteries and veins (straight arrows) and the prominent vascular pulsation ghost artifact (curved arrows)*

cardiac cycle, this will result in different signal intensities within the vessel, depending on the phase of the cardiac cycle at which the signal is measured. This results in a periodic modulation of the signal in voxels within the lumen of the vessel. This also gives rise to ghosts. The intensity of these ghosts is dependent on the signal within the vessel.

When flow is perpendicular to the plane of section, even slowly flowing blood will move completely out of the section between 90° pulses of conventional spin echo sequences (i.e. during the TR interval). Therefore, 'fresh' (or unsaturated) protons will move into the section and be excited by the next 90° pulse. Since these new protons have not been previously excited, they will have maximal longitudinal magnetization. This is equivalent to complete recovery of longitudinal magnetization between 90° pulses. Depending on the rate of flow, this can result in significant intravascular signal. This effect is usually referred to as flow-related enhancement.

If the rate of flow is such that intravascular protons remain within the excited section (following a 90° pulse) until the 180° pulse, then the intravascular signal will be relatively high. On the other hand, if after each 90° pulse the blood completely flows out of the section prior to the 180° pulse (i.e. during the interval of time TE/2), then the vessel will appear as a signal void, since the intravascular protons will not experience the 180° pulse. The effect is usually referred to as a flow-related signal loss.

For a 1-cm thick tissue section, in order to have a signal void, the flow velocity must exceed (1 cm)/(TE/2). For T_1- and proton density-weighted images TE typically is 10–20 ms. For a T_2-weighted image TE typically is 60–80. For example, when TE = 10 ms, TE/2 = 5 ms, and the flow must exceed 1 cm/5 ms (= 200 cm/s) to have a signal void. If TE = 20 ms, the flow must exceed 100 cm/s to have a signal void. If TE = 60 ms, flow must exceed 37.5 cm/s to have a signal void. If TE = 80 ms, flow must exceed 25 cm/s to have a signal void. For 5-mm thick sections these velocities are halved. Thus, for T_1- and proton density-weighted images, even arterial flow will rarely result in a complete signal void.

In reality, for a given value of TE, even if the flow is equal to half of the values given above, half of the excited intravascular blood within a section will move out of the section prior to the 180° pulse and therefore not contribute to the signal. Therefore, most arteries will have little signal, especially on T_2-weighted images. The flow in most veins, however, is such that they may have significant signal if nothing else is done.

Most MRI sequences acquire the data from multiple sections during each TR interval. The 'stack' of sequential sections can be thought of as an imaging volume. To prevent signal in vascular structures with flow perpendicular to the plane of section, 90° excitation pulses are applied above and below the imaging volume immediately prior to each TR interval. These are referred to as saturation pulses. The tissue excited by the saturation pulses (outside the imaging volume), including the vessels they contain, will acquire transverse magnetization. At the same time, they will have complete loss of longitudinal magnetization.

Immediately following application of the saturation pulses (and before the imaging sequence begins) a gradient is applied which causes complete dephasing of the transverse magnetization created by the saturation pulse. This is referred to as a spoiler gradient. This causes the blood flowing into the imaging volume to have no net longitudinal magnetization and not net transverse magnetization. It is said to be 'saturated', so that when it receives an additional 90° excitation pulse (once it is within the sections of the imaging volume) it emits no signal, as it has zero longitudinal magnetization.

These pulses are routinely used to reduce vascular ghost artifacts. Saturation pulses should be routinely employed with both CSE and FSE sequences. They can dramatically reduce the intravascular signal (especially in veins) and thus reduce ghost artifacts (Figure 11).

However, vascular pulsation ghost artifacts can never be completely eliminated. As these artifacts are only visible along the phase-encoding direction, the phase direction is chosen to prevent the ghosts from passing through the structures of most interest. The penalty for using saturation pulses is that it takes time to turn the pulses on and off. This can slightly reduce the total number of sections that can be acquired for a given TR.

When flow is within (rather than perpendicular to) the plane of section, the situation is different. All or most of the protons within such vessels will remain in the section between the 90° and 180° pulses. Some fresh protons will enter the section between 90° pulses (i.e. during the TR interval). However, the flowing protons will be moving in the section during application of the frequency- and phase-encoding gradients. Motion during gradient application causes dephasing and therefore signal loss. This dephasing is sufficient to result in signal void for most in-plane vascular flow.

Even vessels with signal void can given rise to pulsation ghost artifacts. As the vessels expand and contract, their motion will still result in periodic variations of signal intensity within voxels immediately adjacent to the vessels. This effect is rarely seen in pelvic imaging, but can be seen to arise from small vessels within the liver.

Imaging coils

There are three types of imaging coils: linear coils, quadrature coils and multicoils. The simplest type of linear coil configuration is a loop coil. Many small surface coils are of this type. These coils act only as receivers. In order to act as a transmitter, more complex configurations are required. The most commonly used linear coil that can act as both a transmitter and a receiver is the saddle-shaped coil. When used as a transmitter, a linear coil will produce a linearly polarized excitation pulse. Such excitation pulses are less efficient than circularly polarized excitation pulses.

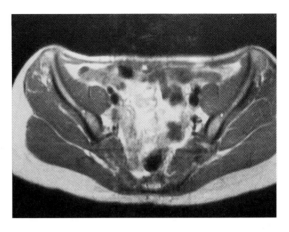

Figure 11 *Otherwise identical parameters and location to those in Figure 10, but with superior and inferior saturation pulses. The intravascular signal is minimal and there is virtual elimination of the vascular pulsation ghost artifact*

A quadrature coil consists of two saddle-shaped linear coils oriented at 90° to one another. When used as a transmitter, these coils can produce a circularly polarized excitation pulse. In addition, quadrature coils provide an improvement in signal/noise ratio by a factor of $\sqrt{2}$ compared to a single linear coil. Virtually all commercially available 'body coils' are quadrature coils. These coils provide a homogeneous excitation of a large volume and allow images to be acquired with a large field of view (FOV). These coils are the most commonly used coils for pelvic imaging.

What about multicoils? For a given region of interest to be imaged, the signal/noise ratio is maximized by using a coil as close as possible to the region of interest, so that the coil diameter equals the distance of the region of interest from the coil. This is achieved by a surface coil, provided that the region of interest is small (and therefore a small FOV can be used). For large regions, it is not practical (or optimal) to use a single surface coil.

In regions close to the coil, local (or surface) coils provide a markedly improved signal/noise ratio compared with body coils. These coils are used as receivers only with the transmitted excitation pulse provided by a body coil. The sensitive region of a local coil is severely limited, typically of the order of the coil diameter. If an object is located within the sensitive region, then it will be in close proximity to the coil and therefore have a high signal.

However, the noise received by the coil will also be limited to noise originating in the sensitive region. The total noise in an image ordinarily comes from the entire object present within the coil. Therefore, when a surface coil is used, only noise originating within the very limited sensitive region of the coil will be of significant amplitude. This markedly reduces the noise within the image, and hence significantly improves the signal/noise ratio of a surface coil.

When used individually, surface coils can provide only small FOV images. If multiple surface coils are used simultaneously, the phase of the signal in each coil will depend on the coil orientation. This is similar to the situation when a quadrature coil is used. Since a quadrature coil consists of two coils oriented at 90° with respect to one another, the signals in the two coils are 90° out of phase. Prior to being fed into the receiver circuit, the signal in one of the coils is phase shifted back by 90° The two signals are then added together (in phase) and fed into a single circuit. The process of phase shifting the two signals prior to their being added will be error-free, provided that the exact difference in orientation of the two coils is known.

Suppose multiple surface coils are used simultaneously in a receive-only mode. Unless the exact orientations of the coils is fixed and known, addition of the signals into a single circuit will result in signal loss, owing to phase differences between the signals. However, suppose the signal from each coil is fed into its own circuit and that the signal from each coil is analyzed separately to reconstruct an image. Each individual image will be identical to the image that would be obtained had the coil been used by itself. Each image will therefore have a relatively small effective field of view.

Suppose we form a composite image by adding together the individual images in each coil. By adding the individual images (rather than the individual signals themselves) we have eliminated the need to know the exact phase relationship of the signals. The addition of the individual images is done on a pixel-by-pixel basis. The effective field of view of the composite image will essentially equal the region spanned by all of the individual coils. This is much greater than the effective field of view of the individual coils alone. Therefore, the composite image will have the signal/noise ratio of a surface coil, but the effective field of view of a much larger coil.

Such an arrangement of individual surface coils acting independently and simultaneously in a receive-only mode is referred to as a multicoil. The number of individual coils that can be used as a multicoil is limited by the fact that each coil requires its own receiver electronics. Such hardware is very expensive. At present, multicoils use a maximum of four separate coils simultaneously.

The improvement in signal/noise ratio of a multicoil compared with a body coil is substantial. There is an approximately two-fold improvement in signal/noise ratio for structures located near the center of the coil array. This results from the fact that n independent coils will provide an improvement in signal/noise ratio of $\sqrt{n}$. For structures located near the individual coils, the improvement in signal/noise ratio is even greater.

The multicoil used in pelvic imaging consists of two adjacent anterior coils and two adjacent posterior coils. The improvement in image quality that can now be obtained using commercially available multicoils is dramatic (Figure 12). All pelvic MRI examinations should now be performed using a multicoil.

COMPUTED TOMOGRAPHY

When conventional radiography is performed, the object being imaged is irradiated by a stationary X-ray source. An X-ray detector is present on the side opposite the source. For plain radiography, the detector consists of a screen–film combination.

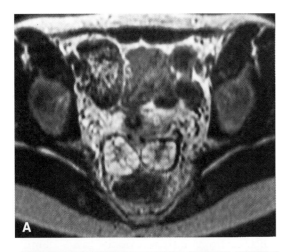

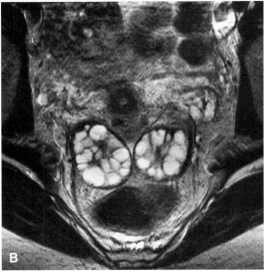

Figure 12 (A) *Fast spin echo T_2-weighted body coil image through the pelvis in a patient with polycystic ovaries. (B) High-resolution fast spin echo T_2-weighted image through the same location as in (A), obtained using a multicoil*

Different portions of the film will be exposed to different amounts of radiation, dependent upon the degree of absorption by the object located between the film and the source.

For example, when a posteroanterior chest radiograph is obtained, the source is fixed in location behind the patient. The cassette containing the film is located in front of the patient. Since air-containing lung tissue absorbs virtually none of the X-rays, the portion of the film beneath the lung will be exposed to a large amount of radiation. On the other hand, since bone absorbs a large amount of the radiation, the portion of film beneath the thoracic vertebrae or ribs will be exposed to only a small amount of radiation. These differences in exposure of the film create the image on a plain radiograph.

Plain radiography has many limitations. When plain radiography is used, a three-dimensional object is projected onto a two-dimensional film. This results in super-imposition of structures. In addition, the contrast differences that can be displayed are severely limited. All soft tissue structures (e.g. heart, blood vessels, liver, spleen, etc.) appear the same and do not have any internal contrast differences. There are essentially four different shades of gray, corresponding to air (black), fat (light gray), soft tissue (dark gray) and bone (white).

Computed tomography (CT) provides a means of imaging individual sections of an object without superimposition of adjacent structures. In addition, it provides markedly improved contrast within and between individual structures compared with plain radiography. The CT scanner contains an X-ray source as well as X-ray detectors. These are housed within the gantry that surrounds the patient. Although CT technology has evolved dramatically since it was first introduced in the mid-1970s, the basic underlying principles have remained the same.

First-generation CT scanners consisted of an X-ray source (which generated a thin pencil-like X-ray beam) and used a single X-ray detector. The source and detector were moved in unison (in both a linear and a rotary fashion) 360° around the patient being scanned. Each exposure was equivalent to obtaining a plain radiograph. By performing multiple exposures with a thin X-ray beam at different angles around an object, a two-dimensional slice (or section) of the object could be accurately reconstructed. By imaging multiple adjacent thin slices, a three-dimensional representation of the object was acquired (one slice at a time). With the use of a first-generation scanner, each section took about 3 min to acquire. The scanner table was advanced between different sections. No exposure was obtained during table movement.

The next generation of CT scanners (second-generation scanners) used a thin fan-shaped X-ray beam (rather than a 'pencil' beam) and a line of multiple detectors rather than a single detector. The size of the fan-shaped beam did not encompass the entire width of the patient. Therefore, both linear and circular movements of the source and detectors were still required. The number of movements were reduced with resultant imaging times of about 10–90 s per section, depending on the precise number of detectors. The table was again advanced between different sections.

Third-generation scanners use a much wider fan-shaped beam and employ a curvi-linear array of multiple detectors. The fan-shaped beam is wide enough to encompass the entire width of the patient. There are no linear-type movements with third-generation scanners. The source moves along a circular arc and the detector array is moved in a corresponding manner. Each 360° rotation corresponds to a single section. Scan times per section for third-generation scanners vary from 2 to 10 s. Once again, the table is advanced between sections. The time to advance the table between sections is of the order of the time required to image each section.

Fourth-generation CT scanners are similar to third-generation scanners. They employ a fixed array of detectors that completely surround the patient. The X-ray source moves and the detectors remain stationary. The main advantage of a fourth-generation scanner compared with a third-generation scanner is its easier detector calibration. The scan time of most fourth-generation scanners is about 2 s per section plus the time required to advance the table between sections.

There are several factors that limit the minimum scan time per section when conventional CT scanners are used. As the X-ray source rotates around the patient, hundreds of short pulses of radiation are produced for each 360° rotation. As multiple exposures are made in rapid sequence, the X-ray source (i.e. the X-ray tube) begins to heat up. Tube cooling can become problematic, as a large number of sections are acquired in rapid succession.

A second factor that limits the minimum scan time per section is related to the circular motion of the X-ray source. The electrical supply of the source is transmitted through electrical cables. As the source rotates, the cables must also rotate. This limits scanning to single 360° turns, alternating in clockwise and counter-clockwise directions. The table is advanced between these alternating turns. In this manner, conventional CT scanners obtain sections by a scan of one section, followed by a small incremental table movement followed by another scan, etc.

The most recent advance in CT technology is helical scanning. Helical scanners use sliding electrical contacts (so-called slip rings) in place of electrical cables. This allows continuous rotation of the X-ray source around the patient. It is unnecessary to use alternate clockwise and counter-clockwise rotations. In addition, helical scanners use improved X-ray tube technology. These tubes have much greater heat capacity, so that exposures can be obtained continuously for longer periods of time. Finally, instead of advancing the scanner table (and hence the patient) between 360° rotations of the source, the table is advanced during a continuous X-ray exposure. Helical scanners can provide imaging times of 1 s per section with no delay between sections.

In helical CT, a single data set is acquired that represents the volume covered during the continuous X-ray exposure. This requires a different approach to image reconstruction from that with conventional scanners, which acquire data one section at a time. The volume of data is interpolated to provide single sections. The great advantage of helical scanning is that sections can be reconstructed at arbitrary locations within the volume and in an overlapping manner, if desired.

When a CT scan is performed, section thickness is determined by the thickness of the fan-shaped X-ray beam. The two-dimensional CT image represents a thin volume of tissue. For most CT applications, section thickness varies from 5 to 10 mm. Section locations are usually specified with respect to an arbitrarily (usually palpable) 'landmark' established prior to the beginning of the examination. For example, when a chest CT scan is performed, the top of the sternum can be selected as the landmark. This position is then assigned as the location 0. All other locations are defined with respect to their distance superior (S) or inferior (I) to the landmark. For example, the position 5 mm below the landmark is specified as I5.

Using a conventional CT scanner with 10-mm thick sections beginning at S0 (section 1) and scanning inferiorly, sequential sections will be located at I10 (section 2), I20 (section 3), etc. Once the scan is completed, these locations are fixed. The 10-mm thick section centered at I10 extends from I5 to I15, and the 10-mm thick section centered at I20 extends from I15 to I25. Suppose a 10-mm diameter lesion is centered at I15 (i.e. the lesion extends from I10 to I20), then half of the lesion will be in section 2 and half of the lesion will be in section 3. This will reduce lesion conspicuousness.

Using a helical CT scanner with 10-mm thick sections, a volume of data is acquired. Individual section locations can be arbitrarily and retrospectively chosen. Initially, section locations may be chosen that start at S0 and are reconstructed in 10-mm increments. In the example above, the section can be retrospectively reconstructed (from the volume of data) centered at location I15, so that a section contains the lesion in its entirety. In addition, overlapping sections can be reconstructed in small increments. For example, 10-mm thick sections can be reconstructed in 1-mm increments at I10, I11, ..., I20. This is a distinct advantage of helical data acquisition.

The CT imaging process results in a representation of a thin slice through an object. Each reconstructed CT image consists of a large number of small picture elements (pixels). Each pixel is assigned a numerical value, based on the degree to which the tissue corresponding to that pixel (within the object being imaged) attenuates the X-ray beam. These numerical (pixel) values are expressed in Hounsfield units (HU, named after the inventor of computed tomography, G. N. Hounsfield). Hounsfield units are normalized with respect to the attenuation of water, where water corresponds to an attenuation of 0 HU.

Each reconstructed CT image consists of digital data, i.e. the intensity of each pixel corresponds to a discrete value. CT images are displayed by means of a gray scale, each pixel being depicted as one of 256 shades of gray, based on its corresponding attenuation value. For display purposes, a level and window are chosen for each image. The level indicates the pixel intensity value around which the gray scale is centered. The window indicates the range of pixel values over which the entire gray scale is displayed.

For example, suppose a CT image is displayed with a level of 50 and a window of 100. All pixels with values greater than or equal to 100 HU will be displayed as white and all pixels with values less than or equal to 0 HU will be displayed as black. All pixels with values between 0 and 100 HU will be assigned one of 256 shades of gray. The same CT image data are often displayed with multiple different level and window settings. Different settings are chosen to maximize contrast for different structures of interest.

For example, a typical liver will have a mean attenuation of 75 HU and will contain values in a relatively narrow range centered around the mean. Therefore, to maximize visualization of liver abnormalities, a level of 75 and a narrow window (e.g. 100–200) are chosen. On the other hand, bone contains pixels with a much wider range of attenuation values. This wide range corresponds to marrow elements, thin trabeculae and dense cortical bone. In order to display such a wide range of pixel values (and therefore visualize the internal architecture of bone), a much wider window must be chosen, centered around the mean attenuation.

For a typical image, soft tissue structures such as the liver or spleen will have an attenuation slightly greater than that of water (e.g. 40 to 80 HU), fat will have an attenuation slightly less than that of water (e.g. −20 to −200 HU), air within the lung or bowel will have an attenuation much less than that of water (e.g. −500 to −1000 HU) and bone will have an attenuation much greater than that of water (e.g. 500 to 1000 HU). Therefore, a typical CT study is photographed several different ways, in order to emphasize different structures of interest.

ULTRASOUND IMAGING

By definition, ultrasound is sound possessing a frequency greater than 20 000 kHz (where 1 kHz = 1 kilohertz = 1000 cycles per second). These are sound waves above the audible range. Sound consists of mechanical waves that are propagated by the vibration of molecules of the material through which the sound is being transmitted. The speed of transmission of sound waves is dependent upon the rigidity of this material. There is a well-defined relationship between the speed of propagation (c), frequency of propagation (f), and wavelength (λ): $c = f\lambda$.

As a sound wave travels through a material, it continually loses a portion of its energy, owing to absorption, deflection and divergence. Absorption results from internal friction within the material through which the sound is being transmitted. Deflection of sound includes reflection, refraction and scattering. Divergence is the spreading out of the sound waves.

If the medium conducting the sound waves is perfectly homogeneous in composition, there will not be significant reflection of the sound waves. However, if the medium conducting the sound is heterogeneous in composition, there will be significant reflection. Acoustic impedance is a measure of the resistance to the conduction of sound

within a given medium. When sound waves reach an interface where there is a change in acoustic impedance, a portion of the sound waves will be reflected. The greater the difference in acoustic impedance, the greater the degree of reflection. Since tissues within the body are homogeneous in composition, there are many interfaces present to serve as reflectors of sound waves.

Modern ultrasound equipment consists of a transmitter, a receiver and a display system. The transmitter emits ultrasound waves into the body of the patient being imaged. The receiver measures the intensity of the reflected sound waves and determines their location. For most modern ultrasound machines, the functions of the transmitter and receiver are served by a single transducer that alternates between transmission and reception. The display depicts the structures being imaged, according to the timing and intensity of the reflected sound waves.

When a voltage is applied to certain crystals (e.g. quartz), they undergo a change in their physical dimensions. This is called the piezoelectric effect and such crystals are referred to as piezoelectric crystals. When a voltage is applied suddenly, a piezoelectric crystal will vibrate. The vibrational motion generates sound waves. Ultrasound transducers contain one or more piezoelectric crystals to generate sound waves. Likewise, when a piezoelectric crystal is exposed to a vibration, it will generate a voltage.

Whereas the speed of sound through air is approximately 330 m/s, the speed of sound through soft tissues of the body is approximately 1540 m/s (which equals 1.54 m/ms or 154 cm/ms). Based on the known speed of transmission of sound, the position of a reflected sound wave can be accurately determined. For example, for a sound wave to travel to a depth of 8 cm and back to the transducer (a total distance of 16 cm) requires about 0.1 ms.

Ultrasound transducers emit short bursts of sound waves (usually referred to as pulses). Following each sound pulse, the transducer acts as a receiver. As reflected sound waves strike the transducer, a voltage is generated. The strength of the voltage is directly proportional to the strength of the reflected sound wave striking the transducer. Based on the time between emission of a sound pulse and the return of a reflected sound wave, the distance of the reflector can be determined (since the speed of sound transmission is constant and known). Therefore, both the intensity and position of a reflected sound wave can be determined.

In this manner, an ultrasound image is generated one line at a time by emission of multiple pulses of sound along adjacent lines of travel. Following each pulse, the reflected echoes are measured and their depth determined. To generate an image with a field of view (i.e. depth) of 8 cm requires about 0.1 ms per line. It therefore takes about 10 ms to generate 100 lines of data. These data are used to generate an image. The entire process of acquiring 100 separate lines of data (and therefore an entire image) can be repeated about 100 times per second. This allows a 'real-time' image to be displayed. The intensity and position of the reflected echoes are displayed on a gray-scale image. Position is displayed with respect to the transducer. Intensity is displayed (by convention) with the strongest echoes being white and the weakest echoes being black on a gray scale.

It is important to remember that, as an ultrasound pulse travels through soft tissue within a patient, the intensity of the pulse decreases owing to absorption as well as reflection. Absorption accounts for the majority of the energy loss and occurs secondary to friction. The ultrasound pulse causes vibration of the soft tissues. As the soft tissues vibrate (at the molecular level), heat is generated because of friction. The greater the frequency of the ultrasound beam, the greater the frictional losses. Therefore, the depth of maximal penetration of an ultrasound beam is inversely proportional to its frequency. It is for this reason that lower-frequency transducers must be used to image deep structures or when imaging very large patients.

On the other hand, the depth resolution of an ultrasound pulse is directly proportional to the physical length of the pulse. Two objects will be resolved as distinct structures if the pulse length is less than twice their separation. Under this circumstance, the echoes generated by the two structures will be separated in time when they reach the transducer.

In general, when an ultrasound pulse is generated, the piezoelectric crystal is made to vibrate a small (but fixed) number of times. The number of vibrations the crystal makes is equal to the number of wavelengths generated. Since the wavelength of ultrasound is inversely proportional to its frequency, the greater the frequency, the smaller the wavelength. Therefore, the greater the frequency of the transducer, the shorter the physical length of the pulse and the better the depth resolution.

Lateral resolution is controlled by the focusing of the ultrasound beam. This is dependent upon many factors, including the type of transducer used (single element or multiple element), the size of the transducer element(s) as well as the frequency of the ultrasound. In general, lateral resolution improves with higher frequency and larger transducers. It is important to note that the lateral resolution of a transducer is not the same at all points. Most ultrasound transducers have a focused beam such that there is a region over which the beam has maximal lateral resolution. This region of optimal focus can usually be selected by the operator.

Most modern ultrasound transducers are arrays that consist of multiple small transducer elements. For example, linear array transducers consist of 50 to 100 (or more) individual elements. Each element is a tiny source of ultrasound. By electronically firing small numbers of multiple adjacent elements in rapid succession, individual 'lines' of ultrasound are used to obtain an image. The beam can also be electronically steered by simple use of a time delay in the firing of adjacent elements.

As already noted, ultrasound imaging is performed by transmission of an ultrasound pulse into a patient and then measurement of the amplitude of the reflected echoes. When sound waves are reflected from a stationary structure, the frequency of the reflected sound wave is equal to the frequency of the original sound wave. However, when sound waves are reflected from a moving structure, the frequency of the reflected sound wave is different from the frequency of the original sound wave. This shift in frequency is usually referred to as the Doppler effect.

Suppose a source emits sound waves into the soft tissues of a patient at frequency f (in units of hertz) and wavelength λ (in units of centimeters). Suppose a stationary reflector of sound is preset. If the sound travels at velocity c within the medium, then sound waves spaced λ cm apart will reach the reflector at frequency $f = (c/\lambda)$ Hz.

However, suppose the reflector is moving away from the source at velocity v (in units of centimeters per second), where $v < c$. As far as the reflector is concerned, sound waves will be travelling towards it at relative velocity $(c - v)$, but will still be spaced λ cm apart. The frequency of the sound waves as they reach the moving reflector (f') will therefore be equal to $(c - v)/\lambda$. Since $\lambda = c/f$, $f' = f(c - v)/c$.

Likewise, suppose the source of sound waves is moving at velocity v away from a stationary reflector as it emits sound waves. The source emits sound waves at a rate of $1/f$ (since the reciprocal of frequency is in units of seconds per cycle). Since the source moves between emission of the sound waves, the distance between the sound waves will change. That is, the sound waves will no longer be spaced λ cm apart, where $\lambda = c/f$.

Since the source moves away from the direction of travel of the sound waves, the spacing between sound waves will be increased by the distance the source travels between waves. Since the time between waves is $1/f$ and the source moves at velocity v, the wavelength will be increased by v/f. The new wavelength will therefore equal $\lambda + v/f$, which equals $(c + v)/f$. Since the sound waves travel at velocity v once they leave the source, the

frequency at the stationary reflector (f'') will equal $c/[(c + v)/f] = fc/(c + v)$.

Similar formulas can be derived when the reflector moves towards a stationary source and when a source moves towards a stationary reflector. These formulas form the basis of the determination of the velocity of a moving reflector in clinical ultrasound. This is usually referred to as Doppler ultrasound.

The red blood cells within blood vessels serve as moving reflectors when a transducer emits ultrasound at frequency f. Suppose blood is flowing away from a transducer at velocity v (relative to the direction of the emission). Furthermore, suppose the transducer emits sound waves at frequency f and denote the speed of sound in soft tissue as c. The sound waves will strike the red blood cells at frequency $f(c - v)/c$. The red blood cells then act as a moving source as they reflect the sound waves back towards the stationary transducer. The frequency of emission by the red blood cells is still $f(c - v)/c$, but this frequency will be shifted by their motion such that the frequency at the transducer will equal $[f(c - v)/c][c/(c + v)]$. This last expression is equal to $f(c - v)/(c + v)$.

The difference between the original frequency f and the above shifted frequency $f(c - v)/(c + v)$ is equal to $2fv/(c + v)$. For clinical ultrasound, c (which equals 1540 m/s) is many orders of magnitude greater than v. Therefore, a good approximation to the frequency shift is $2fv/c$. This is usually referred to as the Doppler shift. If the red blood cells are moving at an angle θ with respect to the line of sight of the transducer, then the component of the velocity along the line of sight will equal $v \cos \theta$. The Doppler shift then becomes $2fv \cos \theta/c$.

The above formula forms the basis of clinical Doppler ultrasound. Based on the frequency shift of reflected ultrasound, the velocity of the reflector can be determined. In addition, depending on whether the frequency shift is positive or negative, flow direction can be determined. Continuous wave Doppler studies use a probe that contains two separate elements: one element that serves as a continuous transmitter and one element that serves as a continuous receiver. In this manner, the Doppler shift (and hence the velocity of motion) of any reflector moving with respect to the line of sight of the transducer can be determined.

Continuous wave Doppler probes do not provide positional information. In order to determine the depth of a reflected sound wave, a short pulse of sound is emitted and the time of reception of the reflected sound is determined. Since the speed of sound in soft tissues is known, the distance travelled by the sound wave (and therefore the depth) can be determined. Since continuous wave probes do not emit pulses of sound, they cannot determine the location of reflectors. They have limited clinical use. For example, when a study of the aorta is performed in patients with aortic stenosis, continuous wave probes are used to determine the maximal velocity of flow within the ascending aorta. In this situation, precise position is not important. The transducer can be aligned so that the line of sight is along the ascending aorta.

Most clinical Doppler studies are carried out using a so-called duplex technique with pulsed Doppler. The transducer is used to generate a real-time gray-scale image. A desired small region is selected along a single line. The transducer then emits short pulses of ultrasound along the selected line only. By determining the time of reception of echoes following each pulse, only those echoes from the desired region are measured. The frequency of the reflected ultrasound is compared with the frequency of the emitted ultrasound and the Doppler shift is determined. The mean velocity of the moving reflectors within the region of interest is then determined. This process is repeated continuously and displayed as a graph of mean velocity (within the small region of interest) vs. time. The gray-scale image can be periodically updated to make sure that the sample is still being obtained from the desired region. The angle between the blood vessel and the line of sight of the transducer is determined manually from the gray-scale image.

There are currently many clinical applications of Doppler ultrasound. An active area of research is the distinction of malignant from benign masses based on Doppler waveforms. Malignant masses release tumor angiogenesis factors in order to maintain their blood supply as they grow in size. However, the tumor-induced small vessels are abnormal in that their walls do not contain smooth muscle. As a result, these abnormal vessels have very low resistance (i.e. low impedance) to blood flow. The resulting waveforms show an abnormally high diastolic flow and/or abnormally high systolic flow. Several different indices (in the form of velocity ratios) have been used to assess the degree and/or presence of abnormal tumor flow within a detected mass. If we denote by S the peak systolic flow velocity, by D the peak diastolic velocity, and by M the mean velocity ($M = [S + D]/2$), then: RI (resistance index) $= (S - D)/S$, PI (pulsatility index) $= (S - D)/M$ and systolic/diastolic ratio $= S/D$. These indices are highly correlated, so that it is unlikely that one index is necessarily 'better' or provides additional information. In published studies, some authors have preferred one index over another in determining the presence or absence of neovascularity within a mass. However, all can be readily calculated from the same data.

Other clinical applications of Doppler ultrasound include evaluation of the carotid arteries and the deep venous systems of the extremities (predominantly the lower extremities). Peak systolic velocities within the internal carotid arteries can be used to assess the presence of hemodynamically significant stenoses. Venous flow can be assessed in the lower extremities to determine the presence or absence of deep venous thrombosis (DVT). However, DVT studies rely heavily on real-time images to determine whether the veins are compressible. Doppler waveforms are complementary to real-time images.

A major advance in Doppler ultrasound is color Doppler imaging. Color Doppler is simply an alternative means of displaying Doppler shift information. Recall that with conventional Doppler imaging, Doppler shift information is determined within a small region along a single line only. By acquiring Doppler shift data along multiple adjacent lines, the velocity of moving reflectors can be determined over a large region. These data are superimposed over a portion of the gray-scale image by color encoding. Blue and red can be used to indicate direction of flow. Different shades of the same color can be used to indicate velocity of flow.

Since the color information takes a relatively long time to acquire (compared with the time needed to acquire the data for the gray-scale image), color Doppler studies superimpose the color data over a gray-scale image that is periodically updated. The rate at which the gray-scale image is updated is dependent upon the size of the region of color data. The larger the region of color data, the slower the rate of update of the gray-scale image. Color flow imaging is extremely useful to identify vessels for standard Doppler evaluation.

Finally, power Doppler imaging has recently achieved much attention. Recall that standard Doppler shift data determine the mean velocity of the reflectors within a small region of interest. The color display then determines color within the image based on the mean velocity of the reflectors within a given region (with higher velocities being assigned more intense color). It does not take into account the number of moving reflectors. Power Doppler imaging takes into account the number of moving reflectors within a given region. Essentially, it computes the power (energy per unit time) of the echoes from moving reflectors within a given region. Power Doppler uses a color display to depict the differences in power of the reflected echoes. The advantage of power Doppler is that it is more sensitive to slow flow and provides better contrast between stationary and moving reflectors. Its clinical utility remains to be determined.

The purpose of this chapter was to provide familiarity with the underlying physical principles of the currently available imaging technologies. Imaging studies play an essential role in the diagnosis and management of female patients with diseases of the pelvis, including reproductive failure. The primary focus was on magnetic resonance technology (the newest of the three), since knowledge of these technical details plays a crucial role in generating and interpreting magnetic resonance images. It is hoped that an understanding of the concepts presented will also improve communication between radiologists and clinicians and foster collaborative research.

References

1. Gordon, A. G., Lewis, B. V. and DeCherney, A. H. (1995). In *Atlas of Gynecologic Endoscopy*, 2nd edn. (Mosby-Wolfe)
2. Tulandi, T., Collins, J. A., Burrows, E. *et al.* (1990). Treatment-dependent and treatment-independent pregnancy among women with periadnexal adhesions. *Am. J. Obstet. Gynecol.*, **162**, 354–7
3. Canis, M., Mage, G., Pouly, J. L. *et al.* (1991). Laparoscopic distal tuboplasty: report of 87 cases and a 4 year experience. *Fertil. Steril.*, **56**, 616–21

ADDITIONAL READING LIST

Magnetic resonance imaging

1. Bailes, D. R., Gilderdale, D. J., Bydder, G. M., Collins, A. G. and Firmin, D. N. (1985). Respiratory ordered phase encoding (ROPE): a method for reducing respiratory motion artifacts in MR imaging. *J. Comput. Assis. Tomogra.*, **9**, 835–8
2. Constable, R. T., Anderson, A. W., Zhong, J. and Gore, J. C. (1992). Factors influencing contrast in fast spin echo MR imaging. *Magn. Reson. Imaging*, **10**, 497–511

3. Constable, R. T. and Gore, J. C. (1992). The loss of small objects in variable TE imaging: implications for FSE, RARE and EPI. *Magn. Reson. Med.*, **28**, 9–24

4. Constable, R. T., Smith, R. C. and Gore, J. C. (1992). Signal to noise and contrast in fast spin echo (FASE) imaging and inversion recovery FASE. *J. Comput. Assis. Tomogra.*, **16**, 41–7

5. Constable, R. T., Smith, R. C. and Gore, J. C. (1993). Coupled spin FSE imaging. *J. Magn. Reson. Imaging*, **3**, 547–52

6. Hayes, C. E., Hattes, N. and Roemer, P. B. (1991). Volume imaging with MR phased arrays. *Magn. Reson. Med.*, **18**, 309–19

7. Hayes, C. E. and Roemer, P. B. (1990). Noise correlations in data simultaneously acquired from multiple surface coil arrays. *Magn. Reson. Med.*, **16**, 181–91

8. Henkelman, R. M. and Bronskill, M. J. (1987). Artifacts in magnetic resonance imaging. *Rev. Magn. Reson. Med.*, **2**, 1–126

9. Hennig, J., Nauerth, A. and Friedburg, H. (1986). RARA imaging: a fast imaging method for clinical MR. *Magn. Reson. Med.*, **3**, 823–33

10. Kier, R., Smith, R. C. and McCarthy, S. M. (1992). Distinction of hemorrhagic from fat containing ovarian tumors using fat and water suppression MR imaging. *Am. J. Roentgenol.*, **158**, 321–5

11. Lange, R. C. and Smith, R. C. (1992). Multicoil arrays boost clinical capabilities. *Magn. Reson.*, **2**, 44–6

12. Melki, P. S., Mulkern, R. V., Panych, L. P. and Jolesz, F. A. (1991). Comparing the FAISE method with conventional dual-echo sequences. *J. Magn. Reson. Imaging*, **1**, 319–26

13. Mulkern, R. V., Melki, P. S., Jakab, N. H. and Jolesz, F. A. (1991). Phase encode order and its effect on contrast and artifact in single-shot RARE sequences. *Med. Phys.*, **18**, 1032–7

14. Mulkern, R. V., Wong, S. T. S., Winalski, C. and Jolesz, F. A. (1990). Contrast manipulation and artifact assessment of 2D and 3D RARE sequences. *Magn. Reson. Imaging*, **8**, 557–66

15. Roemer, P. B., Edelstein, W. A., Hayes, C. E., Souza, S. P. and Mueller, O. M. (1990). The NMR phased array. *Magn. Reson. Med.*, **16**, 192–225

16. Schultz, C. L., Alfidi, R. J., Nelson, A. D., Kopiwoda, S. Y. and Clampitt, M. E. (1984). The effect of motion of two-dimensional Fourier transformation magnetic resonance images. *Radiology*, **152**, 117–21

17. Smith, R. C. (1995). Magnetic resonance imaging of the female pelvis. Technical considerations. *Topics Magn. Reson. Imaging*, **7**, 3–25

18. Smith, R. C., Constable, R. T., Reinhold, C., McCauley, T., Lange, R. C. and McCarthy, S.

19. (1994). Fast spin echo STIR imaging. *J. Comput. Assis. Tomogra.*, **18**, 209–13

19. Smith, R. C. and McCarthy, S. M. (1992). Physics of magnetic resonance. *J. Reprod. Med.*, **37**, 19–26

20. Smith, R. C., Reinhold, C., Lange, R. C., McCauley, T., Kier, R. and McCarthy, S. M. (1992). Fast spin echo MRI of the female pelvis part 1. Use of a whole volume coil. *Radiology*, **184**, 665–9

21. Smith, R. C., Reinhold, C., McCauley, T., Lange, R. C., Constable, R. T., Kier, R. and McCarthy, S. M. (1992). Multicoil high resolution fast spin echo MR imaging of the female pelvis. *Radiology*, **184**, 671–5

22. Wood, M. L. and Henkelman, R. M. (1985). MR image artifacts from periodic motion. *Med. Phys.*, **12**, 143–51

23. Wood, M. L. and Henkelman, R. M. (1986). Suppression of respiratory motion artifacts in magnetic resonance imaging. *Med. Phys.*, **13**, 794–805

Ultrasound

1. Fleischer, A. C., Rodgers, W. H. and Kepple, D. M. (1992). Color doppler sonography of benign and malignant ovarian masses. *Radiographics*, **12**, 879–85

2. Goldstein, A. (1993). AAPM tutorial: overview of the physics of US. *Radiographics*, **13**, 701

3. Goldstein, A. (1993). AAPM tutorial: instrumentation of digital gray scale ultrasound. *Radiographics*, **13**, 1389

4. Hamper, U. M., Seth, S. and Abbas, F. M. (1993). Transvaginal doppler sonography of adnexal masses: differences in blood flow impedance in benign and malignant lesions. *Am. J. Roentgenol.*, **160**, 1225–8

5. Kremkau, F. W. (1993). AAPM tutorial: multiple element transducers. *Radiographics*, **13**, 1163

6. O'Brien, W. D. Jr. (1993). AAPM tutorial: single element transducers. *Radiographics*, **13**, 947

7. Powis, R. L. (1994). AAPM tutorial: color flow imaging. *Radiographics*, **14**, 415

8. Rottem, S., Levit, N. and Thraler, I. (1990). Classification of ovarian lesions by high frequency transvaginal sonography. *J. Clin. Ultrasound*, **18**, 359–63

9. Rubin, J. M. (1994). AAPM tutorial: spectral doppler ultrasound. *Radiographics*, **14**, 139

10. Rubin, J. M., Bude, R. O., Carson, P. L., Bree, R. L. and Adler, R. S., (1994). Power doppler US: potentially useful alternative to mean frequency-based color doppler US. *Radiology*, **190**, 853

11. Taylor, K. J. W. and Holland, S. (1990).

Doppler US I. Basic principles, instrumentation, and pitfalls. *Radiology*, **174**, 297–307

12. Taylor, K. J. W. and Schwartz, P. E. (1994). Screening for early ovarian cancer. *Radiology*, **192**, 1–10

13. Ziskin, M. C. (1993). AAPM tutorial: fundamental physics of ultrasound and its propagation in tissue. *Radiographics*, **13**, 705

Computed tomography

1. Brink, J. A., Heiken, J. P., Wang, G., McEnery, K. W., Schlueter, F. J. and Vannier, M. W. (1994). Helical CT: principles and technical considerations. *Radiographics*, **14**, 887

2. Foley, W. D. and Oneson, S. R. (1994). Helical CT: clinical performance and imaging strategies. *Radiographics*, **14**, 894

3. Kalendar, W. A. (1994). Technical foundation of spiral CT. *Semin. Ultrasound Comput. Tomogr. Magn. Reson.*, **15**, 81

4. Kalendar, W. A., Polacin, A. and Suss, C. (1994). Comparison of conventional and spiral CT: experimental study on the detection of spherical lesions. *J. Comput. Assis. Tomogra.*, **18**, 167

5. Silverman, P. M., Cooper, C. J., Weltman, D. I. and Zeman, R. K. (1995). Helical CT: practical considerations and potential pitfalls. *Radiographics*, **15**, 25

Imaging of the normal female pelvis

2

M. Zawin

Diagnostic imaging of the pelvis in women of reproductive age generally entails ultrasound or magnetic resonance imaging (MRI), since no ionizing radiation is required. Therefore, the normal pelvic anatomy depicted on both modalities will initially be described. Normal anatomy on computed tomography (CT), hysterosalpingography and endoscopy is also reviewed.

ULTRASOUND AND MAGNETIC RESONANCE IMAGING

The uterus

The uterus is the largest and most centrally located reproductive organ, and so it is generally the first to be identified. It is a pear-shaped muscular structure, located posterior to the urinary bladder and anterior to the rectum (Figure 1). It is composed of the upper rounded uterine corpus, and the lower tubular cervix. The upper portion of the corpus is the fundus, and the angle formed by the insertion of the fallopian tubes is called the cornua.

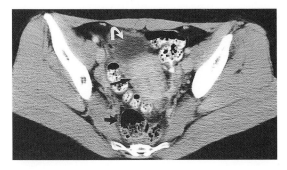

Figure 1 *Normal uterus. Axial CT scan demonstrates the uterus (long black arrow) posterior to the bladder (curved arrow), and anterior to the rectum (short black arrow)*

The size and appearance of the uterus are dependent on a woman's hormonal environment. In the female of reproductive age, the maximal uterine dimensions are 4 × 7 cm, with a corpus length of 4–4.5 cm and a cervical length of 2.5–3 cm[1,2]. The corpus/cervical ratio is 2 : 1[3].

The corpus

The corpus is composed of the inner endometrium, the outer myometrium and an intermediate region, the exact nature of which has been controversial. It has been called the subendothelial myometrial layer on histology, the myometrial halo on ultrasound, and the junctional zone on MRI. The endometrium appears as a linear echogenic stripe on ultrasound (Figure 2). Its echogenicity is due to the two apposing layers and the presence of mucus within the canal. During the early proliferative phase of the menstrual cycle, when only the terminal portions of the glands remain (the zona basalis), the endometrium is almost isoechoic with normal myometrium, and measures 4–8 mm in thickness. With the development of the zona functionalis, the endometrium is slightly more hyperechoic centrally and measures 6–10 mm in the preovulatory stage. In the secretory phase, the endometrium is homogeneously echogenic and measures 7–14 mm[4].

The myometrium can be divided into the myometrium proper or stratum vasculare, and the outer subserosal layer; these are separated by the arcuate venous and arterial plexes. These two layers can be distinguished by ultrasound. The myometrium appears as a layer that is hypoechoic relative to the endometrium (Figure 3). The arcuate vessels are visible with Doppler ultrasound (Color plate A).

There is a hypoechoic region located between the endometrium and the myometrium termed the myometrial halo (Figure 4)[5–7], the exact etiology of which, and its MRI correlation, remain controversial. It has been postulated to represent a subendothelial layer of myometrium consisting of densely packed longitudinally oriented muscle fibers. Their concentration results in a high nuclear area per high-power field[8], and a low water content[9]. These properties contribute to its appearance on both ultrasound and MRI. On ultrasound, it is poorly reflective, and so is hypoechoic.

On T_1-weighted magnetic resonance images, the uterus is homogeneously isointense to striated muscle, and hypointense to the pelvic fat (Figure 5A). The internal anatomy of the uterus, like all the reproductive organs, is optimally visualized on T_2-weighted scans (Figure 5B)[4,10–12]. The endometrium is hyperintense, and its thickness varies during the menstrual cycle, corresponding to the changes seen on ultrasound[1,13,14]. However, the overall endometrial thickness on MRI has been reported to be less than on ultrasound: 6.5 mm vs. 7.9 mm early, and 9.9 mm vs. 11.3 mm late in the cycle, respectively[15].

The myometrium is relatively isointense to striated muscle on T_2-weighted images. The overall thickness ranges from 1.5 to 2.5 cm[4,10], increasing at an average rate of 3.2% per day in the follicular and 1.8% in the luteal phase[14]. Myometrial signal intensity also increases during the menstrual cycle, reaching its maximum in the secretory phase[4].

The junctional zone is hypointense relative to both the endometrium and the myometrium (Figure 5B). In an effort to elucidate the nature of this layer, Brown and colleagues[16] correlated the MRI appearance with histology. They determined that it is composed of two sublayers: an inner compact

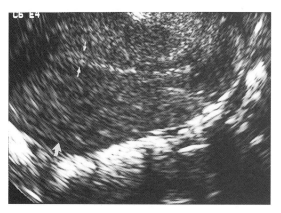

Figure 2 *Normal uterus. Sagittal transvaginal ultrasound scan in the early proliferative phase. The endometrial stripe (small arrows) is thin and echogenic relative to the myometrium (large arrow)*

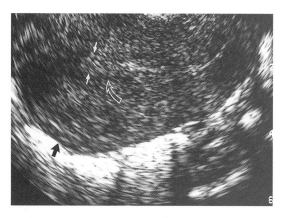

Figure 3 *Normal uterus. Sagittal ultrasound scan in the secretory phase. The endometrial stripe (small arrows) is thicker and is more echogenic than the myometrium (large black arrow). Note the myometrial halo (curved arrow)*

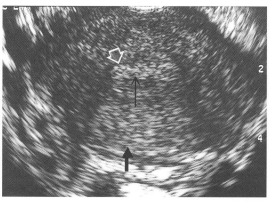

Figure 4 *Normal uterus. Transverse transvaginal ultrasound scan reveals the hypoechoic myometrial halo (long arrow) located between the echogenic endometrial stripe (clear arrow) and the myometrium (short arrow)*

layer, which they theorized corresponds to the myometrial halo seen on ultrasound, and a looser, less well-demarcated outer transitional layer. These layers are indistinguishable on current imaging modalities.

The arcuate vessels appear as signal voids on T_2-weighted scans and are also visualized on gradient echo images (Figure 5B).

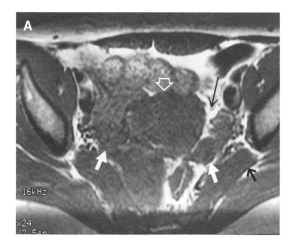

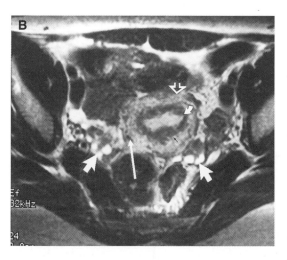

Figure 5 *Normal uterus. Axial T_1-weighted (A) and corresponding T_2-weighted fast spin echo (B) scans. (A) The uterus (clear arrow) is homogeneously hypointense to adjacent fat (long black arrow) and isointense to muscle (short black arrow). (B) The internal architecture is visualized: endometrium (curved arrow), junctional zone (small black arrow), myometrium (clear arrow), and arcuate vessels (long white arrow). Note the ovaries in both (A) and (B) (short white arrows)*

The cervix

The uterine corpus and cervix are delineated by the internal os. The cervix measures approximately 2.5 cm in length and is divided into supravaginal and vaginal portions. The supravaginal portion is covered anteriorly by the parametrium and posteriorly by the peritoneum; the latter continues inferiorly, covering the posterior vagina and reflecting onto the rectum, forming the rectouterine pouch[17].

The cervix is the closest segment of the uterus to the transvaginal probe. The closed cervix appears as a tubular, homogeneous, moderately echogenic structure. Like the uterus, it contains a central hyperechoic stripe corresponding to the endocervical canal, which is composed of mucus and cervical mucosa (Figure 6).

On T_1-weighted magnetic resonance scans, the cervix is homogeneously isointense to striated muscle. Three cervical layers are visualized on T_2-weighted images. These include: a central hyperintense stripe, which is composed of endocervical glands and mucus and is contiguous with the endometrium; a hypointense layer of dense fibromuscular stroma, contiguous with the junctional zone; and an outer layer of looser

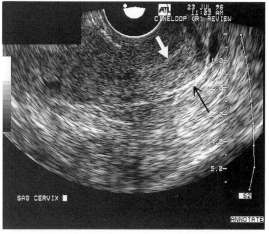

Figure 6 *Normal cervix. Sagittal transvaginal ultrasound image demonstrates a linear echogenic endocervical stripe (white arrow) and the peripheral wall (black arrow)*

stroma with intermediate signal intensity, which is contiguous with the myometrium (Figure 7). Scoutt and co-workers[18] have described high-signal linear structures on high-resolution MRI, extending from the endocervix into the middle layer, corresponding to the plica palmatae. No changes in signal intensities and thickness of the layers have been observed during the menstrual cycle. The endocervix measures 2–3 mm, the middle layer 3–8 mm and the outer layer 2–8 mm in thickness on MRI.

The fallopian tubes

The fallopian tubes are located in the mesosalpinx of the broad ligament. Each originates from the uterine cornua, extends laterally to the inferior pole of the ovary, rises along the anterior ovarian surface and ends at the free border (median) aspect of the ovary. They are approximately 10 cm long, and are divided into four segments: the intrauterine segment, the isthmus, the ampulla and the infundibulum or fimbriated segment[17].

The fallopian tubes are not often visible on ultrasound or MRI. On ultrasound, they may be detected in the presence of abdominal ascites. When enlarged or obstructed, they can be visualized on both modalities. The fallopian tubes are best visualized on hysterosalpingography.

The ovary

The ovaries descend into the true pelvis at puberty. They have a characteristic ovoid shape and contain numerous superficial cysts of varying sizes. Although mobile, they are generally located lateral to the uterus in the ovarian fossa, which is bordered anteriorly by the broad ligament, the mesovarium and ovarian hilus (containing the ovarian vessels, lymphatics and nerves); medially by the ovarian ligaments; and posteriorly by the internal iliac vessels and ureter (Figure 8)[17].

A relatively wide range of normal ovarian dimensions in women of reproductive age have been reported. In the ultrasound literature, Leopold[19] described the normal ovarian measurements as 3 cm × 2 cm × 1 cm. More recently, Hall reported dimensions of

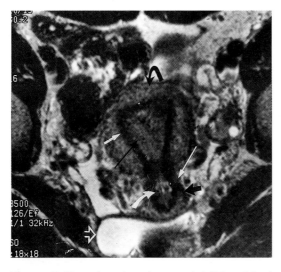

Figure 7 *Normal cervix and uterus. Axial T_2-weighted fast spin echo scan reveals the central stripe (curved white arrow), contiguous with the endometrium (long black arrow), the dense middle fibrous layer (long white arrow) contiguous with the junctional zone (short white arrow), and the outer layer (short black arrow) contiguous with the myometrium (curved black arrow). Note the fluid in the cul-de-sac (clear arrow)*

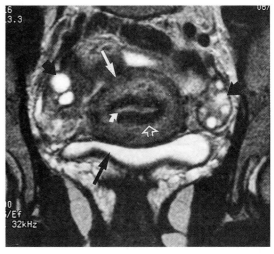

Figure 8 *Normal ovaries and uterus. Coronal T_2-weighted fast spin echo image demonstrates the ovaries containing several hyperintense follicles (short black arrows) on either side of the uterus. Note the endometrium (curved arrow), junctional zone (clear arrow), myometrium (long white arrow) and bladder (long black arrow)*

2.5–5 cm in length, 1.5–3 cm in width and 0.6–1.5 cm in thickness[20]. Volumetric determinations have been used, based on the formula of a prolate ellipse: length × width × thickness × 0.523, with a maximum normal volume, which had classically been 6 ml[21]. More recently, Cohen and associates[22] reported a mean volume of 9.8 ml. On MRI, Outwater and Mitchell[23] reported a mean ovarian size of 2.7 cm × 2.9 cm × 1.9 cm, corresponding to an ovarian volume of 7.8 cm³. To date, there has been no correlative study of measurements obtained on both state-of-the-art ultrasound and MRI equipment.

Most ovaries are visualized with transvaginal ultrasound in women of reproductive age. Possible exceptions include women with markedly enlarged uteri, where the mobile ovaries may be displaced out of the true pelvis. The ovaries undergo changes during the menstrual cycle, and these can be detected on both ultrasound and MRI. On ultrasound, cysts as small as 1–2 mm in size are detectable (Figure 9)[24]. During the follicular phase, under the influence of follicle stimulating hormone (FSH), the single dominant Graafian follicle develops, and is visible by days 8–12 in the cycle. It measures approximately 1.7–2.9 cm in size and is homogeneously anechoic with enhanced through transmission, compatible with simple fluid, and bordered by thin, well-defined walls.

The follicle ruptures following ovulation, which may be accompanied by fluid in the cul-de-sac seen on ultrasound. The corpus luteum then forms, measuring 1.6–2.4 cm in diameter at maturity. Its walls are more irregular, owing to collapse of the Graafian follicle, and its fluid may contain internal echoes secondary to hemorrhage[20,25,26]. If no conception occurs, the corpus luteum involutes in 14 days, forming the corpus albicans, which is not visible on ultrasound or MRI.

On MRI, the ovaries are homogeneously hypointense on T_1-weighted images. Their zonal anatomy is best visualized on the T_2-weighted scans. The cortex contains reticular fibers and fusiform cells, which behave like non-striated muscle and so are hypointense, whereas the medulla is of higher signal intensity, owing to the presence of numerous blood vessels and loose connective tissue. The cortical cysts generally appear of low to intermediate signal on T_1-weighted scans and high signal on T_2, as they contain simple fluid (Figure 10)[3,23]. The development and evolution of the ovarian follicle can be followed on MRI as well as ultrasound[3,27,28].

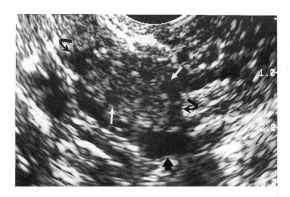

Figure 9 *Normal ovary. Transverse transvaginal ultrasound scan of an ovary (curved arrows) containing multiple anechoic follicles (small white arrows), anterior to the internal iliac vessel (large black arrow)*

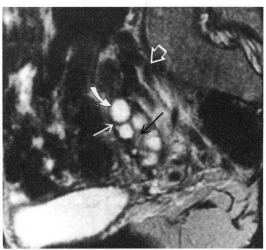

Figure 10 *Normal ovary. Sagittal T_2-weighted fast spin echo scan demonstrates a hypointense cortex (short white arrow), and the higher signal medulla (long black arrow). Several follicles are present (curved arrow). Note the internal iliac vessels (clear arrow)*

The vagina

The vagina is a fibromuscular tubal structure that surrounds the cervix superiorly, and is bordered inferiorly by the vestibule (the cleft between the labia minora), anteriorly by the bladder and urethra, and posteriorly by the rectum and anus (Figure 11A and B)[17]. It is divided into thirds according to its landmarks: the upper by the vaginal fornices, the middle by the bladder base and the lower by the urethra. Owing to its location, low within the pelvis, it is more accessible to MRI and CT than transvaginal ultrasound.

The vaginal length measures 7.5 cm anteriorly and 9.0 cm posteriorly[17]. The vagina contains estrogen and progesterone receptors and so is subject to hormonal variations.

On MRI, it appears as a homogeneously hypointense structure on T_1-weighted scans. On T_2, the central lumen is hyperintense, owing to mucus, and the outer wall is hypointense. Hricak and co-workers[29] have reported an overall increase in signal intensity of both the wall and the stripe during the late proliferative and mid-secretory phases, presumably because of edema. The vaginal stripe also thickens during the mid-secretory phase. A high-signal area is noted surrounding the periphery of the vaginal wall; this is attributed to slow-flowing blood in the perivaginal vessels and areolar tissues[29].

The bladder

The appearance of the urinary bladder depends on the degree of distension. When empty, it appears as a somewhat triangular structure in the mid-pelvis. Adequate distension is necessary for optimum transabdominal ultrasound visualization. It is pear-shaped, and predominantly hypoechoic secondary to urine, with thin well-defined linear echogenic walls (Figure 12). The transvaginal approach, on the other hand, is better tolerated with an empty bladder.

On MRI, the bladder is homogeneously hypointense on T_1, owing to the urine, which has a long T_1 value. The bladder wall, when normal, is generally not distinctly visible. On T_2-weighted images, the urine is very hyperintense, owing to its short T_2 properties, and the wall is more hypointense, similar to striated muscle (Figure 11A and B)[1].

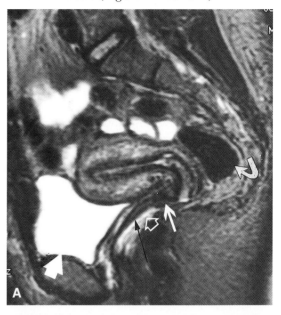

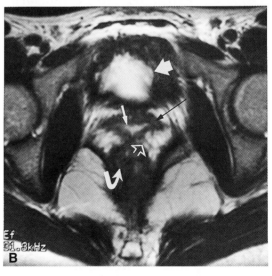

Figure 11 *Normal vagina. Sagittal (A) and axial (B) T_2-weighted images reveal the central vaginal stripe (straight white arrows), the outer wall (long black arrows) and the perivaginal venous plexus (clear arrows). The hyperintense bladder is anterior (short white arrows) and the rectum is posterior (curved arrows)*

The urethra

The urethra is a tubular structure originating from the bladder. It is situated anterior to the vagina. It is composed of muscular, erectile and mucous layers with a central lumen, and measures approximately 2–4.5 cm in length[17].

Owing to its location low within the pelvis, the transvaginal probe must be withdrawn to the vaginal entry to examine the urethra. In the absence of fluid, its apposed mucosal wall can be seen as a linear echogenicity[24]. On transabdominal images, the urethra has a 'bull's eye' appearance in the transverse plane, with a central echogenic lumen and a more hypoechoic outer wall. Just beyond the bladder base, the urethra measures 1–1.5 cm in the anteroposterior dimension and is slightly larger transversely[30].

Its MRI appearance is similar. It has homogeneously low signal on T_1, but demonstrates a target-like appearance on T_2-weighted scans, with a central high signal representing the lumen, and a more hypointense outer muscular wall (Figure 13)[31].

The rectum

The rectum lies posterior to the uterus. Its caliber and appearance varies in accordance with its distension by fecal material or gas. It often has a heterogeneous echotexture on ultrasound, owing to its mixed intraluminal contents (Figure 12). On MRI, it is predominantly of low to middle signal intensity and is well demarcated from its surrounding higher-signal pelvic fat (Figure 13)[1].

COMPUTED TOMOGRAPHY

Normal pelvic structures have been better visualized with the advent of high-resolution CT scanning and improved bolus delivery of intravenous contrast[32]. The uterus appears as a soft tissue structure centrally. The myometrium is enhanced, revealing a lower attenuation endometrial canal (Figure 14). The round ligaments are frequently seen as linear soft tissue structures which arise from the lateral aspect of the uterine fundus, cross anterior to the external iliac vessels and enter the internal iliac canal. They are often visible on MRI as well. The broad ligament is not usually visible in the absence of ascites.

The cervix consists of a moderately enhancing outer layer presumed to correlate with fibrous stroma, and a markedly enhancing inner layer, which probably corresponds to the cer-

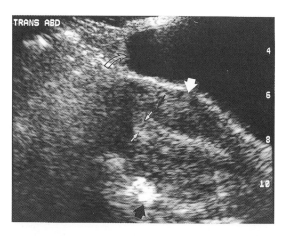

Figure 12 *Normal bladder, uterus and rectum. Sagittal transabdominal ultrasound scan with a distended bladder (curved arrow) anterior to the uterus. Note the endometrial stripe (small arrows), the myometrial halo (longer black arrow), the myometrium (short white arrow), and the rectum (short black arrow)*

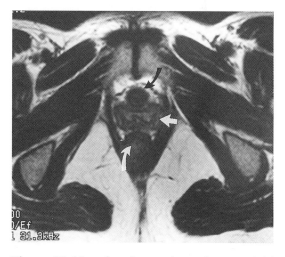

Figure 13 *Normal urethra, vagina and rectum. Axial T_2-weighted fast spin echo scan demonstrating the urethra (curved black arrow), vagina (straight white arrow) and rectum (curved white arrow)*

vical epithelium. The cardinal ligaments appear as triangular soft tissue densities, their bases oriented towards the lateral aspect of the cervix, and their apicies extend laterally to the pelvic side walls. The uterosacral ligaments are thinner, and like the cardinal ligaments originate at the level of the internal os and course posteriorly towards the sacrum (Figure 15).

The ovaries are often visualized in the female of reproductive age, owing to the presence of numerous cysts of varying sizes

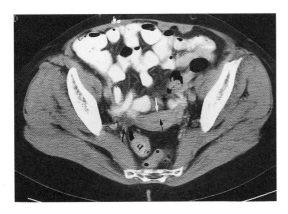

Figure 14 *Normal uterus. Axial CT scan reveals the uterus with the enhancing myometrium (white arrow) and central hypointense canal (short black arrow). Note the right ovary (longer black arrow)*

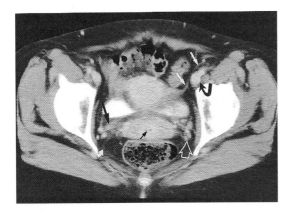

Figure 15 *Normal uterus and cervix. Axial CT scan demonstrates the round ligament (straight white arrows) extending anterior to the external iliac vessels (curved black arrow). The cervical epithelium enhances (short black arrow) as does the pericervical vascular plexus (clear arrow). Note the right cardinal (larger straight black arrow) and uterosacral (curved white arrow) ligaments*

(Figure 16). Because of their mobility, they may be seen lateral to the uterus, posterior and inferior to it in the cul-de-sac, or high in the false pelvis, if the uterus is markedly enlarged.

The vagina contains a poorly enhancing outer wall and a central region of marked enhancement corresponding to the mucosa. The ureters, bladder (Figure 17) and urethra (Figure 18) are also visible.

Pelvic vessels are now more apparent with dynamic scanning techniques. The uterine arteries appear as enhancing linear structures lateral to the uterus, and extend anteriorly over the ureters (Figure 19). The cervico-vaginal vascular plexus is visualized laterally, within the pelvic fat on both CT and MRI (Figure 20).

HYSTEROSALPINGOGRAPHY

Unlike the other imaging modalities, hystero-salpingography is more invasive. Contrast is introduced via the cervical os, outlining the endocervical and endometrial canals, rather than the outer wall of the cervix and uterus. The fallopian tubes are best visualized with hysterosalpingography, and their patency is evaluated.

Hysterosalpingography is generally performed during the preovulatory phase, when the endometrium is thick and smooth. The uterus has been reported to be in the midline in 62% and lateral in 38% of normal patients.

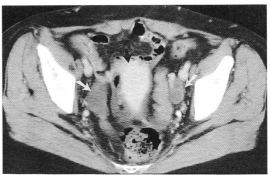

Figure 16 *Normal ovaries. Axial CT scan reveals both ovaries with hypointense follicles (white arrows) on either side of the uterus with the enhancing myometrium (black arrow)*

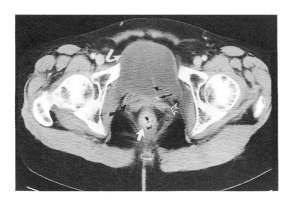

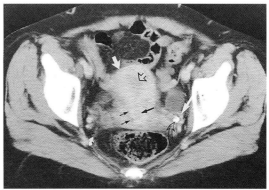

Figure 17 *Normal vagina. Axial CT scan demonstrates the vagina (clear arrow) with the perivaginal vascular plexus (curved black arrow). Note the contrast-filled left ureter (longer black arrow), its ureteral jet (short black arrow), the urine-filled bladder (curved white arrow) and rectum (straight white arrow)*

Figure 20 *Normal uterus and cervix. Axial CT image reveals enhancing myometrium (short white arrow) and cervical epithelium (short black arrows) outlining the endometrial (clear straight arrow) and the endocervical canal (long black arrow). Note the cervicovaginal venous plexus (long white arrow), left ureter (curved clear arrow), and the uterosacral ligament (curved white arrow)*

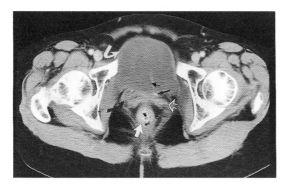

Figure 18 *Normal urethra. Axial CT image of the urethra (curved white arrow), the vagina (black arrow) and posterior rectum (curved clear arrow)*

The normal intrauterine cavity appears as an inverted triangle, the base being formed by the fundus, and the apex by the internal os. The normal fundus may appear straight (83%), concave (14%), or convex (3%) (Figure 21). The normal concavity may be up to 1 cm, as measured by a perpendicular line drawn from a horizontal line extending between the cornua. The endometrial cavity measures 1.2–6 cm in height, with an intercornual distance of 1.8–6 cm. The outline is usually smooth, although focal (29%) and diffuse (16%) irregularities have been reported in normal patients. The cornual lumen is pear-shaped, and may be separated from the cavity by a linear lucency which may be due to its orientation or to muscular contraction (Figure 22)[33].

The isthmus represents the transition between the uterine body and cervix, and is visualized as an area of narrowing (Figure 23). Its length ranges from 0.2 to 1.2 cm[34]. The internal os is located between the uterine cavity and isthmus and has a variable diameter normally of 1–10 mm.

The endocervical canal tapers at the internal os. The normal canal varies in shape, contour and size. The mucosa consists of the plicae palmatae, which appear as thin stacked

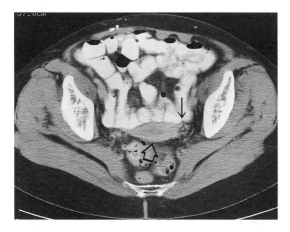

Figure 19 *Normal uterus. Axial CT scan demonstrates the uterus (clear arrow) with adjacent enhancing uterine vessels (black arrow)*

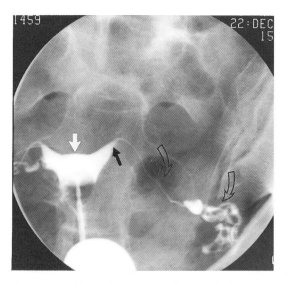

Figure 21 *Normal uterus. Hysterosalpingogram demonstrates a convex superior endometrial contour (white arrow) and a linear lucency at the left cornua (straight black arrow). Note the left fallopian tube (curved arrows)*

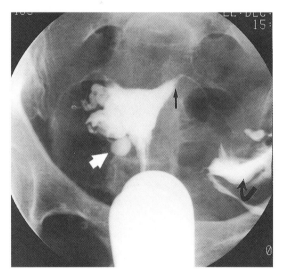

Figure 22 *Normal uterus. Hysterosalpingographic close-up view reveals the cornual lumen (straight black arrow). Note the obstructed right tube (white arrow) and free spillage on the left (curved arrow)*

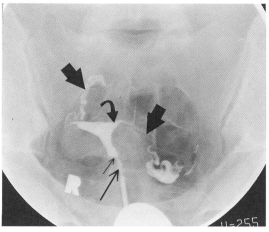

Figure 23 *Normal cervix, uterus and fallopian tubes. Early image from a hysterosalpingogram with a normal endocervical canal (long black arrow), isthmus (short black arrow) and left cornua (curved arrow). Note the bilateral fallopian tubes (wide black arrows)*

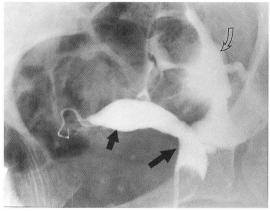

Figure 24 *Normal uterus and cervix. Oblique hysterosalpingographic image reveals normal endometrial (short straight arrow) and endocervical (long straight arrow) canals. Note the unilateral free intraperitoneal spillage on the left (curved arrow)*

folds (Figure 24). During the secretory phase, the contour can appear smooth. The canal measures 3–4 cm in length and 0.5–3.0 cm in width, being widest during the proliferative phase of the menstrual cycle[33].

The fallopian tubes vary in location and course. The lumina of the segments vary in size: the intraluminal portion is thread-like, that of the isthmus measures 1–2 mm and the ampulla ranges from 2 to 12 mm. The fimbriated portion is not separately visualized[33]. Tubal patency is determined by spillage of contrast material into the peritoneum (Figure 25).

The ovaries are not normally seen on hysterosalpingography.

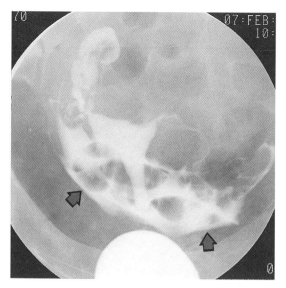

Figure 25 *Fallopian tubal patency. Hysterosalpingogram reveals free intraperitoneal spillage of contrast (arrows)*

ENDOSCOPY

Although more invasive, laparoscopy and hysteroscopy are the procedures of choice for definitive evaluation of the pelvis of the infertile patient. After the umbilical laparoscopic port is placed, the anterior peritoneum is viewed through the laparoscope and the lower operating ports are inserted lateral to the epigastric arteries (Color plate B). Through the laparoscope, the uterus and ovaries are well visualized (Color plate C). Chromopertubation is performed to evaluate the patency of the fallopian tubes by inserting blue dye transcervically. Tubal patency is documented by visualization of free flow of blue dye from the fimbriated ends of the fallopian tubes (Color plate D). Hysteroscopy allows for visualization of the normal endometrium and tubal ostia (Color plate E).

SUMMARY

There are a number of imaging modalities currently available to evaluate the female pelvis. Ultrasound and MRI offer the advantage of lacking ionizing radiation. Computed tomography, although not routinely used, is capable of depicting pelvic organs and the adjacent lymph nodes and urinary structures. Hysterosalpingography is complementary and is indicated for specific purposes, both diagnostic and therapeutic, including documenting and promoting tubal patency. Endoscopy is the procedure of choice for definitive evaluation of the pelvis of the infertile patient, but is more invasive than other imaging modalities available.

References

1. McCarthy, S., Tauber, C. and Gore, J. (1986). Female pelvic anatomy: MR assessment of variations during the menstrual cycle and with the use of oral contraceptives. *Radiology*, **160**, 119–23
2. Davis, G. (1981). *Applied Anatomy*, p. 457. (Philadelphia: Lippincott)
3. McCarthy, S. (1992). Magnetic resonance imaging of the normal female pelvis. *Radiol. Clin. North Am.*, **30**, 769–75
4. Heiken, J. P. and Lee, J. K. T. (1988). MR imaging of the pelvis. *Radiology*, **166**, 11–16
5. Lyons, E. A., Gratton, D. and Harrington, C. (1992). Transvaginal sonography of normal pelvic anatomy. *Radiol. Clin. North Am.*, **30**, 663–75
6. Sample, W. R., Lippe, B. M. and Gyepes, M. T. (1977). Grey scale ultrasonography of the normal female pelvis. *Radiology*, **125**, 477
7. Fleischer, A. C., Kalemeris, G., Entman, S. *et al.* (1986). Sonographic depiction of abnormal endometrium with histopathologic correlation. *J. Ultrasound Med.*, **5**, 445
8. Scoutt, L. M., Flynn, S. D., Luthringer, D. J. *et al.* (1991). Junctional zone of the uterus: correlation of MR imaging and histologic examination of hysterectomy specimens. *Radiology*, **179**, 403–7
9. McCarthy, S., Scott, G., Majumdar, S. *et al.* (1989). Uterine junctional zone: MR study of water content and relaxation properties. *Radiology*, **171**, 241–3

10. Hricak, H., Alpers, C., Crooks, L. E. *et al.* (1983). Magnetic resonance imaging of the female pelvis: initial experience. *Am. J. Roentgenol.*, **141**, 1119–28

11. Bryan, P. J., Butler, H. E. and LiPuma, J. P. (1984). Magnetic resonance imaging of the pelvis. *Radiol. Clin. North Am.*, **22**, 897–915

12. Lee, K. T., Gersell, D. J., Balfe, D. M. *et al.* (1985). The uterus: *in vitro* MR–anatomic correlation of normal and abnormal specimens. *Radiology*, **157**, 175–9

13. Demas, B. E., Hricak, H. and Jaffe, R. B. (1986). Uterine MR imaging: effects of hormonal stimulation. *Radiology*, **160**, 119–23

14. Haynor, D. R., Mack, L. A., Soules, M. R. *et al.* (1986). Changing appearance of the normal uterus during the menstrual cycle: MR studies. *Radiology*, **161**, 459–62

15. Mitchell, D. G., Schonholz, L., Hilpert, P. L. *et al.* (1990). Zones of the uterus: discrepancy between US and MR images. *Radiology*, **174**, 827–31

16. Brown, H. K., Stoll, B. S., Nicosia, S. V. *et al.* (1991). Uterine junctional zone: correlation between histologic findings and MR imaging. *Radiology*, **179**, 409–13.

17. Gray, H., Williams, P. L., Warwick, R., Dyson, M., Bannister, L. H. (eds.) (1995). *Anatomy of the Human Body*, 38th edn. (New York: Churchill Livingstone)

18. Scoutt, L. M., McCauley, T. R., Flynn, S. D. *et al.* (1993). Zonal anatomy of the cervix: correlation of MR imaging and histologic examination of hysterectomy specimens. *Radiology*, **186**, 159–62

19. Leopold, G. (1987). Pelvic ultrasonography. In Sarti, D. (ed.) *Diagnostic Ultrasound Text and Cases*, 2nd edn., pp. 684–7. (Chicago: Year Book Medical)

20. Hall, D. A. (1983). Sonographic appearance of the normal ovary, of polycystic ovary disease, and of functional ovarian cysts. *Semin. Ultrasound*, **4**, 149–65

21. Sample, W., Lippe, B. and Gyepes, M. (1977). Gray-scale ultrasonography of the normal female pelvis. *Radiology*, **125**, 477–83

22. Cohen, H. L., Tice, H. M. and Mandel, F. S. (1990). Ovarian volumes measured by US: bigger than we think. *Radiology*, **177**, 189–92

23. Outwater, E. K. and Mitchell, D. G. (1996). Normal ovaries and functional cysts: MR appearance. *Radiology*, **198**, 397–402

24. Lyons, E. A., Gratton, D. and Harrington, C. (1992). Transvaginal sonography of normal pelvic anatomy. *Radiol. Clin. North Am.*, **30**, 663–75

25. Fleischer, A. C., Daniell, J. F., Rodier, J. *et al.* (1981). Sonographic monitoring of ovarian follicular development. *J. Clin. Ultrasound*, **9**, 275–80.

26. Ritchie, W. G. M. (1986). Sonographic evaluation of normal and induced ovulation. *Radiology*, **161**, 1–10

27. Janus, C. L., Bateman, B., Wiczyk, H. *et al.* (1990). Evaluation of the stimulated menstrual cycle by magnetic resonance imaging. *Fertil. Steril.*, **54**, 1017

28. Janus, C. L., Wiczyk, H. P. and Laufer, N. (1988). Magnetic resonance imaging of the menstrual cycle. *Magn. Reson. Imaging*, **6**, 669

29. Hricak, H., Chang, Y. C. F. and Thurnher, S. (1988). Vagina: evaluation with MR imaging. Part I. Normal anatomy and congenital anomalies. *Radiology*, **169**, 169–74

30. Hennigan, H. W. Jr and DuBose, T. J. (1985). Sonography of the normal female urethra. *Am. J. Roentgenol.*, **145**, 839–41

31. Hricak, H., Secaf, E., Buckley, D. W. *et al.* (1991). Female urethra: MR imaging. *Radiology*, **178**, 527–35

32. Forshager, M. and Walsh, J. M. (1994). CT anatomy of the female pelvis: a second look. *Radiographics*, **14**, 51–66

33. Ott, D. J. and Fayez, J. A. (1991). *Hysterosalpingography. A Text and Atlas*, 2nd edn. (Baltimore, Munich: Urban and Schwarzenberg)

34. Siegler, A. (1974). *Hysterosalpingography*, 2nd edn. (New York: Medcom Press)

The peritoneum and infertility

3

D. L. Olive, A. K. Parsons and R. Troiano

The peritoneal cavity houses the reproductive organs and performs a critical function in the reproductive process: it allows the fallopian tubes and ovaries to lie in direct proximity to one another. Such positioning allows the passage of ovulated oocytes from the ovarian surface to the tubal lumen. If, however, this convenient anatomical relationship is disturbed, the journey of the oocyte becomes significantly more difficult, if not impossible. Normal anatomical relationships are crucial to normal fertility, and distorted anatomy can be instrumental in infertility.

Distorted anatomical proximity may occasionally result from a failure of normal reproductive system development; this, however, is an unusual finding. Much more common is physical hindrance as a result of peritoneal adhesion formation. Such adhesions may result from a variety of disorders, both gynecological and non-gynecological. This chapter reviews these causes, the mechanism by which pelvic adhesions are formed and the techniques used to image such abnormalities.

THE PERITONEUM

The peritoneum consists of two layers of tissue: a superficial mesothelial cell layer and the underlying stroma, composed of connective tissue, blood vessels and lymphatics. Disruption of this surface may result from mechanical trauma, ischemia, infection and foreign materials. Removal of the mesothelial surface invokes an immediate release of histamine and vasoactive kinins from resident stromal mast cells. These components increase the permeability of surrounding blood vessels, producing a serosanguinous exudate rich in inflammatory cells[1]. This exudate normally coagulates and within hours forms fibrinous attachments to surrounding tissues[2,3]. If lysis of this fibrin occurs within 3 days, normal healing will occur[4,5]; however, if lysis is delayed, fibroblastic proliferation may result in abnormal attachments between tissue surfaces.

Peritoneal wound healing differs from that of the skin in that the entire surface becomes epithelialized simultaneously, not gradually from the edge of the defect[6]. The time course for regeneration of the mesothelial layer of both visceral and parietal peritoneum appears to be 5–8 days[7,8].

This regeneration involves both the cellular exudate and the proliferation of mesothelial cells. At 24–36 h after injury, the wound surface contains macrophages intertwined in fibrin filaments. The base of the wound is relatively acellular at this time. At 2 days the wound is covered with a single layer of macrophages supported by a fibrin scaffold. Also on the cell surface is the appearance of primitive mesenchymal cells, with no basement membrane beneath them. Their number increases by day 3, although they are still outnumbered by the macrophages. The base of the wound contains mesenchymal cells and some proliferating fibroblasts. By the 4th day, the mesenchymal cells on the wound surface begin to contact one another. By the 5th day, parietal peritoneum is associated with basement membrane formation, although this is not seen with visceral peritoneum. On the 8th day, a continuous layer of mesothelial cells is present, and a continuous basement membrane is seen at day 10.

New peritoneal cells do not arise, to any significant degree, by the centripetal spreading of mesothelial cells surrounding the wounded area. The question of where these cells come from is currently unanswered. Several possibilities exist: (1) transformation of underlying undifferentiated mesenchymal cells into a new peritoneal membrane[9,10]; (2) transformation of perivascular cells into a new peritoneal membrane[10,11]; (3) transplantation of cells from peritoneal surfaces of adjacent viscera[11,12]; or (4) transformation of cells from the peritoneal fluid into peritoneal cells[8].

MECHANISM OF ADHESION FORMATION

The fibrin matrix discussed above spontaneously resolves under normal circumstances, allowing complete healing of any defect. Plasminogen activators located in the mesothelium and underlying stroma are responsible for this fibrinolytic activity. These activators convert plasminogen to plasmin, a fibrin-splitting enzyme. As adhesion formation appears to be directly related to delayed resolution of fibrinous tissue attachments, it follows that factors suppressing plasminogen activators will ultimately suppress fibrinolysis and promote adhesion development.

A common cause of decreased plasminogen activator activity is surface abrasion[3]. Although mechanical abrasion will reduce plasminogen activator activity, such injuries alone often do not result in adhesion formation. When serosal abrasion is combined with fresh, unclotted blood, adhesion formation is the rule[13]. This effect is not seen, however, when defibrinated blood is applied[13,14]. It appears that the combination of decreased plasminogen activator and a relative abundance of fibrin is needed for developing adhesions.

Another suppressor of plasminogen activator is tissue ischemia[2,15–18]. Ischemic tissue inhibits fibrinolysis by adjacent normal tissue[2]. By reducing the tissue oxidation–reduction potential, infection may potentiate the effect of ischemia in suppressing normal fibrinolytic mechanisms. Endometriosis lesions also have low levels of plasminogen activator, probably representing a method by which the disease facilitates adhesion formation[19].

ENDOMETRIOSIS

Endometriosis is defined as the presence of endometrial tissue in an ectopic location, exclusive of the myometrium. Traditionally, the presence of both glands and stroma are required to establish the diagnosis, although the validity of such a requirement has never been established.

The disease appears nearly exclusively in women of reproductive age, with a mean age of diagnosis from 25 to 29 years[20,21], although this figure is largely dependent upon the mechanism by which diagnosis is made. Endometriosis is rarely found in the premenarchal female, and has never been reported to be symptomatic in such women. The rate of occurrence in adolescents is unknown but the condition does not appear to be rare. In two studies of women under age 20 with chronic pelvic pain or dysmenorrhea unresponsive to medical therapy, endometriosis was found at surgery in 47–65% of cases[22,23]. Simply considering the teenage years to be a single entity, however, may be misleading, as most documented cases of endometriosis in girls under age 17 are associated with Müllerian anomalies and outflow tract obstruction[24]. The disease may occur in the menopausal female, but generally this is a sequela to hormone replacement therapy[25].

The true prevalence of endometriosis in the general population is difficult to determine, owing to selection bias in those investigated for the disease; the difficulty in non-invasive diagnosis makes true population-based investigation virtually impossible. A best estimate is roughly 10% of the reproductive age population.

Endometriosis has long been believed to have a racial preponderance, although variation in prevalence rates appear to be due to such confounding factors as availability of health care, access to contraception, cultural differences in childbearing patterns, attitudes towards menses and pain, and incidence of sexually transmitted diseases. A genetic component to the disorder has been recognized, and is most probably via polygenic, multifactorial inheritance[26,27]. A recent initiative to determine key endometriosis genes, the OXEGENE project, is underway and may produce results in the next few years.

Endometriosis is associated with a wide variety of symptoms, although many with the disease are entirely asymptomatic. Although some symptoms may strongly suggest the diagnosis, none is indicative of the disease. One common symptom is infertility, with a rate of endometriosis in the infertile population undergoing surgical evaluation ranging from 4.5 to 33%, with a mean of 14%[28]. Unfortunately, the prevalence of infertility in women with endometriosis cannot be adequately assessed.

Pelvic pain is also a common complaint in the woman with endometriosis. Secondary dysmenorrhea or worsening primary dysmenorrhea is commonly seen among these patients. Dyspareunia is also a frequent complaint and is most often reported with involvement of the uterosacral ligament or rectovaginal septum. Other types of 'pelvic' pain include non-cyclic lower abdominal pain and backaches. In addition, pain symptoms may be site specific when endometriosis is found in unusual locations outside the pelvis.

Physical examination is of variable value in women with endometriosis, as patients with extensive disease may well have minimal findings. Common signs include nodularity or tenderness of the cul-de-sac, parametrial thickening and adnexal masses. A fixed, retrodisplaced uterus may also be seen with extensive disease. Rarely, cutaneous lesions may be present in such locations as the vagina, perineum, umbilicus and within surgical scars. Ascites has also been reported.

Attempts at diagnosis of endometriosis via serum testing has been generally unsuccessful. The monoclonal antibody OC-125, identifying the antigenic determinant CA-125, has been used widely. Unfortunately, extensive evaluation has revealed insufficient sensitivity or specificity for usefulness in diagnostic screening for the disease[29-31]. Other approaches, such as the detection of PP14 or endometrial antibodies, are still termed experimental and have yet to be proved of diagnostic value.

DOES ENDOMETRIOSIS CAUSE INFERTILITY?

As mentioned above, the association of infertility with endometriosis is without question. However, despite the apparent association, the question remains as to whether endometriosis can actually *cause* infertility.

Certainly, when endometriosis produces anatomical distortion of the pelvic viscera or fallopian tube obstruction, the result is often infertility. The efficacy of surgical therapy for treatment of endometriosis-associated infertility with severe disease (i.e. extensive pelvic adhesions) lends credence to this concept[32], as does evidence from animal models[33,34].

A more intriguing question is whether or not endometriotic implants alone, in the absence of adhesions, can cause infertility. Experimental animal models of endometriosis have been used by several investigators to address this question. In both the rabbit[35] and monkey[33] models, transplanted endometrium has been shown to decrease fertility. However, in both experiments this was apparently due to pelvic adhesion formation; in the absence of such anatomical distortion, there was no change in fertility.

Clinical investigation has also addressed this issue. Jensen prospectively analyzed 91 women undergoing artificial insemination with donor sperm and no other apparent infertility factor[36]. All had husbands with azoospermia or severe oligospermia. Of the 91, seven were found to have endometriosis upon screening laparoscopy. Subsequent fertility was significantly lower in the women with early-stage endometriosis. However, problems with this study include (1) a small number of endometriosis patients, enabling small errors in diagnostic accuracy to have a potentially substantial effect; (2) multiple physicians performing the laparoscopies, making diagnosis likely to be non-uniform; and (3) a monthly rate of conception in women with endometriosis of less than 4%, far lower than in most studies[37]. Therefore, this study must be considered suggestive at best.

Conflicting evidence is presented by Rodriguez-Escudero and colleagues[38]. In a population of 21 donor sperm recipients with endometriosis, these investigators demonstrated a monthly probability of pregnancy of more than 20%. A study by Chauhan and associates[39] also investigated women undergoing donor insemination. By including women with either azoospermic or oligospermic husbands and comparing those with endometriosis to those with no identifiable disorder, the monthly probability of pregnancy was 9.3% in the former and 9.9% in the latter. Finally, a comprehensive multivariate investigation into potential pathogenetic factors affecting fertility in 731 infertile women determined that endometriosis without adhesions did not alter the cumulative conception rate[40]. These studies, along with a lack of efficacy among treatments of early-stage endometriosis in enhancing the fertility rate, seriously question the concept that implants alone can be a primary cause of infertility.

OTHER SOURCES OF INFLAMMATION

Pelvic inflammatory disease (PID) is caused by micro-organisms ascending to the upper genital tract. Inflammation may be present at any point along a continuum that includes endometritis, salpingitis and peritonitis. Most cases of PID are caused by sexually transmitted micro-organisms, namely *Neisseria gonorrhoeae* and *Chlamydia trachomatis*[41–43]. Less frequently, respiratory pathogens such as *Haemophilus influenzae*, Group A streptococci and pneumococci can cause this disorder. Endogenous micro-organisms found in the vagina are also often isolated from the upper genital tract of women with PID. These include anaerobic organisms such as *Prevotella* and peptostreptococci as well as *Gardnerella vaginalis*.

Diagnosis of PID in the acute stage is based on a triad of symptoms and signs including pelvic pain, cervical motion and adnexal tenderness, and fever. However, the presentation may be highly variable and diagnosis may well be delayed.

Evaluation of lower genital tract secretions, both vaginal and endocervical, is a crucial part of the workup of the patient with PID. An increased number of polymorphonuclear leukocytes may be detected in a wet mount of the vaginal secretions or in the mucopurulent discharge.

Post-surgical inflammation can also cause peritoneal adhesion formation. Denuding of the peritoneal surface, ischemia, or toxic effects of gas or other materials may result in peritoneal defects. The mechanisms for repair were mentioned above. Although laparoscopic surgery is less likely to produce adhesions than laparotomy, damage and scarring can certainly be a sequela of either.

The development of an abscess in the pelvis or abdomen is uncommon after gynecological surgery, but may be considerably more common following other surgical procedures. It is most likely to occur in cases with contamination, in which the surgical site is not adequately drained, or as a secondary complication of hematomas. The causative pathogens are usually polymicrobial in nature, and are generally derived from the vagina or gastrointestinal tract.

IMAGING OF PERITONEAL DISORDERS

Ultrasound

Endometriosis

Vaginal ultrasound provides unambiguous confirmation of the presence of persistent ovarian masses, some of which are due to subcortical entrapment of degenerating blood from variably functioning endometriotic glands. These collections are termed endometriomata, and are identifiable as smooth-walled ovarian cysts filled with particulate fluid. Because of the effects of repetitive bleeding, however, they may contain bizarre formations of detritus that suggest tumors, and can provide a never-ending variety of appearances (Figure 1). Since they contain no

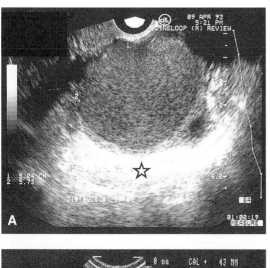

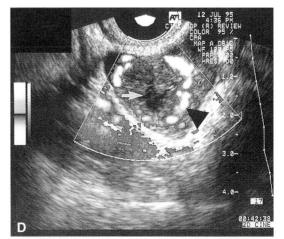

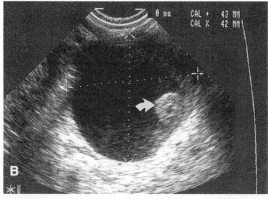

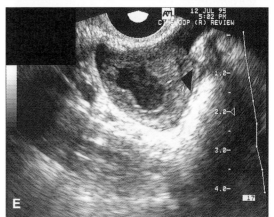

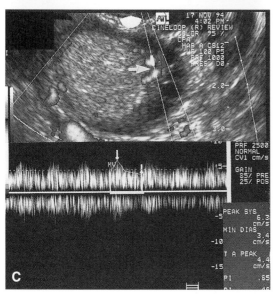

Figure 1 (A) *Typical 5 × 5.7 cm endometrioma filled with homogeneous particulate fluid. The bright enhancement of bowel (starred) beyond the ovary reveals the cystic nature of the mass. There is only a thin rim of normal ovary seen inferior to it. This asymptomatic cyst occurred in a cycling 32-year-old woman who had been treated with tamoxifen for 2 years for breast cancer. (B) Bizarre endometriotic cyst with thin walls, particulate fluid and an apparent papillation (arrow), which consisted of debris. This was interpreted before surgery as a dermoid papilla in a cystic teratoma. (C) Homogeneous endometrioma with typical focal low-impedance ovarian vessel flow in the peripheral ovarian stroma (arrow). There is no flow in the cyst itself and no circumferential flow. (D) Typical circular vessel pattern of the thecal blood flow (arrowhead) surrounding a corpus luteum, shown by 'power' Doppler. The wreath-like arteriole is difficult to image in a single plane. The central clot (white arrow) is present in all corpora lutea, and is surrounded by the thick corrugated granulosa lutein layer. Evaluation of the vascular pattern confirmed this to be a corpus luteum rather than an endometrioma. (E) Same corpus luteum as in (B) (arrowhead), without color power Doppler, demonstrates the simple small central clot surrounded by a thick echogenic wall*

intrinsic vasculature, any vessels associated with them are those of the surrounding ovary. Kurjak and Kupesic[44] described a typical focal stromal or 'hilar' vessel configuration rather than the circumferential ultra-low impedance vasculature of the corpus luteum. They found that the addition of Doppler provided a sensitivity and specificity of over 99% each for the (vaginal) sonographic diagnosis of 103 endometriomata in a group of 656 ovarian masses. Positive preoperative diagnosis of endometriomata assists in surgical planning; however, the persistence of a complex ovarian cyst without decrement in size for more than one complete cycle is an indication for cystectomy, since at this time the treatment of both ovarian tumors and endometriomata is surgical. Needle drainage of complex or blood-filled cysts has not been curative[45,46], and may result in worsening pain or abscess formation[47].

At this time, peritoneal endometriosis cannot be imaged with ultrasound. The importance of detection of superficial asymptomatic endometriosis is probably negligible[48]. Invasive lesions signal their presence by producing adhesions (Figure 2), organ fixation (Figure 3), collections of blood between peritoneal surfaces (Figure 4), hematosalpinges (Figure 5) and/or pain, and these are demonstrable during pelvic examination assisted by vaginal ultrasound.

Adhesions

There are two types of adhesions: those that virtually eradicate peritoneal surfaces by causing their adherence to each other, and those that are attached between surfaces and may restrict or alter the functional movement

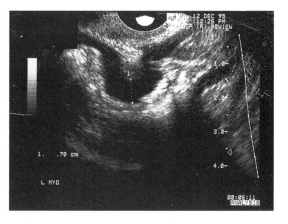

Figure 3 *A painful fixed hairpin-turn point of fixation of the rectosigmoid, with dramatically thickened muscularis measuring 7 mm in a patient with chronic left-sided pain who had undergone a left oophorectomy for severe endometriosis years before. Identification of this site suggested that surgical treatment was required for lysis of adhesions and that preparation of the bowel should be carried out preoperatively. Dense fixation of the sigmoid to the pelvic floor and sidewall was found and pain was relieved following adhesiolysis*

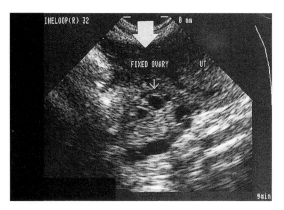

Figure 2 *Ovarian fixation: a right ovary that cannot be brought into contact with the probe at the vaginal wall (at the region of the wide arrow) because the ovary is adhering to the uterine fundus (UT)*

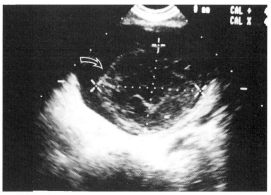

Figure 4 *Retroperitoneal endometrioma in the midline vaginal cuff. This patient had undergone a hysterectomy and unilateral oophorectomy 3 years earlier. Sonographic evaluation for dyspareunia demonstrated this small endometriotic cyst, surrounded by bloody fluid (clear arrow). No ovarian tissue was identified*

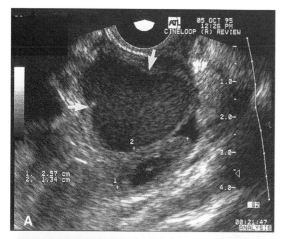

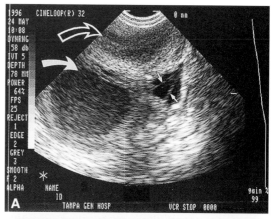

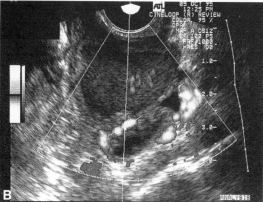

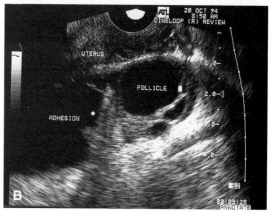

Figure 5 (A) *Hematosalpinx filled with typical thin particulate fluid still showing remnants of two endosalpingeal folds (arrows). It is contiguous with an ovary containing an ovoid corpus luteum, measuring 2.57 × 1.34 cm. The tubal endometriosis occurred in a 43-year-old asymptomatic woman. (B) Positive identification of the corpus luteum vascular pattern with power Doppler, indicating that the blood-filled tube was clearly extraovarian*

Figure 6 (A) *Sagittal view of the posterior cul-de-sac with a tiny pocket of fluid across which filmy adhesions (small arrows) run between the pelvic floor, the ovary in the rectosigmoid, which adhere to each other, and the posterior cervix. The clear arrow indicates the cervical internal os. The white curved arrow points to a 3-cm luteinized unruptured follicle ('hemorrhagic corpus luteum'), the prevention of ovulation caused by the adhesions that plaster this ovary into the cul-de-sac (B) Sagittal view of adhesions around a left ovary that contains a normal follicle. The ovary is adherent to the posterior cardinal ligament lateral to the (marked) uterus*

of organs. Using palpatory vaginal ultrasound, the first type can be discerned by distortion and fixation of pelvic organs. The second type are detectable only when they are outlined by surrounding fluid (Figure 6).

The inability to contact an ovary through the vaginal wall despite bimanual manipulation suggests that it is fixed in a way that keeps it off the pelvic floor, or that the vagina is abnormally non-compliant. Causes of this difficulty include: massive obesity with thick retroperitoneal fat; peritoneal adhesions

fixing the ovary, intervening masses, radiation fibrosis of the vagina, a Müllerian anomaly associated with failure of descent of the ovary, or a combination of these. All of these causes can be identified during the ultrasound-assisted pelvic examination, with gentle bimanual palpation of the ovary or uterus by both the abdominal hand and the ultrasound probe, which is used as the vaginal digits.

Timor-Tritsch and Rottem introduced the

'sliding organ sign' as a means of determining organ mobility to infer the presence of significant adhesions[49]. As Zimmer and colleagues described it, it is the same invaluable maneuver used to discern foci of pain during the ultrasound-assisted pelvic examination: gentle pressure with the vaginal transducer on the organ of interest[49]. The direction of pressure is chosen to provide the maximal excursion of the organ over a contiguous peritoneal surface, under sonographic observation. There have been no prospective trials published comparing the use of this technique with surgical findings. However, using this same principal and abdominal ultrasound transducers, attempts have been made to discern bowel adhesions to the anterior abdominal wall. This technique seems most accurate in patients with previous scars, when performed by those with a working knowledge of surgical anatomy. Kolecki and colleagues[50] found that natural respiratory movements allowed demonstration of anterior abdominal wall adhesions in the upper and middle abdomen much more accurately than in the pelvis. They found the sensitivity and specificity of the technique to be 90% and 92%, respectively, in 110 unselected preoperative patients. Of the ten inaccurate predictions, nine were due to misinterpretation of images of the pelvis. Uberoi and colleagues[51] reported that neither manual compression of the abdominal wall nor observation of its excursion with exaggerated respiration reliably detected all 'fibrinous' abdominal adhesions in 48 unselected patients before surgery, although failure of the bowel to slide freely under the abdominal wall was more specific for dense 'fibrous' abdominal wall adhesions. Caprini and co-workers[52] evaluated 30 patients previously operated on before laparoscopy for the presence of adhesions beneath the umbilicus and surgical scars and elsewhere, to direct the best site for trocar placement. Assessing spontaneous visceral slide during respiration while scanning longitudinally, as well as induced visceral slide during palpatory scanning in transverse or longitudinal

directions, they identified all four periumbilical adhesions and all 16 adhesions beneath old surgical scars.

They defined the normal spontaneous excursion distance as 2–5 cm, and normal induced excursion as at least 1 cm, and recommended this technique be used 'on a highly selective basis by the operating surgeon to guide initial trocar insertion'.

Optimal sonographic imaging of intimately related peritoneal surfaces in the pelvis requires that they be separated by a contrast medium. The clever and observant I. F. Stein, of Stein–Leventhal fame[53], championed the use of intraperitoneal carbon dioxide as a distension medium and contrast to outline the pelvic organs using radiography. He then infused lipiodol transcervically for positive contrast of the reproductive lumen for evaluation of infertile women, terming this 'gynecography'[54–56]. The use of culdoscopy in addition to gynecography provided a direct view of the pelvis, and retention of the gas required for the culdoscopy obviated the requirement for insufflation through the abdominal wall[57]. These techniques have now given way to the use of laparoscopy and vaginal ultrasound with contrast.

The sonographic effect of clear fluid provides stark negative contrast for soft tissue surface demonstration, and is easily detected. Many sonologists have observed the intraperitoneal accumulation of a small amount of transcervically infused fluid to be an indicator of tubal patency[58–60]. The presence of ascites renders even Fitz-Hugh–Curtis adhesions of the liver assessable by abdominal ultrasound[61]. The presence of a small amount of pelvic fluid in the dependent posterior cul-de-sac is found in almost all cycling women, and it is maximal around (not necessarily after) the event of ovulation. Steinkampf and colleagues[62] demonstrated the sensitivity of vaginal ultrasound for intraperitoneal fluid by monitoring saline infused through the umbilical port in patients anesthetized for laparoscopy. Sonographic detection of pelvic fluid was possible at a mean volume of 25.8 ± 6.4 ml (SD). They then measured the ambient pelvic fluid at laparoscopy in 19 infertile women, after estimating the volume and location using preoperative vaginal ultrasound. Peritoneal fluid and its location were accurately identified sonographically in every patient in whom 0.8 ml or more of fluid was aspirated[63].

Davison and Leeton[64] had described the use of vaginal ultrasound and clear fluid to outline the peritoneal surfaces for evaluation of adhesions in an infertile patient in 1988; 500 ml of Hartmann's solution was infused through the umbilicus with a Verres needle immediately preceding laparoscopy, while more fluid was instilled transcervically with a Rubin's cannula. Unilateral tubal patency and damage as well as periovarian adhesions were accurately demonstrated, and the authors were the first to observe that sonography with contrast, or echogynecography, could replace the use of hysteroscopy, hysterosalpingography and laparoscopy in the evaluation of infertility.

Their findings corroborated those of Maroulis and co-workers[65] in a study in which sterile saline was infused through patent tubes by means of a cervical balloon catheter (Table 1). Thirty-eight women were evaluated before laparoscopy for infertility or pelvic pain. They found that a volume of at least 150 ml was required for adequate visualization, and correctly predicted the presence and location of adhesions in 13 women. In the 25 women in whom pelvic adhesions were not identified sonographically, four proved to have adhesions at laparoscopy. One had high fixation of the uterine fundus to the anterior abdominal wall, and three had fixating adhesions between the ovary and the pelvic sidewalls. Two paratubal cysts and two hydrosalpinges were also correctly described. The inability to outline the ovarian surface after instilling pelvic fluid is an important indicator of dense ovarian adhesions, which themselves cannot be delineated. Failure of instilled fluid to pool in the posterior cul-de-sac when there is no mass present is likewise indicative of its obliteration by adherent organ surfaces[66].

A second-look laparoscopy has been advocated for eradication of recurrent adhesions following surgical treatment of severe endometriosis or adhesions, for optimal restoration of function. A recent method to enhance the limited view of office-based endoscopy with imaging was described by Steege[67], who left Tenckhoff catheters in eight women following extensive laparoscopic lysis of adhesions for pelvic pain. He then performed repetitive laparoscopies in the office with a 2-mm laparoscope for assessment and treatment of new adhesions, using the catheters for access. Under office conditions, the deep pelvis was often obscured below the mid-uterus, but he found that tubo-ovarian and pelvic floor adhesions were well imaged with vaginal ultrasound after instillation of normal saline.

Table 1 *Findings in a comparison between a number of patients with vaginal ultrasound and laparoscopic identification of pelvic adhesions from a total of 38 patients. From reference 65*

	Vaginal ultrasound	*Laparoscopy*
Low pelvic adhesions	9	9
High pelvic adhesions	0	1
Fixating ovarian adhesions	0	3
Tubal pathology	2	2
Paraovarian cysts	2	2
No adhesions	29	25

Peritoneal cysts

Various types of benign mesothelial cysts occur throughout the pelvis and retroperitoneum; some are free floating. These may form spontaneously or as reactive responses to chemical or physical irritation (Figure 7), or they may be congenital remnants of embryonic structures, such as paratubal and paraovarian cysts (Figure 8). These are sonographically identifiable as being extra-ovarian, thin-walled simple cysts and are usually insignificant unless they are large enough to distort and obstruct the tube. The occurrence of central echoes and complex

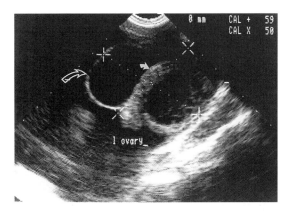

Figure 7 *An ovary with a corpus luteum in a woman with urinary ascites due to a ureteral injury 6 weeks earlier at hysterectomy. Irritation of the ovarian surface by the urine has produced a reactive cyst (clear arrow) and thickened indurated ovarian peritoneum (white arrow). From reference 82, with permission*

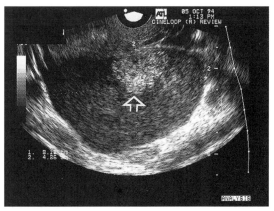

Figure 9 *A 4 × 8 cm paratubal cyst that contained a tumor of low malignant potential in the form of a papillation (arrow), surrounded by thick mucus. The separate ovary was clearly visible, but is not shown here*

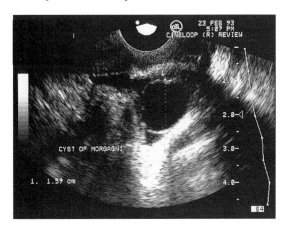

Figure 8 *Fluid outlining a typical paratubal cyst (cyst of Morgagni)*

vessels in an extraovarian cyst is associated with the histological features of neoplasia with low malignant potential, and excision is indicated (Figure 9). These epithelial tumors are filled with thick secretions and may have papillations similar to those of their ovarian counterparts.

Magnetic resonance imaging

Only pigmented hemorrhagic endometriotic lesions can be detected with magnetic resonance imaging (MRI). Large implants behave as ovarian endometriomas. Although the signal characteristics are variable depending on the age of associated hemorrhage, classically these demonstrate hyperintensity on T_1-weighted images with hypointense shading on T_2-weighted images[68–71] (Figure 10). These changes reflect the presence of deoxyhemoglobin and methemoglobin, which shorten T_1 and T_2 relaxation times. However, hypointensity on both T_1- and T_2-weighted images may be seen with acute hemorrhage, whereas hyperintensity on both sequences may reflect older bleeds. Multiplicity of hyperintense cystic lesions correlates highly with endometrial implants[68]. Secondary signs include the presence of a hematocrit effect and the presence of adhesions[69,70].

Several studies have addressed the ability to document pelvic endometriosis. Most studies have examined large lesions with reported sensitivities ranging from 64% to 90%, and specificities from 60% to 98% using conventional T_1- and T_2-weighted sequences[1,2,4,5] (Figure 11). One study[72] showed that the addition of fat-saturation T_1-weighted sequences to conventional imaging increased the sensitivity from 82% to 91%, and the specificity from 91% to 94% (Figure 12).

Small endometrial implants (<1 cm) are more difficult to document, especially when examined without fat-saturation techniques.

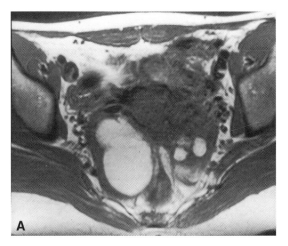

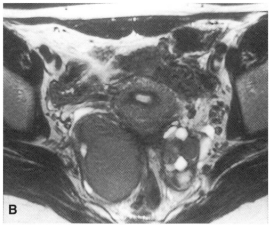

Figure 10 *Bilateral endometriosis with adhesions. T_1-weighted (A) and fast spin echo (FSE) T_2-weighted (B) axial images of the pelvis demonstrating bilateral high signal foci within and on the serosa of the ovaries, which are hyperintense on the T_1-weighted image and hypointense on the FSE T_2-weighted image. Note the low signal band between the sigmoid and the uterus with loss of a clear interface from the right ovary, consistent with adhesions*

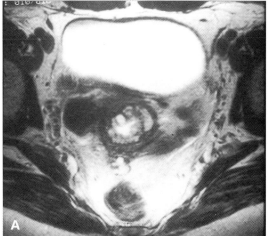

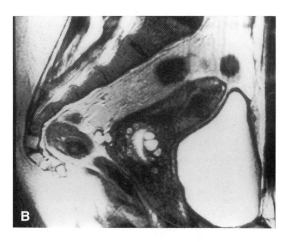

Figure 11 *Endometrial implant in the cul-de-sac. Axial (A) and sagittal (B) fast spin echo T_2-weighted images, showing a small cluster of high signal endometrial implants on the posterior uterine serosa. The hyperintensity of the foci indicates a chronic process*

Implants as small as 3 mm have been seen with the addition of fat-suppressed images, and a reported 64% of lesions of <1.5 cm have been detected[73]. One study showed that use of fat-suppression sequences increased the sensitivity of documenting small implants from 11% to 47%, while the specificity remained stable at approximately 97%[72]. A more recent study demonstrated a sensitivity of 62% in detecting small implants[73].

Although fat-saturation imaging has good contrast resolution and a high signal to noise ratio, detection of small implants may be hindered by field heterogeneities, as well as blurring from bowel peristalsis. Blood vessels and intraluminal intestinal contents may also be hyperintense and mimic small implants. These limitations generally restrict detection of small implants to the serosa of the pelvis.

MRI may have a role as a screening modality in patients suspected of having endometriosis[73]. Additionally, it is useful in monitoring response to treatment and in

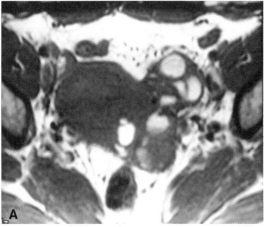

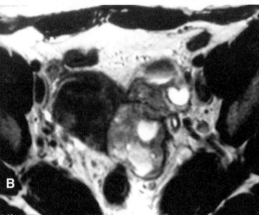

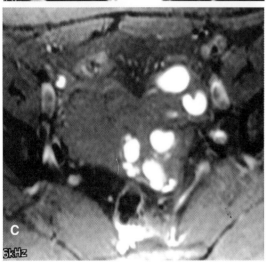

Figure 12 *Diffuse pelvic endometriosis. Axial T_1-weighted (A), fast spin echo T_2-weighted (B) and T_1-weighted fat-suppressed (C) images demonstrate multiple foci at different stages of hemorrhage. Note the increased conspicuity of the hemorrhagic lesions on the fat-suppression image*

evaluating patients with extensive scarring and adhesions that preclude laparoscopic visualization of disease[71]. Most authors remain sceptical of the ability of MRI to stage endometriosis, given its limitations in fully defining the extent of disease. However, one study has proposed that hyperintense implants less than 5 mm in maximum diameter are indicative of early disease, and cystic implants larger that 15 mm are suggestive of advanced disease. Lesions between 5 and 15 mm are equivocal and require further investigation[70]. However, MRI cannot replace laparoscopy in the evaluation of endometriosis. Not only is the MRI appearance of endometriosis not pathogno-monic, but diffuse tiny plaque-like lesions cannot be identified, and exact staging is not possible[68,69,71].

Adhesions are difficult to document by MRI, unless they are extensive. They may be seen as linear low signal bands on both T_1- and T_2-weighted images, lying between organs and/or pelvic sidewalls. Loss of a clear interface between an endometrioma and adjacent organs is also suggestive[69]. Angulation and fixation of bowel loops may also be seen (Figure 10).

Peritoneal mesothelial proliferations, such as benign cystic mesothelioma (peritoneal inclusion cysts) are well characterized on MRI (Figure 13). Thin-walled, unilocular or multilocular cysts are seen distributed within the pelvis and can extend throughout the peritoneum in advanced cases. MRI may be preferable for evaluating the extent of disease, given its larger field of view. The cysts are seen as hypointense on T_1-weighted images, and hyperintense on T_2-weighted images (Figure 13).

Diffuse peritoneal processes, such as disseminated peritoneal leiomyomatosis, which are manifest as small peritoneal nodules, are elusive of diagnosis by an imaging modality.

LAPAROSCOPY

Laparoscopic examination of the pelvis and abdomen affords the simplest and most direct method of inspecting the peritoneal cavity for endometriosis, adhesions and other abnormalities. However, to obtain optimal information with this viewing method, a systematic and thorough approach must be applied. For example, a second puncture for manipulation of pelvic/abdominal structures is essential, particularly in viewing the complete ovarian surface, ovarian fossae, deep cul-de-sac and appendix. Aspiration of the peritoneal fluid may reveal hidden pathology below the surface. Ovaries that are adherent should be mobilized for examination and often have endometriosis hidden from view.

Despite the advantages of directly viewing the peritoneal surface, laparoscopy can have limitations. Extensive adhesion formation may obscure key areas, inhibiting complete evaluation. Endometriosis may also lurk below the visible surface, such as within the rectovaginal septum, and be overlooked on casual inspection. Finally, a lack of experience by the operator may result in lesions being unrecognized.

Sampson first recognized the variety of appearances of endometriosis, describing the chocolate cyst, blebs, nodules, adherent surfaces, red raspberries, blueberries and peritoneal pockets[74–76]. More recently, up to 16 different appearances have been described, many of which encompass the so-called atypical lesions[77–80]. In addition to the traditional black, blue or red lesions, non-pigmented peritoneal lesions as well as a variety of other abnormal shades may represent endometriosis; these forms of the disease are not rare and may well represent the majority of the manifestations of this disorder (Color plate F). In one series, 56% of women with endometriosis had only non-pigmented lesions[77]. Yellow and yellow–brown pigmented lesions as well as adhesions and peritoneal pockets may also contain endometriosis[78]. In addition to being more common, the non-pigmented lesions appear to be more metabolically active[81].

In lesions appearing as typical endometriosis, histological evaluation has revealed hemangiomas, carbon, old suture material,

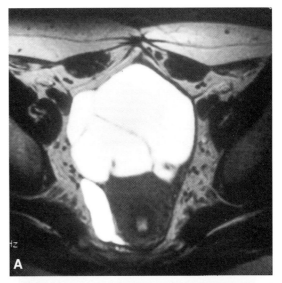

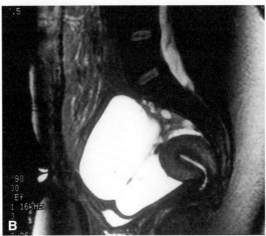

Figure 13 *Benign cystic mesothelioma. Axial (A) and sagittal (B) fast spin echo T_2-weighted images demonstrate multilocular, thin-walled cysts within the pelvis, consistent with peritoneal inclusion cysts*

trophoblastic proliferation, necrotic ectopic pregnancies, adrenal rests, breast cancer, ovarian cancer and peritoneal inflammatory cysts[77,78]. Therefore, biopsy with histological evaluation is essential in evaluating the presence or absence of endometriosis.

Adhesions, too, may be missed at laparoscopy by the too-casual observer. Subtle filmy adhesions covering the ovary may cause an inability of oocytes to reach their ultimate destination, and small adhesions of the tube or ovary may prevent full organ mobility. It is critical during the evaluative process to check the full mobility of each pelvic structure, to ensure that there is no inhibition of normal movement.

Traditional laparoscopy is performed in the operating room under general anesthesia, but the time and expense of this procedure often makes it prohibitive. A recent alternative has been the advent of office laparoscopy under local anesthesia (OLULA). This approach, using local anesthesia with intravenous sedation and new, small fiberoptic endoscopes, enables the procedure to be truly minimally invasive. Costs are decreased by as much as 80%, and recovery is rapid. The procedure appears to be tailor-made for diagnostic evaluation of the pelvis in the infertile female, and early data suggest that such women do well with the procedure. The ultimate role of OLULA in evaluating the peritoneum of infertile women awaits further investigation.

References

1. Trompke, R. and Siegner, R. (1956). Ein Beitrag zu den Verhutungsmaßnahmen postoperativer interabdomineller Verwachsungen. *Arch. Klin. Chir.*, **281**, 323
2. Gazzaniga, A. B., Jares, J. M., Shobe, J. and Oppenheim, E. S. (1975). Prevention of peritoneal adhesions in the rat. *Arch. Surg.*, **110**, 429
3. Gervin, A. S., Puckett, C. L. and Silver, D. (1973). Serosal hypofibrinolysis: a cause of postoperative adhesions. *Am. J. Surg.*, **125**, 80
4. Buckman, R. F., Buckman, P. D., Hufnagel, H. U. and Caldwell, R. (1976). A physiologic basis for the adhesion free healing of deperitonealized surfaces. *J. Surg. Res.*, **21**, 67
5. Raftery, A. T. (1979). Regeneration of peritoneum: a fibrinolytic study. *J. Anat.*, **129**, 659
6. Hertzler, A. E. (1919). *The Peritoneum.* (St. Louis: CV Mosby)
7. Glucksman, D. (1966). Serosal integrity and intestinal adhesions. *Surgery*, **60**, 1009–11
8. Eskeland, G. and Kjaerheim, A. (1966). Regeneration of parietal peritoneum in rats. I. A light microscopical study. *Acta Pathol. Microbiol. Scand.*, **68**, 353–78
9. Robbins, G. F., Brunschwig, A. and Foote, F. W. (1949). Deperitonealization: clinical and experimental observations. *Ann. Surg.*, **130**, 466–79
10. Ellis, H., Harrison, W. and Hugh, TB. (1965). The healing of peritoneum under normal and pathological conditions. *Br. J. Surg.*, **52**, 471–6
11. Johnson, F. R. and Whitting, H. W. (1962). Repair of parietal peritoneum. *Br. J. Surg.*, **49**, 653–60
12. Cameron, G. R., Hassan, S. M. and De, S. N. (1957). Repair of Glisson's capsule after tangential wound of the liver. *J. Pathol. Bact.*, **73**, 1–10
13. Ryan, G. B., Grobety, J. and Majno, G. (1971). Postoperative peritoneal adhesions. *Am. J. Pathol.*, **65**, 117
14. Nisell, H. and Larsson, B. (1978). Role of blood and fibrinogen in development of intraperitoneal adhesions in rats. *Fertil. Steril.*, **30**, 470
15. Ellis, H. (1962). The aetiology of postoperative abdominal adhesions: an experimental study. *Br. J. Surg.*, **50**, 10
16. Buckman, R. F., Woods, M., Sargent, L. and Geruin, A. S. (1976). A unifying pathogenetic mechanism in the etiology of intraperitoneal adhesions. *J. Surg. Res.*, **20**,1
17. Myhre-Jensen, O., Larsen, S. B. and Astrup, T. (1969). Fibrinolytic activity in serosal and synovial membranes. *Arch. Pathol.*, **88**, 623
18. Porter, J. M., McGregor, F. H., Mullen, D. C. and Silver, D. (1969). Fibrinolytic activity of mesothelial surfaces. *Surg. Forum*, **20**, 80
19. Ohtsuka, N. (1980). Study of pathogenesis of adhesions in endometriosis. *Acta Obstet. Gynecol. Jpn.*, **32**, 1758
20. Norwood, G. E. (1960). Sterility and fertility in women with pelvic endometriosis. *Clin. Obstet. Gynecol.*, **3**, 456
21. Olive, D. L. and Haney, A. F. (1986). Endometriosis. In DeCherney, A. H. (ed.) *Reproductive Failure*, pp. 153–201. (New York: Churchill Livingston)
22. Goldstein, D. P., deCholnoky, C., Emans, S. J. and Leventhal, J. M. (1980). Laparoscopy in the diagnosis and management of pelvic pain in adolescents. *J. Reprod. Med.*, **24**, 251
23. Chatman, D. L. and Ward, A. B. (1982). Endometriosis in adolescents. *J. Reprod. Med.*, **27**, 156
24. Huffman, J. W. (1981). Endometriosis in young teenage girls. *Pediatr. Ann.*, **10**, 44

25. Djursing, H., Peterson, K. and Weberg, E. (1981). Symptomatic postmenopausal endometriosis. *Acta Obstet. Gynecol. Scand.*, **60**, 529

26. Simpson, J. L., Elias, S., Malinak, L. R. and Buttram, V. C. Jr (1980). Heritable aspects of endometriosis. I. Genetic studies. *Am. J. Obstet. Gynecol.*, **137**, 327

27. Malinak, L. R., Buttram, V. C. Jr and Elias, S. (1980). Heritable aspects of endometriosis. II. Clinical characteristics of familial endometriosis. *Am. J. Obstet. Gynecol.*, **137**, 332

28. Pauerstein, C. J. (1989). Clinical presentation and diagnosis. In Schenken, R. S. (ed.) *Endometriosis: Contemporary Concepts in Clinical Management*, pp. 127–44. (Philadelphia: J. B. Lippincott)

29. Malkasian, G. D. Jr, Podratz, K. C., Stanhope, C. R. *et al.* (1986). CA-125 in gynecologic practice. *Am. J. Obstet. Gynecol.*, **155**, 515

30. Patton, E. P., Field, C. S., Harms, R. W. and Coulam, C. B. (1986). CA-125 levels in endometriosis. *Fertil. Steril.*, **45**, 770

31. Gurgan, T., Kisnisci, H., Yarali, H. *et al.* (1990). Serum and peritoneal fluid CA-125 levels in early stage endometriosis. *Gynecol. Obstet. Invest.*, **30**, 105

32. Olive, D. L. and Lee, K. L. (1986). Analysis of sequential treatment protocols for endometriosis-associated infertility. *Am. J. Obstet. Gynecol.*, **154**, 613–19

33. Schenken, R. S., Asch, R. H., Williams, R. F. and Hodgen, G. D. (1984). Etiology of infertility in monkeys with endometriosis. *Fertil. Steril.*, **41**, 122

34. Werlin, L. B., DiZerega, G. S. and Hodgen, G. D. (1981). Endometriosis: effect of ovulation, ovum pickup, and transport in monkeys: an interim report (abstr.). *Fertil. Steril.*, **35**, 263

35. Kaplan, C. R., Eddy, C. A., Olive, D. L. and Schenken, R. S. (1989). Effect of ovarian endometriosis on ovulation in rabbits. *Am. J. Obstet. Gynecol.*, **160**, 40

36. Jansen, R. P. S. (1986). Minimal endometriosis and reduced fecundability: prospective evidence from an artificial insemination by donor program. *Fertil. Steril.*, **46**, 141

37. Olive, D. L. and Haney, A. F. (1986). Endometriosis-associated infertility: a critical review of therapeutic approaches. *Obstet. Gynecol. Surv.*, **41**, 538

38. Rodriguez-Escudero, F. J., Neyro, J. L., Corcostegui, B. and Benito, J. A. (1988). Does minimal endometriosis reduce fecundity? *Fertil. Steril.*, **50**, 522

39. Chauhan, M., Barratt, C. L. R., Cooke, S. M. S. and Cooke, I. D. (1989). Differences in the fertility of donor insemination recipients – a study to provide prognostic guidelines as to its success and outcome. *Fertil. Steril.*, **51**, 815

40. Dunphy, B. C., Key, R., Barratt, C. L. R. and Cooke, I. D. (1989). Female age: the length of involuntary infertility prior to investigation and fertility outcome. *Hum. Reprod.*, **4**, 527

41. Soper, D. E., Brockwell, N. J. and Dalton, H. P. (1992). Microbial etiology of urban emergency department acute salpingitis: treatment with ofloxacin. *Am. J. Obstet. Gynecol.*, **167**, 653–60

42. Sweet, R. L., Draper, D. L., Schachter, J., James, J., Hadley, W. K. and Brooks, G. F. (1980). Microbiology and pathogenesis of acute salpingitis as determined by laparoscopy: what is the appropriate site to sample? *Am. J. Obstet. Gynecol.*, **138**, 985–9

43. Wasserheit, J. N., Bell, T. A., Kiviat, N. B., Wolner-Hanssen, P., Zabriskie, V., Kirby, B. D. *et al.* (1986). Microbial causes of proven pelvic inflammatory disease and efficacy of clindamycin and tobramycin. *Ann. Intern. Med.*, **104**, 187–93

44. Kurjak, A. and Kupesic, S. (1964). Scoring system for prediction of ovarian endometriosis based on transvaginal color and pulsed Doppler sonography. *Fertil. Steril.*, **62**, 81–8

45. Vercellini, P., Vendola, N., Bocciolone, L., Colombo, A., Rognoni, M. T. and Bolis, G. (1992). Laparoscopic aspiration of ovarian endometriomas. *J. Reprod. Med.*, **37**, 577–80

46. Trio, D., Pittelli, M. and Rangoni, G. (1995). Ultrasound-guided aspiration of endometriomas: possible applications and limitations. *Fertil. Steril.*, **64**, 709–13.

47. Padilla, S. L. (1993). Ovarian abscess following puncture of an endometrioma during ultrasound-guided oocyte retrieval. *Hum. Reprod.*, **8**, 1282–3

48. Koninckx, P. R., Oosterlynck, D., D'Hooghe, T. and Meuleman, C. (1994). Deeply infiltrating endometriosis is a disease whereas mild endometriosis could be considered a non-disease. *Ann. NY Acad. Sci.*, **734**, 333–41

49. Zimmer, E. Z., Timor-Tritsch, I. E. and Rottem, S. (1991). The technique of transvaginal sonography. in Timor-Trisch, I. E. and Rottem, S. (eds.) *Transvaginal Sonography*, 2nd edn. (New York: Elsevier)

50. Kolecki, R. V., Golub, R. M., Sigel, B., Machi, J., Kitamura, H., Hosokawa, T., Justin, J., Schwartz, J. and Zaren, H. A. (1994). Accuracy of viscera slide detection of abdominal wall adhesions by ultrasound. *Surg. Endosc.*, **8**, 871–4

51. Uberoi, R., D'Costa, H., Brown, C. and Dubbins, P. (1995). Visceral slide for intraperitoneal adhesions? A prospective study in 48 patients with surgical correlation. *J. Clin. Ultrasound*, **23**, 363–6

52. Caprini, J. A., Arcelus, J. A., Swanson, J., Coats, R., Hoffman, K., Brosnan, J. J. and Blattner, S. (1995). The ultrasonic localization

of abdominal wall adhesions. *Surg. Endosc.*, **9**, 283–5

53. Stein, I. F. and Leventhal, M. (1935). Amenorrhea associated with bilateral polycystic ovaries. *Am. J. Obstet. Gynecol.*, **29**, 181

54. Stein, I. F. (1931). Eight years' experience with roentgen diagnosis in gynecology: pneumoperitoneum and lipiodol in pelvic diagnosis. *Am. J. Obstet. Gynecol.*, **21**, 671

55. Stein, I. F. and Arens, R. A. (1926). Pneumoperitoneum in gynecology. *Radiology*, **7**, 326

56. Stein, I. F. and Arens, R. A. (1930). Visualization of the pelvic vescera. *Radiology*, **15**, 85

57. Spellacy, W. N. and Tobin, J. A. (1964). Gynecography: a neglected adjuvant to culdoscopy. *Obstet. Gynecol.*, **24**, 286

58. Richman, T. S., Viscomi, G. N., DeCherney, A., Polan, M. L. and Alcebo, L. O. (1984). Fallopian tubal patency assessed by ultrasound following fluid injection. *Radiology*, **152**, 507–10

59. Randolph, J. R., Ying, Y. K., Maier, D. B., Schmidt, C. L. and Riddick, D. H. (1986). Comparison of real-time ultrasonography, hysterosalpingography and laparoscopy/hysteroscopy in the evaluation of uterine abnormalities and tubal patency. *Fertil. Steril.*, **46**, 828–32

60. Parsons, A. K., Cullinan, J. A., Goldstein, S. R. and Fleischer, A. C. (1996). Sonohysterography, sonosalpingography and sonohysterosalpingography. In *Principles and Practice of Ultrasonography in Obstetrics and Gynecology*

61. van Dongen, P. W. (1993). Diagnosis of Fitz-Hugh–Curtis syndrome by ultrasound. *Eur. J. Obstet. Gynecol. Reprod. Biol.*, **50**, 159–62

62. Steinkampf, M. P., Blackwell, R. E. and Younger, J. B. (1994). Visualization of free peritoneal fluid with transvaginal sonography. *J. Reprod. Med.*, **24**, 729–30

63. Nichols, J. E. and Steinkampf, M. P. (1993). Detection of free peritoneal fluid by transvaginal sonography. *J. Clin. Ultrasound*, **21**, 171–4

64. Davison, G. B. and Leeton, J. (1988). A case of female infertility investigated by contrast-enhanced echo-gynecography. *J. Clin. Ultrasound*, **16**, 44–7

65. Maroulis, G. B., Parsons, A. K. and Yeko, T. R. (1992). Hydrogynecography: a new technique enables vaginal sonography to visualize pelvic adhesions and other pelvic structures. *Fertil. Steril.*, **58**, 1073–5

66. Rasmussen, F., Larsen, C. and Justesen, P. (1986). Fallopian tube patency demonstrated at ultrasonography. *Acta Radiol. Diagn.*, **27**, 61–3

67. Steege, J. F. (1994). Repeated clinic laparoscopy

68. Togashi, K., Nishimura, K., Kimura, I. *et al.* (1991) Endometrial cysts: diagnosis with MR imaging. *Radiology*, **180**, 73–8

69. Arrive, L., Hricak, H. and Martin, M. (1989). Pelvic endometriosis: MR imaging. *Radiology*, **171**, 687–92.

70. Nyberg, D. A., Porter, B. A., Olds, M. O. *et al.* (1987). Imaging of hemorrhagic adnexal masses. *J. Comput. Assist. Tomogr.*, **7**, 257–64

71. Zawin, M., McCarthy, S., Scoutt, L. *et al.* (1989). Endometriosis: appearances and detection at MR imaging. *Radiology*, **171**, 693–6

72. Suimara, K., Okizuka, H., Imaoka, *et al.* (1993). Pelvic endometriosis: detection and diagnosis with chemical shift MR imaging. *Radiology*, **188**, 435–8

73. Ha, H. K., Lim, Y. T., Kim, H. S. *et al.* (1994). Diagnosis of pelvic endometriosis: fat-suppressed T_1-weighted vs. conventional MR imaging. *Am. J. Roentgenol.*, **163**, 127–31

74. Sampson, J. A. (1921). Perforating hemorrhagic (chocolate) cysts of the ovary. *Arch. Surg.*, **3**, 245

75. Sampson, J. A. (1940). The development of the implantation theory for the origin of peritoneal endometriosis. *Am. J. Obstet. Gynecol.*, **40**, 549

76. Sampson, J. A. (1924). Benign and malignant endometrial implants in the peritoneal cavity and their relationship to certain ovarian tumors. *Surg. Gynecol. Obstet.*, **38**, 287

77. Jansen, R. P. S. and Russell, P. (1986). Nonpigmented endometriosis: clinical, laparoscopic, and pathologic definition. *Am. J. Obstet. Gynecol.*, **155**, 1154

78. Martin, D. C., Hubert, G. D., Vander Zwaag, R. *et al.* (1989). Laparoscopic appearances of peritoneal endometriosis. *Fertil. Steril.*, **51**, 63

79. Stripling, M. C., Martin, D. C., Chatman, D. L. *et al.* (1988). Subtle appearance of endometriosis. *Fertil. Steril.*, **49**, 427

80. Stripling, M. C., Martin, D. C. and Poston, W. M. (1988). Does endometriosis have a typical appearance? *J. Reprod. Med.*, **33**, 879

81. Vernon, M. W., Beard, J. S., Graves, K. *et al.* (1986). Classification of endometriotic implants by morphologic appearance and capacity to synthesize prostaglandin. *Fertil. Steril.*, **46**, 801

82. Gleeson, N. C., Parsons, A. K., Hoffman, M. S. and Cavanagh, D. (1993). Urinary ascites with pelvic urinoma presenting as ovarian neoplasm: clinical and ultrasonographic features. *Obstet. Gynecol.*, **82**, 644–6

for the treatment of pelvic adhesions: a pilot study. *Obstet. Gynecol.*, **83**, 276–9

Diagnostic imaging in ovarian dysfunction   4

J. M. Brown and L. B. Schwartz

Normal adult ovaries typically have a volume of approximately 6 to 10 cm^3 [1-3], although up to 18 cm^3 is normal in premenopausal women[4]. Typically each is located in a recess along the pelvic sidewall, although their position is variable. This recess is bounded posterolaterally by the internal iliac vessels and ureter, and anteriorly by the obliterated umbilical artery. The arteries, veins and lymphatics supplying the ovary run in a suspensory ligament attached to the parietal peritoneum. The primary function of the ovary is the cyclic release of mature oocytes. This process of follicular development, maturation and release, as well as the subsequent formation and regression of the corpus luteum, requires the continuous repetitive production of hormones by the ovary itself as well as interaction with pituitary gonadotropins, especially follicle stimulating hormone (FSH) and luteinizing hormone (LH). The pituitary is not innately cyclic in its production, but depends on stimulation from the hypothalamus in addition to reciprocal interaction with the ovary. The monthly release of oocytes therefore requires functionally normal ovarian tissue and also the complex and precise participation of other neuroendocrine tissues. The ovary orchestrates this process by providing feedback signals to the hypothalamic–pituitary axis and through the production and direct action of ovarian hormones, most importantly estrogen. Ovarian hormones are produced cyclically as a consequence of follicular maturation, which involves three phases: follicular, ovulatory and luteal. Morphological and physiological changes occur repetitively within the ovary as the process occurs and monitoring of these changes is important in the evaluation of the infertile patient.

Ultrasound is well accepted as the examination of choice for ovarian screening and allows visualization of the ovaries in most patients. Cohn and associates[3] examined 762 consecutive patients in their clinic and obtained visualization adequate for measurement in 725 (95%), although other series have shown less satisfactory results. DeSantis and colleagues[5] identified only 76% of normal ovaries in premenopausal patients and even fewer of those with masses. Differences in equipment affect results and the technique is highly operator dependent, especially when an endovaginal approach is used. The advent of endovaginal ultrasound probes has, however, enabled the use of higher frequencies, which provide improved lateral and axial resolution and reduce the incidence of imaging artifacts. As the penetration of these high-frequency probes is limited, endovaginal scanning is combined with transabdominal imaging when a larger field of view or visualization of deeper structures is indicated.

Normal-sized adult ovaries are not always seen on computed tomography (CT), although the adnexal tissue is seen lateral to the uterus[6]. Unless it is well opacified, adjacent bowel may be difficult to separate from ovarian tissue. If the ovaries contain cysts or tumors, they may be seen discretely and measurement of attenuation values used to characterize fluid, hemorrhage or calcification. Even when an ovary is enlarged by a mass, however, detailed characterization of the tissue and architecture may be difficult[7]. In addition, if the pelvic anatomy is significantly distorted, origin of a mass may be difficult to determine[7]. Magnetic resonance imaging (MRI), with its multiplanar capabilities, large field of view and improved soft tissue contrast, is able to visualize ovaries of normal size in 87 to 96% of adult, cycling women[8], and is able to localize ovaries that may be in atypical positions owing to the presence of an enlarged leiomyomatous uterus, a full urinary bladder or loops of bowel[9]. Each of these three major imaging modalities plays a specific role in the evaluation of the dysfunctional ovary. This chapter examines the various causes of ovarian dysfunction and the imaging procedures and protocols used to optimize diagnosis.

ENDOCRINE AND METABOLIC ABNORMALITIES

Hormonal abnormalities produce a spectrum of reproductive disorders that usually require laboratory analysis for differentiation. These may originate in the ovary itself, in the adrenal glands or in the pituitary, and are often difficult to sort into discrete clinical entities. Polycystic ovary disease is a relatively common, occasionally familial, endocrine disorder said to affect over 35% of the female population[1] and results in chronic anovulation. Although the cause has not been established, the absence of a midcycle LH surge along with an abnormally elevated LH/FSH ratio suggests the diagnosis, and patients frequently have elevated androgens as well[10]. The syndrome originally described by Stein and Leventhal presents with the triad of obesity, hirsutism and amenorrhea[11]; however, the spectrum of clinical, laboratory and imaging findings associated with polycystic ovaries is much broader. Morphologically polycystic ovaries are common, being identified sonographically in 22% of the normal population[12] and in up to 80% of women with recurrent first-trimester abortion[13].

Endovaginal scanning has improved the sonographic diagnosis of polycystic ovary disease. Patient discomfort and anatomical distortion associated with a full urinary bladder are eliminated and the higher-frequency transducers improve visualization and resolution. Obese patients are easily examined and evaluation of follicle number and size as well as the characteristics of ovarian stroma can be assessed. The typical sonographic appearance shows bilaterally enlarged spherical ovaries with multiple peripheral follicles, usually more than five in each ovary (Figure 1). The follicles are small (5–8 mm), oval and immature; maturing follicles of >1 cm are seen much less often than in normal individuals[14,15]. Pache and co-workers[16] reported a median ovarian volume of 9.8 ml in patients with polycystic ovary disease compared with 5.9 ml in controls. Others have suggested that the typical volume in these patients approaches 14 cm^3 [17]. Mean size and number of follicles in the patients of Pache and colleagues was 3.8 mm and 9.8 compared with 5.1 mm and 5.0, respectively, for controls, and patients tended to have increased stromal echogenicity. Follicle size and ovarian volume provided the best discrimination, with sensitivity of 92% and specificity of 97% when used in combination. In addition, endovaginal ultrasound may be used to monitor ovarian volume in patients undergoing hormonal therapy[14]. Sonographic findings cannot be taken in isolation to make the diagnosis, however, as the findings are variable and probably non-specific. At least 30% of patients have normal-sized ovaries[15], and this group may be in the early stage of the disease.

CT can often diagnose polycystic ovary disease by observing bilateral enlarged ovaries with multiple small cysts[18]. These small cysts may be below the resolving power of CT, however, and patients will appear to have bilateral solid adnexal masses[19,20]. CT, therefore, is not routinely used in the workup of patients suspected of having polycystic ovary disease.

MRI depicts the characteristic findings of small peripheral cysts and stromal hyperplasia (Figure 2). The cysts have low signal intensity on T_1-weighted images and high signal on T_2-weighted sequences. The cellular central ovarian stroma has low to intermediate signal intensity on both[21]. Although MRI has been found to be superior to transabdominal ultrasound in identifying

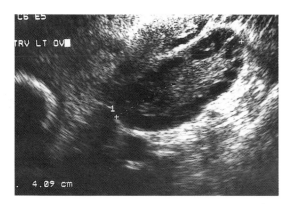

Figure 1 *Transvaginal ultrasound demonstrates the multiple peripheral follicles typical of polycystic ovary disease*

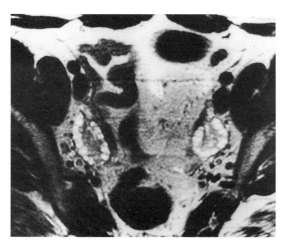

Figure 2 *Both ovaries are seen on this T_2-weighted axial magnetic resonance image. The central stroma is low to intermediate in signal intensity and that of the peripheral follicles is high*

polycystic ovaries[22], endovaginal scanning has improved the resolution of small subcapsular cysts and remains the method of choice to confirm a clinical and endocrinological diagnosis of polycystic ovary disease[23].

Although anovulation and the triad of oligomenorrhea, obesity and hirsutism are commonly seen in patients with polycystic ovary syndrome due to intrinsic ovarian disease, diseases of other endocrine organs can produce similar clinical symptoms. This triad can also be caused by Cushing's syndrome, adrenal hyperplasia or adrenal tumors. In addition to hirsutism, adrenal tumors and androgen-secreting ovarian tumors also usually present with virilization. Therefore, although the ovaries of most women with polycystic ovary syndrome are enlarged and contain numerous small cysts, the appearance is not pathognomonic. These anatomical findings have also been noted in some women with acromegaly, hyperprolactinemia or adrenal hyperplasia, and adrenal lesions may therefore need to be excluded as part of the diagnostic workup in patients with findings of polycystic ovary syndrome.

Computed tomography has been the principal technique for imaging the adrenal glands for many years[24–26]. This is still an excellent modality for the identification of adrenal masses, but it often lacks the ability to characterize these masses and provide a specific diagnosis. Recent developments in MRI offer the prospect of good anatomical information as well as increased tissue specificity based on signal intensity differences.

Early reports focused on the signal intensity of the adrenal mass relative to liver or fat on spin-echo images[27–29]. Significant overlap in findings between different types of masses was seen, however, particularly with high field strength magnets[30,31], and calculation of T_2 values was proposed[32,33]. Recently two new techniques have been employed to differentiate adrenal lesions. Different gadolinium enhancement patterns on fast gradient echo (GRE) images were reported by Krestin and co-workers[34] when adenomas and non-adenomas were compared. Mitchell and associates[35] reported that use of chemical shift imaging could identify lipid frequently present in adenomas, thereby excluding malignancy. A number of series using these techniques have reported results. Reinig and colleagues[36] evaluated 53 masses using T_1-, T_2- and T_{2^*}-weighted sequences as well as calculated T_2 values, chemical shift imaging and gadolinium enhancement. Although chemical shift imaging and T_{2^*}-weighted GRE sequences provided the best differentiation between adrenal adenomas, metastases and pheochromocytomas in their patient population, there was still a significant overlap between individual patients. In a study of 51 masses reported by Korobkin and co-workers[37] chemical shift, dynamic enhancement or both were employed and opposed and in-phase GRE images compared (Figure 3). This resulted in a specificity of 100% and sensitivity of 81% for the diagnosis of adenoma, although pathological documentation was not always obtained. Investigation with MRI is continuing and it is reasonable to expect improved accuracy as experience increases (Figure 3).

In summary, CT may continue to be used in the evaluation of adrenal hyperplasia and in the identification of hyperfunctioning adenomas, which are often suspected on the basis of clinical presentation. If low attenuation values are documented, indicating the presence of fat, no further workup is required, as these have been shown to be adenomas[38]. If the appearance is typical, CT can also reliably diagnose an adrenal cyst or myelolipoma. MRI is indicated when CT findings are equivocal and in the patient with a history of cancer who is found to have an adrenal mass. Metaiodobenzyl guanidine scintigraphy is helpful if a pheochromocytoma is suspected, although it is not always readily available. Percutaneous biopsy is still required for definitive characterization of indeterminate lesions.

Abnormalities of corpus luteum function with insufficient progesterone production are known as luteal phase defects and have been reported to occur in 1– 3% of women with infertility[39] and in up to one-third of patients with recurrent pregnancy loss[40]. The corpus luteum produces progesterone, which is necessary for maintaining an endometrium receptive to embryo implantation. Inadequate quantity or duration of progesterone production, and the abnormal endometrium that results, may lead to unsuccessful implantation or early pregnancy loss. The precise and predictable histological changes occurring in the endometrium under hormonal stimulation allow accurate dating relative to the time

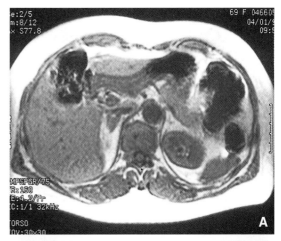

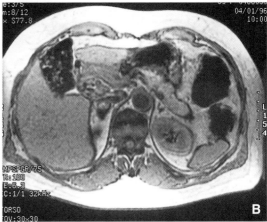

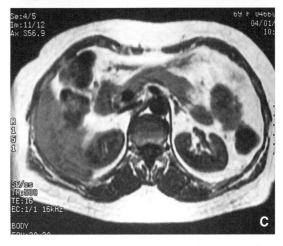

Figure 3 *Change in signal intensity between in-phase (A) and out-of-phase (B) images can confirm the presence of fat in an adrenal lesion, and therefore the diagnosis of adenoma as seen in this left adrenal mass. For comparison, an image of the normal right adrenal gland is provided (C)*

of ovulation. The diagnosis of luteal phase insufficiency depends on evaluating a late luteal phase (day 26) endometrial biopsy and demonstrating a discrepancy of 2 or more days between the expected degree of maturation and that observed with comparison to the onset of the next menses in two or more cycles[41]. Although the length of the follicular phase varies, the luteal phase is a constant 14 days and a decrease in progesterone production or in total rate of production will be reflected in endometrial abnormalities seen at biopsy. It is important that at least two cycles be evaluated, as up to 20% of women with normal fertility will show an out-of-phase endometrium in isolated cycles[39]. The cause of luteal insufficiency may be related to any of several defects in the hypothalamic–pituitary axis or, less commonly, to inability of the endometrium to respond to progesterone stimulation. In addition, at least two causes are related directly to ovarian function. Development of inadequate or defective LH receptors may result in poor corpus luteum function and inadequate progesterone production. This in turn reflects insufficient FSH stimulation, which is necessary to induce normal LH receptors[42]. Deficient response to gonadotropins may also be responsible, leading to poor follicular development or to premature follicular atresia.

These changes are inconsistently seen with ovarian imaging, and findings on ultrasound, CT and MRI do not contribute reliably to diagnosis. Sonography may demonstrate replacement of the follicle with an echogenic structure, reflecting invasion by blood clot and fibroblasts, and a cystic corpus luteum may or may not be seen[43,44]. Most often, a small irregular cyst with echogenic walls is seen, but a mature corpus luteum is identified in only about 50% of normally cycling women[45]. When it is seen, the corpus luteum should remain present and without significant change throughout the luteal phase of the cycle, disappearing near the onset of menses or within 72 h thereafter. When the corpus luteum is isoechoic and not seen, its presence may be detected by the typical color Doppler pattern of high-velocity, low-impedance flow[45] (Figure 4 [see also Color plate G]). A well-defined cyst may develop and reach several centimeters in size.

Luteinization of an unruptured ovarian follicle has been reported as a cause of infertility in women with apparently normal ovulatory cycles. Diagnosis of this luteinized unruptured follicle (LUF) syndrome required laparoscopic visualization of the ovaries and/or recovery of an oocyte from the unruptured follicle until the sequential changes of ovulation and luteinization were demonstrated with high-resolution ultrasound[46–49]. Decrease in follicular size and the appearance of free fluid in the cul-de-sac indicate ovulation, whereas loss of the clearly

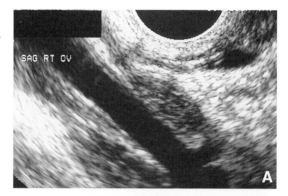

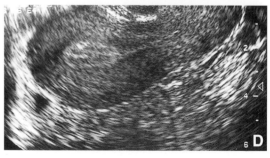

Figure 4 *The corpus luteum may be isoechoic to the surrounding ovarian parenchyma and difficult to visualize on gray-scale sonography (A). The presence of prominent peripheral vascularity on color flow imaging (B) and low-impedance flow on spectral Doppler (C) are typical and aid in identification (see Color Plate G(i) and G(ii), page x for (B) and (C), respectively. Typical midcycle endometrium confirms the stage of cycle (D)*

demarcated follicular margin and the appearance of low-density internal echoes are taken as signs of luteinization[44]. The follicular margin in LUF may be 4–7 mm thick and probably represents the hypertrophied granulosa cell layer[45]. Progesterone levels in these patients are normal and the luteal phase is of normal length. Kerin and colleagues[47] observed this phenomenon in 4.9% of cycling women, and suggested that it represents a sporadic and infrequent event. Other studies found an incidence of up to 57% of cycles in patients with unexplained infertility or endometriosis[48]. The frequency remains uncertain, however, as correlation with laparoscopic findings of ovulation stigmata suggest significant rates of false-positive and false-negative diagnosis with the use of ultrasound criteria. The syndrome may be intermittent or may occur continuously and may account for some cases of infertility not explained by other clinical or laboratory findings.

A related and possibly associated syndrome, the empty follicle syndrome, in which no ovum is found within the dominant follicle, was defined sonographically by Hilgers and co-workers in 1989[50]. They demonstrated absence of the cumulus oophorus by trans-abdominal sonography. In a subsequent study of 152 infertile patients they used transvaginal sonography, finding an overall incidence of 43.4%, which increased with age but was unrelated to follicular rupture[51]. They described the cumulus as a crescent-shaped, hyperechoic rim with an internal hypoechoic area, and identified an empty follicle by the absence of the cumulus in both longitudinal and transverse planes. The majority of their patients had confirmed pelvic disease, usually endometriosis or pelvic adhesions, but there was no correlation of empty follicles with the type of synchronous pathology. They propose that this syndrome may be a significant etiological factor in infertility and that transvaginal ultrasound provides an accurate non-invasive means of evaluation[51]. To our knowledge, other imaging modalities have not been used in its assessment.

Ovarian hyperstimulation disorder is unique to patients undergoing ovulation induction and represents its most serious complication. It occurs to a mild degree in most patients receiving gonadotropins. Clinically the presentation ranges from mild abdominal discomfort to severe electrolyte imbalance with ascites and pleural effusion. The likelihood of clinically significant hyperstimulation has been correlated with the number and size of follicles, being more likely when there are many small follicles (≤ 10 mm) than a smaller number of large (> 15 mm) follicles[52]. Ovarian hyperstimulation syndrome (OHSS) is suggested by the sonographic visualization of bilaterally enlarged ovaries that contain multiple small follicles. An estrogen level exceeding 3000 pg/ml is also an accurate predictor[14]. The full-blown clinical syndrome is fortunately uncommon and is in fact rare unless pregnancy occurs[45]. Ultrasound demonstrates markedly enlarged ovaries, often over 10 cm in diameter, with multiple thin-walled cysts (Figure 5). Free fluid is usually seen within the pelvis. The clinical and imaging findings typically resolve by the end of the cycle unless the patient becomes pregnant, in which case resolution may take several weeks. Because the ovarian enlarge-ment puts these patients at increased risk of torsion, ultrasound studies should include documentation of normal perfusion.

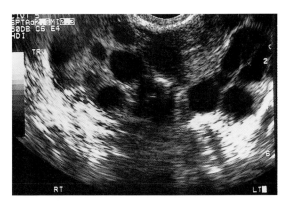

Figure 5 *Multiple cysts are seen in both ovaries in this patient undergoing chemical ovarian stimulation*

CONGENITAL AND DEVELOPMENTAL ABNORMALITIES

Disorders of ovarian function may reflect a chromosomal or genetic defect that results in failure of normal gonadal development. Random meiotic or mitotic events leading to chromosome disorders are not inherited. However, absent gonadal development occuring with a normal karyotype, called pure gonadal dysgenesis, may reflect a gene disorder and can occur in siblings. These patients are phenotypically female and of normal stature. They seldom present before puberty. Karyotype is 46,XX or 46,XY. Although most patients have no functioning ovarian tissue, some may have a few ovarian follicles, may show some breast development, and can menstruate spontaneously for a few years. It has been proposed[53] that development of gonadal malignancy is increased in this group.

At least two X chromosomes are necessary for normal ovarian development. Patients with an absent or structurally abnormal X chromosome fail to develop ovaries and may have fibrous tissue known as gonadal streaks present in the normal anatomical position of the ovary. Although the development of secondary sexual characteristics may be absent or reduced, external genitalia are typically female, since estrogen is not required for the development of Müllerian duct or regression of Wolffian duct structures. The absence of estrogen feedback via the hypothalamic–pituitary axis leads to elevated gonadotropin levels, which can be used to confirm the diagnosis of hypergonadotropic hypogonadism. Goldenberg and colleagues[54] demonstrated that all patients with primary amenorrhea and FSH levels of > 40 mIU/ml lacked any functioning ovarian follicles.

The most common form of primary gonadal dysgenesis is Turner's syndrome, which occurs in about one in 2000 to 3000 live births. Physical manifestations include short stature, 'shield' chest, webbed neck, wide carrying angle, short fourth metacarpals and hypoplastic or spoon-shaped nails. Renal anomalies and aortic coarctation are common.

About half of these patients have an absent X chromosome (45,XO) and the remainder have one normal X and one abnormal X chromosome, owing to partial deletion or ring formation[55]. A wide variety of chromosomal mosaics have also been identified with varying proportions of abnormal cells in different tissues. Studies with DNA probes suggest that mosaicism is much more common than has been thought from conventional chromosome analysis[56]. Although it is usually possible to diagnose these patients well before the age of puberty, inadequate growth monitoring or lack of typical dysmorphism may delay diagnosis. Patients with mosaicism generally have fewer anatomical abnormalities than those with a 45,XO karyotype. Some may have a few ovarian follicles and about 20% produce enough estrogen to menstruate and even achieve pregnancy, but eventually premature ovarian failure ensues.

Patients presenting with primary amenorrhea or oligomenorrhea are imaged with sonography for assessment of uterine size, shape and maturity. The presence and development of the ovaries is used in conjunction with physical and laboratory findings to establish the diagnosis. Patients with a pure 45,XO karyotype have a prepubertal uterus and non-visualized ovaries. Genetic mosaics (45,XO/46,XX) have variable findings. The uterine configuration varies from prepubertal to intermediate, but will be shorter and have a lower fundal/cervical length ratio than in the normal adult female. Ovaries may be absent, small or normal in appearance[57] (Figure 6). In pure gonadal dysgenesis absent or streak ovaries are identified. Mixed gonadal dysgenesis is a mosaic of karyotypes 45,XO/ 45,XY with a streak ovary on one side and a contralateral intra-abdominal testis. Patients in both groups have an increased risk of gonadal tumors, thought to be related to the presence of the Y chromosome. Pseudo-Turner's or Noonan's syndrome is characterized by phenotypic changes of Turner's syndrome with normal ovaries on sonographic examination and normal ovarian function.

If ovarian follicles are damaged by

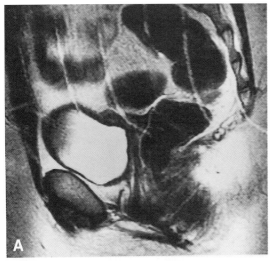

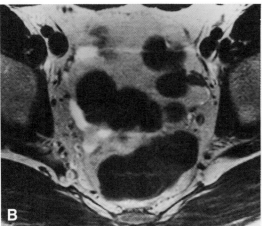

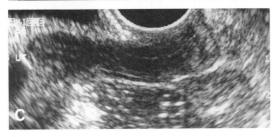

Figure 6 *Prepubertal uterus (A) and small ovaries (B) were seen on MRI in this patient with gonadal dysgenesis. Prepubertal uterus with an increased cervical length to fundal ratio in a patient with primary amenorrhea (C)*

infection, radiation, medication, ischemia or surgery, they may fail to produce adequate estrogen for endometrial growth and normal cyclic menstruation. These patients present with secondary amenorrhea after medical treatment for tubo-ovarian abscess, after radiation or chemotherapy, or after surgery that directly damages the ovaries or interferes with their normal blood supply. When ovarian estrogen production fails in the setting of hypergonadotropism before the age of 40, it is termed premature ovarian failure (POF). Coulam and colleagues[58] estimated that up to 1% of women have POF with an incidence that increases steadily from age 15 to 39. The etiology is multifactorial and may be the result of a reduced number of primordial follicles or an increased rate of atresia. Significant evidence suggests that specific genetic defects may be responsible[59]. Antiovarian antibodies have been isolated and, along with the association of POF with other immunological endocrine disorders including Hashimoto's thyroiditis, Addison's disease and hypoparathyroidism, suggest that it may be an autoimmune disorder. Thirty to fifty per cent of chromosomally normal patients without a history of radiation or chemotherapy have an associated auto-immune disease, usually thyroid disease[60]. Up to 92% of these women have non-organ-specific antibodies, usually antinuclear antibodies or rheumatoid factor[61], although most have no clinical evidence of autoimmunity.

The clinical presentation of POF is variable. Patients present at different ages with symptoms of amenorrhea or infertility. Ovarian failure may be temporary or intermittent. Symptoms of menopause, including mood swings, hot flushes and vaginal dryness, may be present. The diagnosis is confirmed by documenting elevated gonadotropin levels. Once the diagnosis is established, patients should be screened for associated endocrine disorders and have chromosomal analysis to detect the presence of a Y chromosome, which would predispose them to gonadal malignancy.

When the ovaries of patients with POF are examined, two histological patterns are seen. The majority have generalized sclerosis similar to a typical postmenopausal ovary. In up to 30%, primordial follicles are identified which have not progressed beyond the antral stage. This is termed gonadotropin-resistant ovarian syndrome, and these patients usually menstruate for months to years before ovarian failure and secondary amenorrhea occur.

A subgroup of patients with unexplained infertility was described recently by Toner and co-workers[62] as having decreased functional ovarian reserve and a poor prognosis for future fertility. This group had normal, ovulatory menstrual cycles, but showed elevated FSH levels (> 20 mIU/ml) on day 3 of the spontaneous cycle.

Imaging findings in these patients depend on the type and severity of disease. Decrease in ovarian size or in number of follicles is easily assessed with transvaginal ultrasound or MRI. Perfusion can be assessed with duplex Doppler interrogation. The impedance to uterine artery blood flow has been shown to be significantly higher in women with infertility, including those with POF, than in women of normal fertility[63–65]. Although there is overlap of pulsatility index values in the two groups, up to 50% of infertile women have values outside the normal range[63]. Endometrial thickness is also decreased in the infertility group, correlating with estradiol levels[66]. It is likely that subnormal hormone levels are responsible for both findings. Many patients will have morphologically normal ovaries despite clinical evidence of dysfunction, and diagnosis is based on clinical presentation and endocrine studies.

OVARIAN AND ADNEXAL MASSES

Ovarian factors in infertility are usually associated with an endocrine imbalance. Ovarian masses, if large, can distort the anatomical relationship between the ovary and tube and an inflammatory process may lead to distortion and subsequent decreased fertility. Most commonly, however, the problem is interference with ovulation. The majority of ovarian masses seen in women of childbearing age are cystic and, of these cystic masses, most are physiological. Neoplastic lesions both benign and malignant do occur, but are most often complex or solid.

CYSTIC MASSES

Functional, non-neoplastic ovarian lesions occur commonly. The majority are follicular cysts or corpus luteal cysts, depending on their origin (Figure 7 [see also Color plate H]). Normal ovaries characteristically contain several follicles that vary in size from 2 to 15 mm. A follicle that matures but fails to ovulate or regress may become distended with fluid and enlarge to several centimeters in size. Except for size, they cannot be differentiated from normal follicles; the term follicular cyst is usually given to those greater than 3 cm in diameter[67]. Corpus luteum cysts result from similar lack of regression and tend to be larger and more often symptomatic than follicular cysts, presenting with pelvic pressure, pain or a palpable mass.

Occasionally, functional cysts may rupture, causing a hemoperitoneum and requiring emergency surgery to control bleeding. Strict criteria for ultrasound diagnosis of these lesions requires that they be anechoic, round or oval and thin-walled, and produce posterior acoustic enhancement. Hemorrhage within them generates internal echoes. This produces a variable appearance, which may be similar to that of an endometrioma, cystic teratoma, ovarian neoplasm or abscess (Figure 8). Enhanced through-transmission

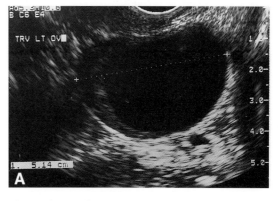

Figure 7 *Purely cystic masses in the ovary are common and virtually always physiological, non-neoplastic lesions, although they may be large and occasionally produce symptoms. Follicular (A) and corpus luteal (B) cysts are similar in appearance, but the latter will show typical, peripheral vascularity (see Color Plate H, page xi for (B))*

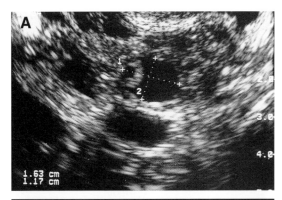

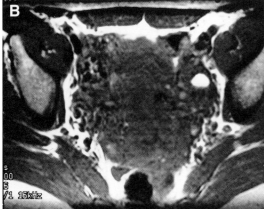

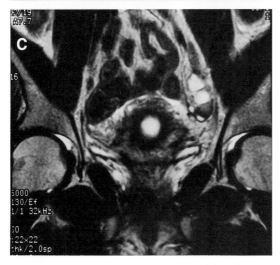

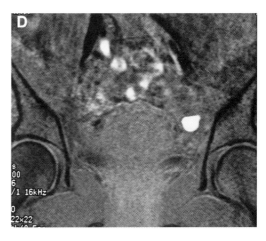

Figure 8 *Hemorrhage into an ovarian cyst may produce an appearance suspicious for neoplasia (A). Confirmation of the presence of blood products can be obtained using MRI. A combination of pulse sequences is required; shown here are T_1-weighted (B), T_2-weighted (C) and fat saturation images (D). Hemorrhage does not decrease in signal intensity with fat saturation techniques*

remains an important sonographic characteristic reported in more than 90% of hemorrhagic cysts[68]. Both follicular and corpus luteal cysts usually resolve during the next cycle without intervention. Therefore, unless symptoms preclude a conservative approach, a follow-up ultrasound examination should be performed within 6–8 weeks.

If the cyst persists, hormonal suppression may be considered, although some women find the side-effects unpleasant. If there is doubt as to the diagnosis of simple functional cyst, laparoscopy is often performed. Endovaginal aspiration is a less invasive alternative if there is no suspicion of malignancy, and evaluation of aspirated cyst contents can aid in differentiation of lesions, as described below. Color Doppler interrogation of corpus luteal cysts may reveal the prominent peripheral low-impedance flow typically seen in an active corpus luteum[69–71] (Color plate I). This flow pattern is also seen in some neoplastic lesions and there is considerable overlap in values of peak velocity and pulsatility index[72]. Doppler interrogation of adnexal masses is performed with increasing frequency and the significance of the findings is controversial. This subject will be examined more completely in the sections dealing with complex and solid masses.

When seen on CT, functional ovarian cysts are non-enhancing, well-circumscribed structures with attenuation values within the range of water[18,73]. Thin septations or focal wall thickening is seen in up to one-third and in one study malignancy could not be excluded in 22%[73]. When hemorrhage has occurred, high-attenuation blood products may be seen layering dependently[7].

MRI shows functional cysts to have a thin, well-defined wall. As with cysts elsewhere, these lesions demonstrate low signal on T_1-weighted images which becomes high with increased T_2 weighting. Following contrast administration, cysts remain of low signal while the surrounding ovarian tissue enhances, increasing visibility. The cyst wall may enhance, especially if the lesion is hemorrhagic. Hemorrhagic cysts demonstrate signal characteristics typical of blood products and, as with other imaging modalities, may have an appearance similar to that of endometriomas[74]. If cysts contain proteinaceous or mucinous material, they may demonstrate high signal on T_1-weighted images.

Theca lutein cysts are the least common of the functional ovarian cysts. They are believed to occur secondary to an elevated circulating level of human chorionic gonadotropin (hCG). These lesions are frequently associated with gestational trophoblastic disease and have been reported with multiple gestations, diabetes and fetal hydrops. Iatrogenic theca lutein cysts are not uncommon in patients undergoing ovulation induction. These patients are at risk of ovarian hyperstimulation syndrome, which may produce severe clinical manifestations including hydrothorax, ascites and coagulopathy.

Unlike other physiological cysts, theca lutein cysts are almost always bilateral and may produce massive ovarian enlargement. Sonographically they are multilocular cystic masses containing cysts of variable size with multiple septations. When gonadotropin levels normalize, the cysts regress, although this may take several months. Serial hCG assays and endovaginal scans can be used to monitor their course.

Aspiration or biopsy of ovarian lesions, for therapy as well as diagnosis, can be performed under imaging guidance. The transgluteal approach using CT has been employed[75,76], but poses at least a theoretical risk of sciatic nerve injury and is not optimal for an abscess collection in which a drain must be left in place. Endovaginal biopsy with transabdominal ultrasound guidance can be used[77–79], but visualization of the needle is not as good as with direct endovaginal guidance. Cyst aspiration by a device mounted directly on the endovaginal transducer provides a close approach to these lesions and detailed visualization. This approach can be used when cysts exhibit no signs of malignancy or when patients are not surgical candidates. Although this method is simple and rarely produces complications, recurrence of the cyst is not unusual. Bret and co-workers[80] reported 68 transvaginal ultrasound-guided aspirations or biopsies of which 48 were ovarian cysts. Their series included cyst aspirations in 23 premenopausal and 13 postmenopausal women with recurrence rates of 48% and 80%, respectively. Granberg and colleagues[81] reported a 1-year recurrence rate of 73% in women under 40 and found recurrence least likely in well-defined unilocular cysts. In a series of 88 patients reported by de Crespigny and associates[82] 52% had no recurrence after 14 months of follow-up. Alcohol sclerosis of cysts which recur has been suggested, and Bret and co-workers[83] reported a series of seven such patients. Sclerosis was achieved following a procedure in which 100% alcohol was left within the cyst cavity for 20 min and then the cyst fluid was aspirated. Four cysts had not recurred at follow-up of 2–12 months.

In addition to relief of symptoms, pathological evaluation of cyst fluid can provide diagnostic information. We routinely send aspirated fluid for analysis. Evaluation of the aspirated fluid in the series of Bret and colleagues[80] assisted in the diagnosis of hemorrhagic cysts, endometriomas, one dermoid cyst and one cystoma. Granberg and co-workers[84] found cytological evaluation less helpful in predicting malignancy. They examined fluid aspirated from cystic tumors in 50 patients and found positive and negative predictive values for malignancy of 100% and 81%, compared with 73% and 100%, respectively, from ultrasound findings alone. They concluded that cytological evaluation, when compared to endovaginal ultrasound, does not significantly increase accuracy in diagnosis of malignancy. For 136 cyst aspirations, Pinto and associates[85] reported that the addition of a tumor antigen assay to the cytological examination of aspirated fluid was helpful in differentiating follicular and lutein cysts from epithelial cysts and endometriosis. CA-125 was consistently elevated in serous cysts and in endometriomas, but low in functional cysts. High carcinoembryonic antigen levels were found in mucinous lesions, whereas levels were low in functional cysts and variable with endometriosis. Cytological analysis remained essential, as values from benign and malignant epithelial cysts overlapped significantly.

Therefore, in premenopausal patients, symptomatic or persistent cysts may be aspirated for relief of symptoms and/or for diagnosis, but it should be remembered that up to half of these may recur. Biopsy of complex or solid lesions remains controversial, because of the risk of spreading a potentially malignant lesion; treatment is usually surgical. An exception to this practice may be made for patients with a history of cancer if the purpose is to confirm metastatic disease or recurrence.

COMPLEX AND SOLID MASSES

Tubo-ovarian abscess

Pelvic inflammatory disease (PID) is one of the most widespread gynecological problems occurring in young women. It is estimated that approximately 1 million cases occur annually in American women between 15 and 44 years of age[86]. Follow-up of women with laparoscopically proven PID suggests that approximately 20% of these women will become infertile[86]. The incidence of infertility increases with repeated infection. Westrom[87] reported an incidence of 11.4% after one episode of PID, 23.1% after two and 54.3% following three or more. The term in not precisely defined and is used to refer to inflammation occurring anywhere in the upper genital tract. Most long-term sequelae, including infertility, result from destruction of tubal architecture. In virtually all cases, acute PID results from ascending infection from the vagina and cervix. The most common pathogens are *Chlamydia trachomatis* and *Neisseria gonorrhea*, although the condition is often polymicrobial[88]. In less than 1% of cases, acute PID results from transperitoneal spread of infectious material from a perforated appendix or intra-abdominal abscess[89]. Patients with acute PID present with a wide range of non-specific clinical symptoms. Fever, leukocytosis and lower abdominal pain occur without classic features to differentiate acute PID from other inflammatory conditions such as appendicitis, endometriosis or inflammatory bowel disease. Physical findings of cervical motion tenderness, vaginal discharge and adnexal mass help in establishing the proper diagnosis. Hager and colleagues[90] established clinical criteria for acute PID which have been adopted by the Obstetrical and Gynecological Infectious Disease Society. On the basis of a review of symptoms, signs and laboratory findings in 414 patients with proven PID, Hager and colleagues established a mathematical model which correctly predicted 87% of cases and had an overall correct classification rate of 76%[91]. However, given the incidence of the disease and the significance of the sequelae, there remains a clinically important degree of inaccuracy in establishing the diagnosis.

Pelvic ultrasound examination is the first imaging study obtained in women suspected of having acute PID. Although the study is of limited value in mild disease, these patients may have a thickened endometrial stripe and fluid is occasionally seen within the uterus. When the disease invades the fallopian tubes, fluid is seen in and around them as well as in the cul-de-sac. Bilateral involvement is typical, although it is often asymmetric. Ovarian involvement is less common, occurring in severe cases. Delayed or inadequate treatment can result in abscess formation.

Typical tubo-ovarian abscesses are complex masses with ill-defined, irregular margins and thickened walls. They may be uni- or multilocular. Hypoechoic or anechoic areas usually represent collections of purulent fluid (Figure 9). Echogenic foci with acoustic shadowing are suggestive of air. In severe or widespread infection, the pelvic organs may be fixed and tissue planes effaced. These patients usually find the examination painful, a sign that helps in confirming the diagnosis of acute infection. Transvaginal sonographic guidance is useful for aspiration of fluid collections for diagnosis and for placement of drainage catheters if indicated. Serial scans should be obtained to monitor response to therapy once the diagnosis is made.

Endometriosis

Endometriosis is a benign but often progressive disease resulting from heterotopic foci of endometrium located outside the uterus. It is generally believed that the incidence is increasing, although both incidence and prevalence are difficult to quantify, as the diagnosis is often made incidentally during laparoscopy or imaging studies performed for unrelated reasons. Endometriosis has been reported in 5–25% of all laparotomies performed in females of reproductive age, and in 30–45% of those performed in infertile patients[92–94]. Although this is a chronic, inflammatory condition which may mimic PID, clinical history, presenting symptoms and physical and laboratory examinations help in differentiation. Patients are typically somewhat older than those with PID, usually 25–35 years, constitutional symptoms are less common and dysmennorrhea and dyspareunia are frequent findings.

Several theories have been proposed to explain the histogenesis of endometriosis, but none is universally accepted. By definition, endometriosis involves the presence of endometrial glands and stroma in an aberrant or ectopic location. The most popular theory

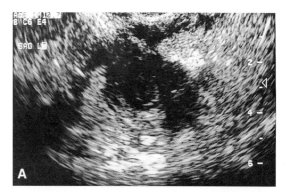

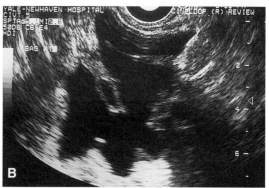

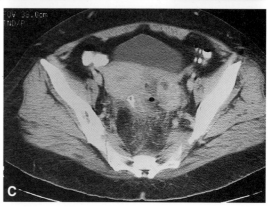

Figure 9 *Complex ovarian masses can be diagnosed as tubo-ovarian abscesses in the appropriate clinical setting. On ultrasound they appear as ill-defined, often multilocular lesions (A), often associated with hydrosalpinx (B) and free fluid. On CT, a complex adnexal mass is seen with surrounding inflammatory change and effacement of tissue planes (C)*

is of retrograde menstruation initially proposed by Sampson in 1927[95]. Other possible etiologies include metaplasia of the colonic epithelium, lymphatic or vascular metastasis, defects of the immune system and iatrogenic dissemination. There may be a genetic predisposition to the development of endometriosis as well. An investigation by Sampson and colleagues[94] demonstrated a seven-fold increase in the incidence of endometriosis in women with affected relatives. Whatever the cause, functioning endometrial tissue adheres to the ovaries, the fallopian tubes and the pelvic peritoneum. The bladder and rectum are less frequently involved and disease in areas remote from the pelvis occurs rarely.

Olive and Martin[96] reported that 65% of otherwise normal women with mild endometriosis conceived without treatment. With moderate or severe disease, pregnancy rates in their patient group without therapy were much lower – 25% and 0%, respectively. The causal relationship between severe endometriosis and infertility is well established; although medical therapy may be helpful, surgery is often necessary.

Endometrial deposits are most commonly small and widely dispersed, therefore pelvic sonography may be normal. In a study by Friedman and co-workers[97], ultrasound depicted endometriosis in only four of 37 patients, for a sensitivity of 10.8%. Even with direct correlation with known areas of disease, there were 33 false-negative results. Repeated episodes of proliferation and bleeding may lead to complex, predominantly cystic endometriomas commonly referred to as chocolate cysts. When the characteristic appearance of a thick-walled mass with diffuse low-level echoes is present, and the clinical setting is appropriate, the diagnosis can be made (Figure 10). However, the lesions may contain echogenic nodular clot or debris and occasional septations, making the appearance less specific. With severe or long-standing disease, adhesions and scar tissue produce immobility of the pelvic organs, obscure pelvic tissue planes and obstruct the fallopian tubes. Endometriotic deposits by definition contain glandular endometrial tissue. It is logical, therefore, that tumors of endometrial cell origin can develop within them; several histologic types have been reported[98]. We

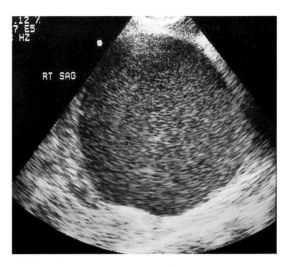

Figure 10 *A thick-walled mass with diffuse low-level echoes is diagnostic of an endometrioma*

have seen several cases of clear cell carcinoma originating within endometriomas. These lesions were identified by the development of echogenic nodular soft tissue with variable patterns of vascularity (Figure 11). Although this is not common, and the presence of clots within endometriotic cysts may be confusing, one should be alert for such changes, particularly if they are fixed, persistent and vascular, and if they are associated with changing symptoms.

Computed tomography is of little help in the diagnosis of endometriosis. Contrast resolution may be inadequate to distinguish endometriomas, even from normal adnexal tissue, and there is no typical CT density[99]. Although previously used in conjunction with ultrasound for diagnosis and disease monitoring, CT with its ionizing radiation has been largely replaced by MRI. Because of its tissue characterization ability, MRI is more sensitive and specific in the detection of endometriosis than either ultrasound or CT. This is particularly true for patients with small deposits or diffuse disease who often have normal ultrasound scans. Zawin and associates[100] found a sensitivity of 71% and specificity of 82% in the identification of endometriosis by MRI using laparoscopy as the gold standard. In a more recent series,

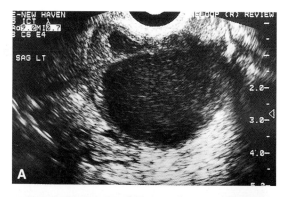

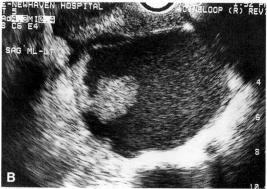

Figure 11 *The diagnosis of endometrioma can be made on ultrasound, but atypical appearances should raise suspicion. This patient presented with a typical endometrioma (A), which was found to contain a solid nodule with internal vascularity a year later (B). The lesion was resected and a diagnosis of clear cell carcinoma was made*

sensitivity and specificity of 90% and 98%, respectively, were reported by Togashi and colleagues[101]. The MRI appearance of endometriosis can be quite varied. Ectopic endometrium has the same signal intensity characteristics as normal endometrium; is intermediate on T_1-weighted images and high on T_2-weighted images. Because endometriosis is a chronic process with cyclic bleeding over many years, hemorrhage of varying age is commonly present. Endometriotic cysts are typically multilocular and walls with low signal intensity are seen, probably reflecting either a fibrous capsule or a hemosiderin ring[100,102]. Signal intensity characteristics of the cysts depend on the state of the blood breakdown products. Togashi and co-workers[101] reported that hyperintense signal

on T_1-weighted images and shading on T_2-weighted images is the most common MRI appearance. The study by Zawin and colleagues described a second frequent pattern, that of hypointensity on both T_1- and T_2-weighted images. In their series, the signal intensities ranged from hyperintense on all sequences to hypointense on all sequences. Patterns of signal intensity corresponding to acute, subacute and chronic hemorrhage were identified. Varying signal intensity from different lesions within the same patient is frequently reported[100,102], with at least one area having high signal intensity on T_1-weighted images[103]. The appearance of endometriomas on T_2-weighted images is often heterogeneous, and posterior shading is a typical finding. Lesion multiplicity is common[100,102–104] and helps to distinguish endometriomas from hemorrhagic cysts.

Most authors agree that the MRI appearance of endometriosis is not pathognomonic, although it is the best modality currently available[100,103,105–107]. Identification of adhesions and small foci or intraperitoneal implants may be limited and differentiation from other hemorrhagic lesions difficult[100,104,106]. In some cases MRI can visualize areas not visible to the laparoscopist, as dense adhesions can limit pelvic inspection; it is clearly useful in monitoring the response to treatment once the diagnosis is made. Because adhesions reportedly occur in 100% of patients following surgery[108] and recur in more than 70% after lysis[109], a non-invasive means of monitoring disease is of obvious clinical benefit.

Adnexal torsion

Torsion of the ovary or entire adnexa is an acute condition requiring emergency surgery. It is an unusual cause of lower abdominal or pelvic pain, accounting for 3% of gynecological surgical emergencies in a review by Hubbard[110]. Torsion is most common during the first three decades of life but is also seen in older women with benign ovarian tumors. Probably because of the tendency for adhesion to adjacent tissues, torsion is less common in patients with ovarian malignancies. Pregnancy appears to predispose women to torsion. Approximately 20% of patients with torsion are pregnant at diagnosis, and ovaries enlarged by ovulation induction are most susceptible[111].

The most common etiology of adnexal torsion is ovarian enlargement by a benign mass. Torsion of a normal ovary is possible and occurs more frequently in children. Paraovarian cysts, solid benign tumors and serous cyst are frequently associated. Dermoid cysts are the tumor most frequently reported in patients with torsion, probably because of their prevalence[110].

Patients with adnexal torsion present with acute severe unilateral lower abdominal or pelvic pain, often associated with anorexia, nausea and vomiting. Leukocytosis and a palpable mass are present in the majority[112]. In the early stages there is venous stasis. As edema develops, arterial compromise and hemorrhagic infarction ensues. Prompt surgical therapy offers the only means of organ salvage. However, because the clinical presentation is confusing, diagnosis may be delayed and salvage is uncommon[110].

Ultrasound is the imaging modality of choice for patients with suspected adnexal torsion. Although there is no specific appearance and both cystic and solid masses are seen, the most common diagnostic finding is unilateral ovarian enlargement with multiple peripheral cystic structures of uniform size[113] (Figure 12A). These cystic structures are thought to reflect transudation of fluid into ovarian follicles; free fluid is also found in approximately one-third of cases[112–114]. The addition of color Doppler sonography has been helpful in the diagnosis of adnexal torsion, although the presence of a dual blood supply and anatomic mobility make this more difficult to apply to the ovary than to the testis. Findings with color Doppler sonography are variable, however, and depend on the extent and duration of torsion. In addition, color Doppler sonography is an operator-dependent modality and false-positive results may be obtained if suboptimal

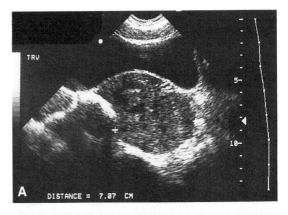

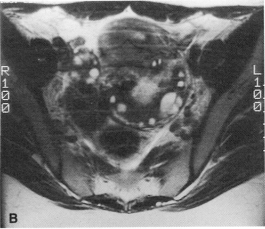

Figure 12 *Ultrasound demonstrated unilateral ovarian enlargement (A) in this patient with ovarian torsion. Because the presentation was atypical, MRI was used to confirm the diagnosis and more clearly demonstrates the peripheral cysts (B)*

technique or machine settings are employed. Rasado and colleagues[115] reported three cases of surgically proven torsion in which normal arterial flow was identified within the affected ovary. In a larger series, Fleischer and co-workers[116] reported that ovarian viability could be predicted preoperatively by the presence of central venous flow. All ten non-viable ovaries lacked central venous flow, whereas it was present in all three found to be viable at surgery. Increased likelihood of viability was also found in smaller ovaries. Correlation with clinical and laboratory findings is important, as lack of central flow may be seen in other lesions, such as intraovarian hemorrhage[117]. Further study of both arterial and venous flow in patients with torsion is clearly necessary to determine its role in diagnosis. Power Doppler, now available on many ultrasound machines, provides a perfusion map without regard to direction or velocity of flow. Because of its increased sensitivity, it may improve accuracy in ultrasound studies.

CT and MRI is usually not required for diagnosis of adnexal torsion but may be helpful in atypical cases (Figure 12B). Kimura and colleagues[118] reported common findings in ten patients with proven torsion of an adnexal tumor. These findings included deviation of the uterus to the twisted side, engorgement of blood vessels, a small amount of ascites and obliteration of adjacent fat planes. Patients in whom infarction had occurred demonstrated lack of enhancement, thick blood vessels draping around the mass and protrusion of the lesion towards converging vessels. These findings may be unexpectedly seen in patients with a subacute course, but can be helpful in identifying patients with benign lesions who nonetheless require surgery to remove necrotic tissue.

Ovarian dermoid cysts

Ovarian dermoid cysts or cystic teratomas are benign neoplasms accounting for up to 44% of all ovarian neoplasms[119]. Malignant transformation occurs, but is rare[120]. However, since dermoid cysts are usually removed at diagnosis to prevent torsion or rupture, little is known about the progression of this disease. They are bilateral in approximately 15%[121] and most are less than 10 cm in diameter[122]. Dermoid cysts arise from all three germ layers and the resulting variety of tissues contained can lead to different imaging appearances. Sebum is commonly present and, if homogeneous, is anechoic. When mixed with hair, the numerous tissue interfaces produce a highly echogenic appearance (Figure 13A). Hair and

fat within a dermoid cyst are highly echogenic and produce posterior shadowing, as do fragments of bone or teeth[123]. Strongly echogenic tissue may obscure deeper structures; this has been called the 'tip of the iceberg' sign. An echogenic focus within a predominantly cystic mass is a characteristic finding. Called a dermoid plug or Rokitansky nodule, this protuberance from the inner cyst wall has been reported in 33–90% of lesions[124–128]. Because sebum is liquid at body temperature, a fat fluid level is a characteristic finding when serous fluid is also present. This has been clearly demonstrated with CT[129–131], but is less commonly seen sonographically.

The presence of fat in an adnexal mass is diagnostic of a cystic teratoma. On CT fat is identified by its characteristic Hounsfield density. Interestingly, the fat within a dermoid cyst may have a lower Hounsfield number than the subcutaneous fat, probably a reflection of its liquid nature[18]. A fat fluid level and mural calcification are also characteristic as described and are easily seen with CT. MRI is probably the most accurate test available for diagnosis, although it is usually not the first study obtained. Chemical shift imaging and fat saturation techniques provide high sensitivity and specificity for intralesional fat, the most important finding in diagnosis[132]. Morphological findings of gravity-dependent layering, floating fat and dermoid plugs may be seen with MRI as with other imaging modalities. Contrast enhancement in MRI is not helpful, as both the wall and the solid core may enhance[133]. Because complex and solid ovarian lesions are treated surgically, precise diagnosis of a teratoma may not be necessary preoperatively, although confident diagnosis of a benign lesion allows a less invasive surgical procedure to be performed. Differentiation from cystic hemorrhagic lesions that may be treated non-operatively is, however, important. Using MRI with fat saturation provides an accuracy of 96%[134,135] and is a useful problem-solving technique for lesions that are indeterminate at either ultrasound or CT examination (Figure 13B and C).

Ovarian epithelial neoplasms

Tumors arising from surface epithelial cells represent the majority of ovarian neoplasms. These epithelial neoplasms may be benign (cystadenoma) or malignant (cystadeno-carcinoma), but some 15–20% are borderline or of low malignant potential[17]. Epithelial tumors may produce serous or mucinous material. Serous tumors are more likely to be borderline or malignant (40%) than the mucinous lesions (15%), although the histology cannot be determined preoperatively and both are treated surgically[17]. Ultrasonography and CT have been largely used to detect, characterize and evaluate the extension of these tumors, although MRI is being employed with increasing frequency. In a series of 170 tumors reported by Buy and co-workers[125], CT detected 87% of masses and correctly predicted malignancy in 94%. Ultrasound identified 86% and correctly characterized malignancy in 80%. When ultrasound is compared with MRI, accuracy of 99% for MRI and 68% for ultrasound was reported in one study[136] and 70% vs. 83% in another[137]. The use of color and duplex Doppler to identify malignant flow patterns holds promise, but remains controversial and of undetermined value, as described below.

Lesions containing only simple, cystic loculi and single, thin septations are unlikely to be malignant, whereas those with solid components have an increased malignant potential. This is particularly true if internal structures such as mural nodules, thick septations or irregular, thickened walls are seen. These findings, whatever the modality used, are important in evaluating the likelihood of malignancy, if conservative therapy is contemplated in a patient who is a poor surgical risk or if aspiration is indicated.

Ovarian pregnancy

Ectopic pregnancy frequently presents with a complex adnexal mass. This occurs in the fallopian tubes in the vast majority of cases and is described in the chapter on fallopian

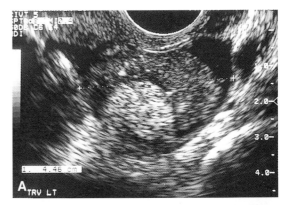
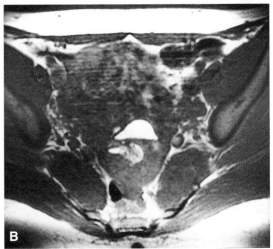
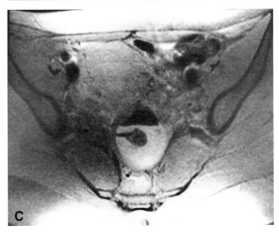

Figure 13 *The large number of tissue interfaces in a dermoid cyst typically produce an echogenic appearance (A). MRI can confirm the presence of fat, thereby making the diagnosis as illustrated with T_1-weighted spin echo (B) and fat saturation (C) images. Note the decreased signal intensity with the fat saturation technique*

tube pathology, but a brief discussion of ovarian pregnancy is included here. In Breen's series[138], over 97% of ectopic pregnancies were tubal and less than 1.7% ovarian. Many patients with ovarian pregnancies are believed to have a ruptured corpus luteum cyst. In Hallat's series of 25 ovarian pregnancies[139], correct diagnosis was made in only 28%, even at surgery. In his series the hemorrhagic mass was found adjacent to but never within the corpus luteum. Hemoperitoneum of > 500 ml was found in 81% of patients. Imaging of these patients is as indicated for any suspected ectopic pregnancy, with ultrasound as the primary modality.

Ovarian remnant syndrome

The ovarian remnant syndrome is a rare entity occurring in patients who previously underwent bilateral oophorectomy. Fewer than 35 cases have been reported since the entity was first described by Kaufman in 1962[140]. Patients typically present with pain weeks to years after oophorectomy and may or may not have a palpable mass. The syndrome represents a complication of oophorectomy, usually occurring in cases in which the ovaries were adherent to the mesentery or pelvic sidewalls and functioning ovarian tissue is left behind. This tissue responds to hormonal stimulation and a cystic or complex mass results. Transabdominal pelvic ultrasound should be employed in addition to endovaginal evaluation, as the mass may be outside the field of view of an endovaginal probe. Because associated ureteral obstruction has been reported[140,141], ultrasound assessment of the kidneys is indicated.

Solid ovarian masses

Solid ovarian masses are relatively uncommon. Granulosa cell tumors, fibromas, thecomas, Sertoli–Leydig tumors and Brenner tumors together comprise less than 7% of all ovarian tumors. These are classified as sex cord–stromal tumors and even the cell of origin is controversial. Histological diagnosis cannot be made by imaging findings: all appear as hypoechoic solid masses which may contain small cystic spaces. They produce variable posterior shadowing and occasionally contain foci of calcification. In some cases, these tumors produce hormones and patients will present with precocious puberty, irregular cycles, menorrhagia or amenorrhea. Androgen production results in virilization or hirsutism. An important differential is a pedunculated uterine leiomyoma which may not require surgical resection. The distinction is difficult to make, unless a vascular pedicle connecting the mass to the uterus can be identified with color Doppler sonography, confirming the diagnosis of leiomyoma. Alternatively, MRI may evaluate the pelvic organs in their entirety and illustrate the anatomical relationship of the lesion to the uterus as well as its tissue characteristics, thereby diagnosing a pedunculated fibroid (Figure 14). Other lesions that may appear solid include metastases, teratomas, dysgerminomas and lymphoma. The patient's age, clinical history and symptoms are often helpful in narrowing the differential diagnosis.

Doppler assessment of ovarian masses

Doppler ultrasound provides assessment of blood flow by depicting the frequency changes that occur in vascular structures. Color Doppler provides a subjective evaluation of perfusion and facilitates placement of the sample volume for specific interrogation and spectral analysis. This technique has been used to assess the relative vascularity and flow patterns of ovarian lesions and can have an impact on decisions regarding appropriate therapy. Complex lesions without internal vascularity suggest hemorrhage. Lesions with similar internal consistency but which demonstrate internal flow do not represent areas of hemorrhage and may require surgery. Initial reports suggested a difference

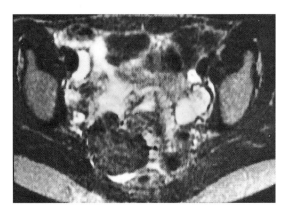

Figure 14 *When an adnexal mass is identified, the tissue of origin may not be clear. This leiomyoma was thought to be an ovarian mass on ultrasound examination, but its true etiology was proven with MRI, which provides a larger field of view and improved tissue characterization. Note the attachment to the uterus and typical low signal intensity on the T_2-weighted image. The ovary is visualized separately above it*

in flow patterns between benign and malignant lesions[142,143]. Malignant lesions tend to have high diastolic flow with lower quantitive pulsatility index.

The value of using flow patterns to predict histology has been tested in many studies with somewhat variable results and the reliability of the technique remains controversial. Fleischer and co-workers[144] described results of color Doppler sonography in 43 patients with surgically proven ovarian masses. Their study demonstrated significant overlap in flow patterns between benign and malignant lesions. With a pulsatility index of < 1.0 considered as indicative of malignancy, the positive predictive value was 73%. Kurjak and colleagues[145] used a resistance index of 0.4 as a cut-off level and found that all 624 benign masses had a higher index, whereas those of 54 of 56 cancers were lower. Hamper and colleagues[146] studied 31 masses and reported a pulsatility index of 0.77 ± 0.3 for malignant and 1.93 ± 1.02 for benign masses, although there was significant overlap. In a study of 50 masses, Jain[147] reported 82% specificity and 80% accuracy for diagnosis of malignancy

using a pulsatility index of < 1.0. Brown and co-workers[148] studied 44 masses and found that, although there was a tendancy towards lower pulsatility and resistance index values in malignant masses, the overlap was such that no cut-off value could be chosen that had both high sensitivity and high specificity. The overlap in appearance, vascularity and impedance estimates reported in these more recent studies makes it clear they cannot be used reliably to differentiate benign from malignant lesions (Figure 15 [see also Color plate J]). Measurement of serum CA-125, an antigen expressed by epithelial ovarian tumors as well as by other tissues of Müllerian origin, has been proposed as a means of increasing reliability of ultrasound findings in the differentiation of benign and malignant lesions. Although CA-125 levels are elevated in 80–85% of women with advanced epithelial ovarian cancer, this finding is non-specific, particularly in premenopausal patients, as levels will be elevated in many benign gynecological and non-gynecological conditions. Minor elevations and fluctuating levels are likely to be associated with benign disease, and measurement of CA-125 levels is of limited usefulness as a screening tool. Rather, its importance lies in sequential testing of women with known disease, as high or increasing levels have a strong correlation with residual or recurrent tumor[149]. Lesion morphology as well as patient age, presentation and family history must be considered in addition to flow patterns; even lack of detectable flow by Doppler ultrasound does not exclude malignancy[148]. Misdiagnosis by Doppler findings is most frequent in hemorrhagic cysts, dermoid cysts and inflammatory and metabolically active benign masses[150].

CONCLUSIONS AND FUTURE DIRECTIONS

Ovarian imaging has become an essential part of the evaluation and treatment of many forms of reproductive failure. This is mostly

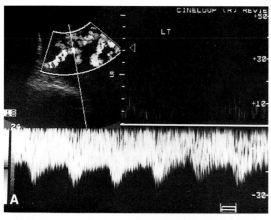

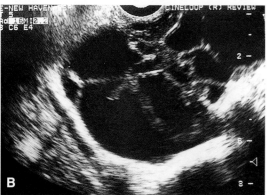

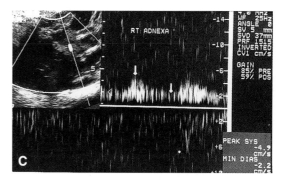

Figure 15 *Although lesions with soft tissue components, thick or vascular septations and low-impedance flow are more likely to be malignant, there is considerable overlap in both appearance and vascularity. Mass (A) with thick, vascular septations proved to be a serous cystadenoma. Another mass with a suspicious gray-scale appearance demonstrated minimal vascularity and was found to be a mucinous cystadenoma (B, C). A primarily cystic mass with mural nodularity and high-velocity, low-impedance flow was resected and diagnosed as an ovarian cancer (D) (see Color Plate J, page xi for (D))*

due to technological advances including the transvaginal ultrasound probe, which allows close proximity to the ovaries, and therefore improved resolution; use of color and duplex Doppler ultrasound enables assessment of perfusion patterns. Pelvic MRI now provides a large field of view with improved soft-tissue contrast and detailed multiplanar visualization of ovarian anatomy and characterization of normal and pathological tissue. The application of these techniques provides improved diagnosis of common physiological ovarian disorders that cause infertility and aids in management of ovulation induction cycles for anovulatory patients. Moreover, these non-invasive pelvic imaging modalities can often differentiate physiological ovarian cysts from pathological benign and malignant masses, thus allowing expedient use of appropriate therapy. Surgical intervention can be reserved for indicated cases, avoiding unnecessary surgeries. This is critically important in this group of women desiring reproductive potential for whom preservation of ovarian function is crucial. Also, the 'thorn in the side' of any pelvic surgery is the development of postoperative adhesions which can, in turn, lead to infertility, and should, therefore, be avoided wherever possible.

References

1. Kurman, R. J. (1987). Anatomy and histology of the ovary. In Kurman, R. J. (ed.) *Blaustein's Pathology of the Female Genital Tract*, 3rd edn. (New York: Springer-Verlag)
2. Birnholz, J. C. (1984). Ultrasonic visualization of endometrial movements. *Fertil. Steril.*, **41**, 157
3. Cohn, H. L., Tice, H. M. and Mandel, F. S. (1990). Ovarian volumes measured by US: bigger than we think. *Radiology*, **177**, 189

4. Higgins, R. V., van Nagell, J. R., Donaldson, E. S., *et al.* (1989). Transvaginal sonography as a screening method for ovarian cancer. *Gynecol. Oncol.*, **34**, 402

5. DeSantis, D. J., Scatarige, J. C., Kemp, G,. Given, F. T., Hsiu, J. G. and Cramer, M. S. (1993). A prospective evaluation of transvaginal sonography for detection of ovarian disease. *Am. J. Roentgenol.*, **161**, 91

6. Bryan, P. J., Cohen, W. N. and Seidelmann, F. E. (1988). The pelvis. In Haaga, J. R. and Alfidi, R. J. (eds.) *Computed Tomography of the Whole Body*, 2nd edn, p. 1116. (St. Louis: CV Mosby)

7. Scoutt, L. M., McCarthy, S. M. and Moss, A. (1983). Computer tomography and magnetic resonance imaging of the pelvis. In Moss, A. A., Gamsu, G. and Genant, H. K. (eds.) *Computed Tomography of the Body with Magnetic Resonance Imaging*, 2nd edn, p. 1215. (Philadelphia: W. B. Saunders)

8. Dooms, G. C., Hricak, H. and Tscholakoff, D. (1986). Adnexal structures: MR imaging. *Radiology*, **158**, 639

9. Zawin, M., McCarthy, S. M., Scoutt, L. M. *et al.* (1990). High field MRI and US evaluation of the pelvis in women with leiomyomas. *Magn. Reson. Imaging*, **8**, 371

10. Chering, A. P. and Chang, R. J. (1990). Polycystic ovary syndrome. *Clin. Obstet. Gynecol.*, **33**, 655

11. Stein, I. F. and Leventhal, M. C. (1935). Amenorrhea associated with bilateral polycystic ovaries. *Am. J. Obstet. Gynecol.*, **29**, 181

12. Polson, D. W., Adams, J., Wadsworth, S. *et al.* (1988). Polycystic ovaries – a common finding in normal women. *Lancet*, **1**, 870

13. Sagle, M., Bishop, K., Ridley, N. *et al.* (1988). Recurrent early miscarriage and polycystic ovaries. *Br. Med. J.*, **297**, 1027

14. Coleman, B. G. (1992). Transvaginal sonography of adnexal masses. *Radiologic Clinics of North America*, **30**, 677

15. Yeh, H. C., Futterweit, W. and Thornton, J. C. (1987). Polycystic ovarian disease: US features in 104 patients. *Radiology*, **163**, 111

16. Pache, T. D., Wladimiroff, J. W., Hop, W. C. J. and Fauser, B. C. J. M. (1992). How to discriminate between normal and polycystic ovaries: transvaginal US study. *Radiology*, **183**, 421

17. Sutton, C. L., McKinney, C. D., Jones, J. E. and Gay, S. B. (1992). Ovarian masses revisited: radiologic and pathologic correlation. *Radiographics*, **12**, 853

18. Ascher, S. M. and Silverman, P. M. (1991). Application of computed tomography in gynecologic diseases. *Urol. Radiol.*, **13**, 16

19. Lee, K. J. T. and Marx, M. V. (1989). Pelvis. In Lee, K. J. T., Sagel, S. S. and Stanley, R. J. B. (eds.) *Computed Body Tomography with MRI Correlation*. pp. 851–97. (New York: Raven Press)

20. Gross, B. H., Moss, A. A., Mihara, K. *et al.* (1983). Computed tomography of gynecologic disease. *Am. J. Roentgenol.*, **141**, 765

21. Carrington, B. M. (1991). The adnexal. In Hricak, H. and Carrington, B. M. (eds.) *MRI of the Pelvis. A Text Atlas.* (London: Martin Dunitz)

22. Faure, N., Prat, X., Bastide, A. *et al.* (1989). Assessment of ovaries by magnetic resonance imaging in patients presenting with polycystic ovarian syndrome. *Hum. Reprod.* **4**, 468

23. Ardaen, Y., Robert, Y., Lemartre, L. *et al.* (1991). Polycystic ovarian disease: contribution of vaginal endosonography and reassessment of ultrasonic diagnosis. *Fertil. Steril.*, **55**, 1062

24. Glazer, G. M., Francis, I. R. and Quint, L. E. (1988). Imaging of the adrenal glands. *Invest. Radiol.*, **23**, 3–11

25. Dunnick, N. R. (1990). Adrenal imaging: current status. *Am. J. Roentgenol.*, **154**, 927–36

26. Francis, I. R., Gross, M. D., Shapiro, B., Korobkin, M. and Quint, L. E. (1992). Integrated imaging of adrenal disease. *Radiology*, **184**, 1–13

27. Reinig, J. W., Doppman, J. L., Dwyer, A. J. *et al.* (1986). Adrenal masses differentiated by MR. *Radiology*, **158**, 81–4

28. Glazer, G. M., Woolsey, E. J. and Borrello, J. (1986). Adrenal tissue characterization using MR imaging. *Radiology*, **158**, 73–9

29. Falke, T. H., Strake, L., Shaff, M. I. *et al.* (1986). MR imaging of the adrenals: correlation with computed tomography. *J. Comput. Assis. Tomogra.*, **10**, 242–53

30. Chang, A., Glazer, H. S., Lee, J. K. T. *et al.* (1987). Adrenal gland: MR imaging. *Radiology*, **163**, 123–8

31. Reinig, J. W., Doppman, J. L., Dwyer, A. J. *et al.* (1986). MRI of indeterminate adrenal masses. *Am. J. Roentgenol.*, **147**, 493–6

32. Baker, M. E., Blinder, R., Spritzer, C. *et al.* MR evaluation of adrenal masses at 1.5T. *Am. J. Roentgenol.*, **153**, 307–12

33. Kier, R. and McCarthy, S. (1989). MR characterization of adrenal masses: field strength and pulse sequence considerations. *Radiology*, **171**, 671–4

34. Krestin, G. P., Steinbrick, W. and Friedmann, G. (1989). Adrenal masses: evaluation with fast gradient-echo MR imaging and Gd-DPTA-enhanced dynamic studies. *Radiology*, **171**, 675–80

35. Mitchell, D. G., Crovello, M., Matteucci, T. *et al.* (1992). Benign adrenocortical masses: diagnosis with chemical shift MR imaging. *Radiology*, **185**, 345–51

36. Reinig, J. W., Stutley, J. E., Leonhardt, C. M. *et al.* (1994). Differentiation of adrenal masses with MR imaging: comparison of techniques. *Radiology*, **192**, 41–6

37. Korobkin, M., Lombardi, T. J., Aisen, A. M. *et al.* (1995). Characterization of adrenal masses with chemical shift and gadolinium enhanced MR imaging. *Radiology*, **197(2)**, 411–18

38. Lee, M. J., Hahn, P. F., Papanicolaou, N. *et al.* (1991). Benign and malignant adrenal masses: CT distinction with attenuation coefficients, size, and observer analysis. *Radiology*, **179**, 415–18

39. Steptoe, P. C. and Edwards, R. G. (1976). Reimplantation of a human embryo with subsequent tubal pregnancy. *Lancet*, **1**, 880

40. Steptoe, P. C. and Edwards, R. G. (1978). Birth after the reimplantation of a human embryo. *Lancet*, **2**, 236

41. Beu-Raphael, Z., Masbrach, S., Dor, J. *et al.* (1986). Treatment of independent pregnancy after *in vitro* fertilization and embryo transfer trial. *Fertil. Steril.*, **45**, 564

42. March, C. M. and Shoupe, D. (1991). Luteal phase defects. In Mishell D.R. Jr, Davajan V. and Lobo R. A. (eds.) *Infertility, Contraception and Reproductive Endocrinology*, pp.793–806. (Boston: Blackwell Scientific Publications)

43. Lenz, S. (1985). Ultrasonic study of follicular maturation, ovulation, and development of corpus luteum during normal menstrual cycles. *Acta Obstet. Gynecol. Scand.*, **64**, 15

44. de Crespigny, L. J., O'Herlihz, C. and Robinson, H. P. (1981). Ultrasonic observations of the mechanisms of human ovulation. *Am. J. Obstet. Gynecol.*, **1939**, 636

45. Ritchie, W. G. M. (1994). In Callen, P. W. (ed.) *Ultrasonography in Obstetrics and Gynecology*. (Philadelphia: W. B. Sanders)

46. Coulam, C. B., Hill, L. M. and Breckle, R. (1982). Ultrasonic evidence for luteinization of unruptured preovulating follicles. *Fertil. Steril.*, **37**, 524

47. Kerin, J. F., Kirby, C., Morris, D. *et al.* (1983). Incidence of luteinized unruptured follicle phenomenon in cycling women. *Fertil. Steril.*, **40**, 620

48. Liukkonen, S., Koskimies, A. I., Tenhunen, A. and Ylostulo, P. (1984). Diagnosis of luteinized unruptured follicle (LUF) syndrome by ultrasound. *Fertil. Steril.*, **41**, 26

49. Killick, S. and Elstein, M. (1987). Pharmacologic production of luteinized unruptured follicles by prostaglandin synthetase inhibitors. *Fertil. Steril.*, **47**, 773–7

50. Hilgers, T. W., Dvorak, A. D., Tamisiea, D. F. *et al.* (1989). Sonographic definition of the empty follicle syndrome. *J. Ultrasound Med.*, **8**, 411

51. Hilgers, T. W., Dip, A., Kimball, C. R. *et al.* (1992). Assessment of the empty follicle syndrome by transvaginal sonography. *J. Ultrasound Med.*, **11**, 313

52. Blankstein, J., Shaler, J., Saadin, T. *et al.* (1987). Ovarian hyperstimulation syndrome: prediction by number and size of pre-ovulatory follicles. *Fertil. Steril.*, **47**, 597

53. Savage, M. O., Lowe, D. G., Ransley, P. G. *et al.* (1986). Germ cell neoplasia in patients with abnormal sexual differentiation (abstr. 131). *Pediatr. Res.*, **20**, 1183

54. Goldenberg, R. L., Grodin, J. M., Aodbard, D. and Ross, G. T. (1973). Gonadotropins in women with amenorrhea. *Am. J. Obstet. Gynecol.*, **116**, 1003

55. Palmer, C. G. and Reichmann, A. (1976). Chromosomal and clinical findings in 110 females with Turner's syndrome. *Hum. Genet.*, **35**, 35–49

56. Connor, J. M. and Loughlin, S. A. R. (1989). Molecular genetics of Turner's syndrome. *Acta Paediatr. Scand.*, **356** (Suppl.), 77–80

57. Deutsch, A. L. and Gosink, B. B. (1982). Non-neoplastic gynecologic disorders. *Semin. Roentgenol.* **17**, 269–83

58. Coulam, C. B., Adamson, S. C. and Annegers, J. F. (1986). Incidence of premature ovarian failure. *Obstet. Gynecol.*, **67**, 604

59. Krauss, C. M. *et al.* (1987). Familial premature ovarian failure due to interstitial deletion of the long arm of the X chromosome. *N. Engl. J. Med.*, **317**, 125

60. Alper, M. M. and Garner, P. R. (1985). Premature ovarian failure: its relationship to autoimmune disease. *Obstet. Gynecol.*, **66**, 27

61. Miguot, M. H., Schoemaker, J., Kleingeld, M. *et al.* (1989). Premature ovarian failure I. The association with autoimmunity. *Eur. J. Obstet. Gynecol. Reprod. Biol.*, **30**, 59

62. Toner, J. P., Philput, C. B., Jones, G. S. and Suheil, J. M. (1991). Basal follicle-stimulating hormone level is a better predictor of *in vitro* fertilization performance than age. *Fertil. Steril.*, **55**, 784–91

63. Steer, C. V., Tan, S. L., Mason, B. A. and Campbell, S. (1994). Midluteal phase vaginal color Doppler assessment of uterine artery impedance in a subfertile population. *Fertil. Steril.*, **61**, 53–8

64. Achiron, R., Levran, D., Swan, E. *et al.* (1995). Endometrial blood flow response to hormone replacement therapy in women with premature ovarian failure: a transvaginal Doppler study. *Fertil. Steril.*, **63**, 550–4

65. Critchley, H. O. D., Wallace, W. H. B., Shalet, S. M. *et al.* (1992). Abdominal irradiation in childhood: the potential for pregnancy. *Br. J. Obstet. Gynaecol.*, **99**, 392–4

66. Adams, J. M., Tan, S. L., Wheeler, M. J. *et al.* (1988). Uterine growth in the follicular phase of spontaneous ovulatory cycles and during luteinizing hormone-releasing hormone induced cycles in women with normal or polycystic ovaries. *Fertil. Steril.*, **49**, 52–5

67. Morrow, C. P. and Townsend, D. F. (1987). Tumor-like conditions of the ovary. In Morrow, C. P. and Townsend, D. E. (eds.) *Synopsis of Gynecologic Oncology.* 3rd edn, p. 305. (New York: Churchill Livingstone)

68. Baltarowich, O. H., Kurtz, A. B., Pasto, M. E. *et al.* (1987). The spectrum of sonographic findings in hemorrhagic ovarian cysts. *Am. J. Roentgenol.*, **148**, 901

69. Hala, K., Hala, T., Senoh, D. *et al.* (1990). Change in ovarian arterial compliance during the human menstrual cycle assessed by Doppler ultrasound. *Br. J. Obstet. Gynaecol.*, **97**, 163

70. Scholtes, M. C. W., Wladimiroff, J. W., Van Rijen, H. J. M. *et al.* (1989). Uterine and ovarian flow velocity waveforms in the normal menstrual cycle: a transvaginal Doppler study. *Fertil. Steril.*, **52**, 981

71. Taylor, K. J. W., Burns, P. N., Wells, P. N. T. *et al.* (1985). Ultrasound Doppler flow studies of the ovarian and uterine arteries. *Br. J. Obstet. Gynaecol.*, **92**, 240

72. Fleischer, A. C., Rodgers, W. H., Kepple, D. M. *et al.* (1992). Color Doppler sonography of benign and malignant ovarian masses. *Radiographics*, **12**, 879

73. Sawyer, R. W., Vick, C. W., Walsh, J. W. *et al.* (1985). Computer tomography of benign ovarian masses. *J. Comput. Assis. Tomogra.*, **9**, 784

74. Arrive, L., Hricak, H. and Martin, M. C. (1989). Pelvic endometriosis: MR imaging. *Radiology*, **171**, 687

75. Butch, R. J., Mueller, P. R., Ferruce, J. T. Jr *et al.* (1986). Drainage of pelvic abscesses through the greater sciatic foramen. *Radiology*, **158**, 487

76. Pardes, J. G., Scheinder, M., Koizumi, J., Engel, I. A. and Anh, Y. H. (1986). Percutaneous needle biopsy of deep pelvic masses: a posterior approach. *Cardiovasc. Intervent. Radiol.*, **9**, 65

77. Dellenbach, P., Nisand, P., Moreau, L., Feger, B., Plumere, C. and Gerlinger, P. (1985). Transvaginal sonographically controlled follicle puncture for oocyte retrieval. *Fertil. Steril.*, **44**, 656

78. Nosher, J. L., Winchman, H. K. and Needell, G. S. (1987). Transvaginal pelvic abscess drainage with US guidance. *Radiology*, **165**, 872

79. Loy, R. A., Gallup, D. G., Hill, J. A., Holzman, G. M. and Geist, D. (1989). Pelvic abscess: examination and transvaginal drainage guided by real time ultrasonography. *South. Med. J.*, **82**, 788

80. Bret, P. M., Laurent, G., Atri, M., Gillett, P., Seymour, R. J. and Senterman, M. K. (1992). Transvaginal US-guided aspiration of ovarian cysts and solid pelvic masses. *Radiology*, **185**, 377

81. Granberg, S., Crona, N., Euk, L., Hammarberg, K. and Wikland, M. (1989). Ultrasound guided puncture of cystic tumors in the lower pelvis of young women. *J. Clin. Ultrasound*, **17**, 107–11

82. de Crespigny, L., Robinson, H. P., Davoren, R. A. M. and Fortune, D. (1989). The simple cyst: aspirate or operate? *Br. J. Obstet. Gynaecol.*, **96**, 1035–9

83. Bret, P. M., Atri, M., Gurband, L., Gillett, P., Seymour, R. J. and Senterman, M. K. (1992). Ovarian cysts in postmenopausal women: preliminary results with transvaginal alcohol sclerosis. *Radiology*, **184**, 661–3

84. Granberg, S., Norstrom, A. and Wikland, M. (1991). Comparison of endovaginal ultrasound and cytological evaluation of cystic ovarian tumors. *J. Ultrasound Med.*, **10**, 9–14

85. Pinto, M. M., Bernstein, U. T., Brogan, D. A., Parikh, F. and Lavy, G. (1990). Measurement of CA-125, carcinoembryonic antigen, and alpha-fetoprotein in ovarian cyst fluid: diagnostic adjunct to cytology. *Diagn. Cytopathol.*, **6**, 160–3

86. Washington, A. E., Arno, P. S. and Brooks, M. A. (1986). The economic cost of pelvic inflammatory disease. *J. Am. Med. Assoc.*, **255**, 17–38

87. Westrom, L. (1980). Incidence, prevalence, and trends of acute pelvic inflammatory disease and its consequences in industrialized countries. *Am. J. Obstet. Gynecol.*, **138**, 880–92

88. Thompson, S. E., Hagar, W. D. and Wong, K. H. (1980). The microbiology and therapy of acute pelvic inflammatory disease in hospitalized patients. *Am. J. Obstet. Gynecol.*, **136**, 179

89. Drogemueller, W. (1992). Upper genital tract infections. In Mishell, D. R., Stellchener, M. A. and Drogemueller, W. (eds.) *Comprehensive Gynecology*, pp. 691–720. (St. Louis: Mosby Year Book)

90. Hager, W. D., Eschenbach, D. A., Spence, M. R. and Sweet, R. L. (1983). Criteria for diagnosis and grading of salpingitis. *Obstet. Gynecol.*, **61**, 113–14

91. Hagdu, A., Westrom, L., Brooks, C. A. *et al.* (1986). Predicting acute pelvic inflammatory

disease: a multivariate analysis. *Am. J. Obstet. Gynecol.*, **155**, 954–60

92. Drogemueller, W. (1992). Endometriosis and adenomyosis. In Mishell, D. R., Stellchener, M. A. and Drogemueller W. (eds.) *Comprehensive Gynecology*, pp. 691–720. (St. Louis: Mosby Year Book)

93. Kilchin, J. D. (1984). Endometriosis. In Sciarra, J. J. (ed.) *Gynecology and Obstetric.* (Philadelphia: Harper and Row)

94. Simpson, J. L., Elias, S., Malinak, L. L. *et al.* (1980). Heritable aspects of endometriosis. *Am. J. Obstet. Gynecol.*, **137**, 327

95. Sampson, J. A. (1927). Peritoneal endometriosis due to menstrual dissemination of endometrial tissue into peritoneal cavity. *Am. J. Obstet. Gynecol.*, **14**, 422

96. Olive, D. L. and Martin, D. C. (1987). Treatment of endometriosis-associated infertility with CO_2 laser laparoscopy: the use of one and two parameter exponential models. *Fertil. Steril.*, **48**, 18

97. Friedman, H., Vogelzang, R. L., Mendelson, E. B. *et al.* (1985). Endometriosis detection by US with laparoscopic correlation. *Radiology*, **157**, 217

98. Heaps, J. M., Nieberg, R. K. and Berek, J. S. (1990). Malignant neoplasma arising in endometriosis. *Obstet. Gynecol.*, **75**, 1023–8

99. Fishman, E. K., Scatarize, J. C., Saksonk, F. A. *et al.* (1983). Computed tomography of endometriosis. *J. Comput. Assis. Tomogra.*, **7**, 257–64

100. Zawin, M., McCarthy, S., Scoutt, L. and Comite, F. (1989). Endometriosis: appearance and detection at MR imaging. *Radiology*, **171**, 693–6

101. Togashi, K., Nishimura, K., Kimura, I. *et al.* (1991). Endometrial cysts: diagnosis with MR imaging. *Radiology*, **180**, 73–8

102. Nishimura, K., Togashi, K., Itoh, K. *et al.* (1987). Endometrial cysts of the ovary: MR imaging. *Radiology*, **162**, 315–18

103. Woodward, P. J., Wagner, B. J. and Farley, T. E. (1993). MR imaging in the evaluation of female infertility. *Radiographics*, **13**, 293–306

104. Nyberg, D. A., Porter, B. A., Olds, M. O. *et al.* (1987). Imaging of hemorrhagic adnexal masses. *J. Comput. Assis. Tomogra.*, **11**, 664–9

105. Dooms, G. C., Hricak, H. and Tscholakoff, D. (1986). Adnexal structures: MR imaging. *Radiology*, **158**, 639–46

106. Mitchell, D. G., Mintz, M. C., Spritzer, C. E. *et al.* (1987). Adnexal masses: MR imaging observations at 1.5T with US and CT correlation. *Radiology*, **162**, 319–24

107. Mitchell. D. G. (1989). Magnetic resonance imaging of the adnexa. *Semin. Ultrasound Comput. Tomogr. Magn. Reson.*, **9**, 143–57

108. Daniell, J. F. and Pittaway, D. E. (1983). Short interval second-look laparoscopy after infertility surgery: a preliminary report. *Reprod. Med.*, **28**, 281–3

109. Webster, B. W., Wentz, A. C. and Maxim, W. S. (1987). Endometriosis. In DeCherney, A. H. and Polan, M. L. (eds.) *Reproductive Surgery*, pp. 221–42. (Chicago: Year Book Medical)

110. Hubbard, L. T. (1985). Adnexal torsion. *Am. J. Obstet. Gynecol.*, **152**, 456

111. Drogemueller, W. (1992). Benign gynecologic lesions. In Mishell, D. R., Stellchener, M. A. and Drogemueller, W. (eds.) *Comprehensive Gynecology*, pp. 691–720. (St Louis: Mosby Year Book)

112. Gray, M. and Itzchak, Y. (1988). Sonographic evaluation of ovarian torsion in childhood and adolescence. *Am. J. Roentgenol.*, **150**, 647

113. Coleman, B. G. (1992). Transvaginal sonography of adnexal masses. *Radiologic Clinics of North America*, **30**, 677–91

114. Grinf, M., Shalev, J., Strauss, S. *et al.* (1984). Torsion of the ovary, sonographic features. *Am. J. Roentgenol.*, **143**, 1331

115. Rosado, W. M., Trambert, M. A., Gosink, B. B. and Pretorius, D. H. (1992). Adnexal torsion: diagnoses by using Doppler sonography. *Am. J. Roentgenol.*, **159**, 1251–3

116. Fleischer, A. C., Stein, S. M., Cullinan, J. A. and Warner, M. A. (1995). Color Doppler sonography of adnexal torsion. *J. Ultrasound Med.*, **14**, 523–8

117. Quillan, S. P. and Siegel, M. T. (1994). Transabdominal color Doppler sonography of the painful adolescent ovary. *J. Ultrasound Med.*, **13**, 549

118. Kimura, I., Togashi, K., Kawakami, S. *et al.* (1994). Ovarian torsion: CT and MR appearances. *Radiology*, **190**, 337–41

119. Koonings, P. P., Campbell, K., Mishell, D. R. and Grimes, D. A. (1989). Relative frequency of primary ovarian neoplasms: a 10 year review. *Obstet. Gynecol.*, **74**, 921–6

120. Mendelson, E. B. and Bohm-Velez, M. (1992). Transvaginal ultrasonography of pelvic neoplasms. *Radiologic Clinics of North America*, **30**, 703–34

121. Fried, A. M., Woodring, J. H. and Loh, F. K. (1985). Ovarian dermoid: side by side presentation of the sonographic differential diagnosis. *Med. Radiogr. Photogr.*, **61**, 32

122. Buy, J. N., Ghossain, M. A., Moss, A. A. *et al.* (1989). Cystic teratoma of the ovary with CT detection. *Radiology*, **171**, 697

123. Dodd, G. D. III., Lancaster, K. T. and Morilton, J. S. Ovarian lipoleiomyoma in a fat containing mass in the female pelvis. *Am. J. Roentgenol.*, **153**, 1007

124. Laing, F. C., van Dalsem, V. F., Marks, W. M. et al. (1981). Dermoid cysts of the ovary: their ultrasonographic appearance. Obstet. Gynecol., 57, 99

125. Buy, J. N., Ghossain, W. A., Sciot, C. et al. (1991). Epithelial tumors of the ovary: CT findings and correlation with US. Radiology, 178, 811

126. Fleischer, A. C., James, A. E. Jr, Millis, J. B. et al. (1978). Differential diagnosis of pelvic masses by gray scale sonography. Am. J. Roentgenol., 131, 469

127. Quinn, S. F., Erikson, S. and Black, W. C. (1985). Cystic ovarian teratomas: the sonographic appearance of the dermoid plug. Radiology, 155, 477

128. Sister, C. L. and Siegel, M. J. (1990). Ovarian teratomas: a comparison of the sonographic appearance in prepubertal and postpubertal girls. Am. J. Roentgenol., 154, 139

129. Cederlund, C. G., Karlsson, S. and Nyman, U. (1981). Computer tomography of ovarian dermoid cysts. Acta Radiol., 22, 435

130. Feldberg, M. A. M., van Waes, P. F. G. M. and Hendriks, M. J. (1984). Direct multiplanar CT findings in cystic teratoma of the ovary. J. Comput. Assis. Tomogra., 6, 1131

131. Skane, P. and Huebner, K. H. (1983). Computed tomography of cystic teratomas with gravity dependent layering. J. Comput. Assis. Tomogra., 5, 837

132. Mitchell, D. G. (1992). Benign disease of the uterus and ovaries: applications of magnetic resonance imaging. Radiologic Clinics of North America, 30, 777–87

133. Hricak, H. and Kim, B. (1993). Contrast-enhanced MR imaging of the female pelvis. J. Magn. Reson. Imaging, 3, 297–306

134. Kier, R., Smith, R. C. and McCarthy, S. M. (1992). Value of the lipid-and-water-suppression MR images in distinguishing between blood and lipid within ovarian masses. Am. J. Roentgenol., 158, 321–5

135. Stevens, S. K., Hricak, H. and Campos, Z. (1993). Teratomas versus cystic hemorrhagic adnexal lesions: differentiation with proton selective fat saturation MR imaging. Radiology, 186, 481–8

136. Komatsin, T., Konishi, I., Mandai, M. et al. (1996). Adnexal masses: transvaginal US and gadolinium-enhanced MR imaging assessment of intramural structure. Radiology, 198, 109–15

137. Jain, K. A., Friedman, D. L., Pettinger, T. W. et al. (1993). Adnexal masses: comparison of specificity of endovaginal US and pelvic MR imaging. Radiology, 186, 697–704

138. Breen, J. L. (1970). A 21 year survey of 654 ectopic pregnancies. Am. J. Obstet. Gynecol., 106, 1004

139. Hallat, J. G. (1982). Primary ovarian pregnancy: a report of twenty-five cases. Am. J. Obstet. Gynecol., 143, 55

140. Kaufman, J. J. (1962). Unusual causes of extrinsic ureteral obstruction. Part I. J. Urol., 87, 319–27

141. Phillips, H. E. and McGahan, J. P. (1982). Ovarian remnant syndrome. Radiology, 142, 487–8

142. Bourne, T., Campbell, S., Steer, C., Whitehead, M. I. and Collins, W. B. (1989). Transvaginal color flow imaging: a possible new screening technique for ovarian cancer. Br. Med. J., 229, 1367

143. Kurjak, A., Zalud, I., Jurkovic, A., Alfirevic, Z. and Miljan, M. (1989). Transvaginal color Doppler assessment of pelvic circulation. Acta. Obstet. Gynecol. Scand., 68, 131–5

144. Fleischer, A. C., Rodger, W. H., Rao, B. K. et al. (1991). Assessment of ovarian tumor vascularity with transvaginal color Doppler sonography. J. Ultrasound Med., 10, 563–8

145. Kurjak, A, Zalud, I. and Alfirevic, Z. (1991). Evaluation of adnexal masses with trans-vaginal color ultrasound. J. Ultrasound Med., 10, 295–7

146. Hamper, U. M., Sheth, S., Abbas, F. M. et al. (1993). Transvaginal color Doppler sonography of adnexal masses: differences in blood flow impedance in benign and malignant lesions. Am. J. Roentgenol., 160, 1225–8

147. Jain, K. A. (1994). Prospective evaluation of adnexal masses with endovaginal gray scale and duplex and color Doppler US: correlation with pathologic findings. Radiology, 191, 63–7

148. Brown, D. L., Fiates, M. C., Laing, F. C. et al. (1994). Ovarian masses: can benign and malignant lesions be differentiated with color and pulsed Doppler US? Radiology, 190, 333–6

149. Taylor, K. J. W. and Schwartz, P. E. (1994). Screening for early ovarian cancer. Radiology, 192, 1–10

150. Fleischer, A. C., Rodgers, W. H., Kepple, D. M. et al. (1992). Color Doppler sonography of benign and malignant ovarian masses. Radiographics, 12, 879–85

Imaging and intervention of the abnormal fallopian tube

5

K. W. Dickey, T. G. Zreik, J. M. Brown and M. G. Glickman

A plug of hardened mucus of the most insignificant character – the merest *debris* of the fallopian secretion – may cut off an illustrious race, or change a dynasty.

Dr Tyler Smith, London, 1849

INTRODUCTION

The fallopian tubes, like other hollow organs, have only a few ways in which they express disease. They can be absent, obstructed and/or ruptured. Ciliary dysfunction may alter the tubal hemodynamics.

As seen in congenital anomalies and post-surgical cases, the tubes can be absent. Obstruction is the most common abnormality of the tube manifest by dilatation, sometimes to huge size. Another abnormality, salpingitis isthmica nodosa, is also common. Salpingitis isthmica nodosa is often associated with infertility and ectopic pregnancy; however, its role in the physiology of tube dysfunction is not known. Space-occupying masses such as tubal pregnancy or neoplasm can cause obstruction and, in the case of tubal pregnancy, tubal rupture and hemorrhage.

Although great advances in imaging technology have occurred in the past two decades, hysterosalpingography (HSG) continues to be the cornerstone of tubal imaging. When performed by an experienced operator, HSG is the only examination that can image both the normal and the abnormal tube. Transvaginal ultrasound, with or without Doppler, has an important role in the diagnosis of ectopic pregnancy.

Although transcervical techniques for re-canalizing fallopian tubes were first described in 1849[1], recent years have seen their rediscovery. The use of transcervical and laparoscopic techniques for diagnosing and treating tubal disease makes infertile women less often dependent on open surgical procedures. Current techniques include transcervical fallopian tube catheterization, fallopian tube recanalization, laparoscopy and hysteroscopy.

IMAGING OF FALLOPIAN TUBE PATHOLOGY

Congenital anomalies

Although congenital anomalies of the uterus are commonly seen in a busy clinical practice, anomalies of the fallopian tubes are rare. They include accessory ostia, multiple lumina, diverticula, tubal duplication or complete agenesis. Accessory tubes are thought to contribute to infertility by capturing oocytes that would otherwise enter the normal moiety. If an oocyte is fertilized and captured by the accessory tube, an ectopic pregnancy may result. These accessory tubes are rarely opacified with contrast on HSG[2,3].

In Müllerian duct anomalies of the uterus, the number of tubes usually correlates with the number of uterine horns (i.e. a unicornuate uterus has one tube, etc.), as both the uterus and fallopian tube are of Müllerian duct origin. Müllerian duct remnants, such as paratubal cysts, can be imaged with magnetic resonance imaging (MRI) or computed tomography (CT), if they are large enough. Although MRI and ultrasound are valuable in the imaging of uterine anomalies, the resolution is not sufficient to image the tube of normal diameter[4]. HSG is the best modality to evaluate the structure and patency of tubes involved in congenital anomalies (Figure 1).

Fallopian tube obstruction

Obstruction can occur anywhere along the course of the tube, from the cornual to the ampullary segment. Tubal obstruction is thought to contribute to female infertility in as many as 30–50% of cases[5]. The fimbriated segment is the most common site of tubal obstruction. Isolated isthmic occlusion owing to any pathological process is uncommon. Obstruction at or near the uterotubal junction is present in as many as 20–25% of patients who have tubal abnormalities on HSG[5-7]. A tube can be effected at more than one site simultaneously, and often by two different disease processes.

The etiology of obstruction may be tubal spasm, cellular debris, pelvic inflammatory disease (PID), polyps, synechiae, peritubal adhesions, previous pelvic surgery including sterilization procedures, primary or adjacent tumors, or tubal pregnancy. The differential diagnosis varies with the location of obstruction; i.e. cornual/proximal obstruction is most likely to result from cellular debris, and distal/fimbrial obstruction is most likely to result from infection and subsequent hydrosalpinx and/or peritubal adhesions.

Many modalities have been used in imaging the fallopian tubes, including HSG, CT, MRI, nuclear medicine and ultrasound with or without color Doppler. With current imaging technology, the proximally obstructed tube is best evaluated with HSG. Tubal segments of normal diameter are not well seen with other modalities. Since the introduction of simple techniques for selective catheterization of fallopian tubes, HSG can be modified to include contrast medium injection directly into the tube; with direct

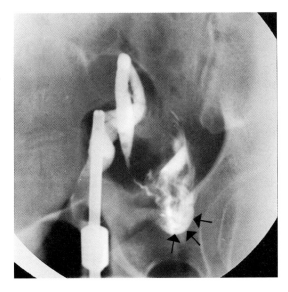

Figure 1 *Hysterosalpingogram of a patient with a unicornuate uterus. The associated fallopian tube was normal. The other tube was absent. The patient also had evidence of peritubal adhesions (arrows)*

injection tubal pathology is more readily seen[8-13]. Animal studies have shown no lasting deleterious effects on tubal epithelium from the direct injection of contrast into the tube[14]. Many reports have described an increased pregnancy rate in patients after undergoing HSG alone[15-19]. It is unknown whether the therapeutic effect is due to the pressure of injection causing opening of obstructed tubes, or a primary effect of the contrast medium. The fluoroscopic demonstration of spillage of contrast from the distal tube and free flow in the peritoneal space is the hallmark of tubal and peritubal patency.

Ultrasound HSG has been described as using real-time imaging during intrauterine injection of a sonographic contrast agent, such as sterile saline. However, this technique can diagnose only tubal obstruction and is not capable of pinpointing the affected segment[20,21]. Gross patency of the tubes can also be demonstrated by chromopertubation at laparoscopy. This involves transcervical injection of colored dye and confirmation of tubal spillage by direct laparoscopic visualization.

At the cornual/proximal segment of the tube, signs of obstruction can be factitiously present on HSG, with or without forceful injection. In one series, laparoscopy revealed patent tubes in more than 17% of patients whose HSG showed tubal occlusions[22]. Such falsely positive hysterosalpingograms are presumed to result from spasm of the utero-cornual portions of the fallopian tube in response to instrumentation. A variety of agents have been used in the treatment of cornual spasm, including sublingual nitroglycerin[23]. Winfield and colleagues[24] suggested the use of intravenous glucagon to treat spasm. However, these systemic methods have not been clearly shown to relieve uterotubal spasm consistently. Another option presently under investigation at our center is the administration of aminophylline, a methyl-xanthene that functions as a phosphodiesterase inhibitor. The drug is diluted with contrast material and is given transcervically, either within the uterine cavity or injected directly into the affected tube. Aminophylline has been shown to relax smooth muscle in the upper urinary tract, serving as an effective means of reversing spasm at the ureteropelvic junction[25]. In reviewing the HSG reports of our pilot series of seven patients in whom aminophylline was used in the presence of proximal tubal occlusion, aminophylline reversed the spasm in three of the seven patients and tubal patency was documented. In the four patients in whom the tubes remained closed after topical application of aminophylline, three required fallopian tuboplasty and one patient went on to have *in vitro* fertilization.

Although many reports dating back as far as 1849[1] cite cellular debris as the most common cause of organic proximal tubal obstruction, no large trials with radiological/pathological correlation support this hypothesis[1]. Undetected submucosal fibroids have been shown to prevent filling of the tubes owing to a ball-valve mechanism at the cornual segment. This has been seen in as many as 15% in one series[15]. The histology of proximal tube occlusion has been studied in patients undergoing proximal tube resection and reimplantation. In one series, 18 patients were studied after diagnosis of proximal obstruction with HSG or laparoscopic chromopertubation. Subsequent evaluation of the resected segment showed no evidence of obstruction in 11 of 18 pathological specimens. Six cases demonstrated amorphous material in the tubal lumen which formed a cast of the lumen. This material may be the 'cellular debris' first described by Smith in 1849 and often described as the most common etiology of proximal tubal occlusion[1,6]. However, another series showed identifiable pathology in 41 of 42 resected tubes (98%)[26]. Similar findings were reported by Letterie and Sakas[5], in which 27 tubes from 15 patients were histologically evaluated after failed attempts at fluoroscopic cannulation. In this population, 93% of the specimens exhibited abnormalities: obliterative fibrosis was found in 61%, chronic salpingitis in 57% and salpingitis isthmica nodosa in 42%. Many of the resected segments had components of more than one disease. These authors suggested that transcervical fallopian tube recanalization is successful in tubes obstructed by the cellular debris, but probably fails in histologically occluded tubes. Other reported causes of proximal obstruction include synechiae, endometriosis and polyps. Although polyps in the cornual portion of the tube have been suggested as a contributor to subfertility, this remains controversial[27,28] (Figure 2).

Mid-tubal occlusion is relatively rare, although the exact incidence is not known. Reported incidence ranges from 2.7 to 13.3%. The disease processes leading to mid-tubal occlusion that have been described are tuberculosis, inflammation, infection, endometriosis, tubal pregnancy, congenital anomalies, adenomatoid tumors, intratubal adhesions and surgical mishaps (Figure 3), e.g. during inguinal hernia repair[29].

Obstruction at the distal end or ampullary segment of the fallopian tube is most often due to previous infection and subsequent adhesion formation in the region of the fimbriae. The process then leads to the

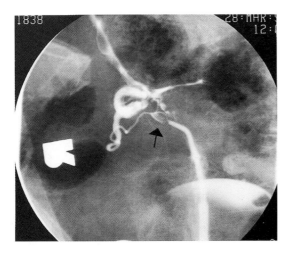

Figure 2 *Selective contrast injection of the right fallopian tube reveals a filling defect within the interstitial region (arrow). Hysteroscopic biopsy confirmed this to be a polyp*

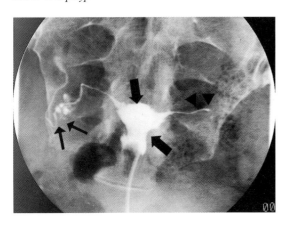

Figure 3 *Hysterosalpingogram of a patient with salpingitis isthmica nodosa after salpingectomy. Contrast injection reveals diverticular outpouchings in the isthmic portion of the right fallopian tube consistent with salpingitis isthmica nodosa (broad arrows). This tube was noted to be patent on later images. The left tube did not fill distal to the mid-isthmic portion, owing to a previous salpingectomy (arrowheads). Incidentally noted are irregularities of the uterine cavity due to scarring (thin arrows)*

development of hydrosalpinx. The distal portion of the tube can become occluded, or may have a very small opening into the peritoneal cavity. This opening may be demonstrated only after delayed filming after HSG. Subclinical pelvic inflammatory disease is thought to be the primary causal factor for postinflammatory abnormalities in the tubes, including hydrosalpinx[30]. *Chlamydia trachomatis* is the most likely bacterium in both clinical and subclinical infection[31,32]. Intrauterine devices (IUDs) have been cited as causative factors in the development of subclinical salpingitis and subsequent hydrosalpinx.

The diagnosis of hydrosalpinx can be made by a number of different imaging modalities, including CT, MRI and ultrasound (Figure 4). However, these modalities cannot show normal tubes and reliably image mild tubal dilatation. HSG remains the most accurate imaging modality for the diagnosis of hydrosalpinx. However, careful technique is important. The tube must be completely filled with contrast material for accurate assessment of the dilated segment (Figure 4A).

Peritubal adhesions may also be demonstrated on HSG, with or without an associated hydrosalpinx. They have been attributed to the same inflammatory processes responsible for other tubal pathology[2]. The diagnosis of peritubal adhesions almost always requires delayed filming of the pelvis after HSG, to demonstrate pooling of contrast in the peritoneal space adjacent to the ampullary or fimbriated portion of the tube (Figure 5, p. 96).

The postsurgical tube

As seen in Figure 3, HSG can depict tubal obstructions caused by previous surgery, including tubal ligation. In patients seeking reversal of tubal ligation, HSG has traditionally been used to demonstrate the length of the uterine end of the affected tube. The value of this measurement for preoperative salpingo-salpingostomy planning has recently been disputed[2,33–35]. After reanastomosis, the tube can also be evaluated with HSG. Often, there is an area of relative narrowing at the anastomotic site.

Salpingitis isthmica nodosa

Salpingitis isthmica nodosa, a tubal disease with classic radiological and pathological findings, was first described by Chiari in

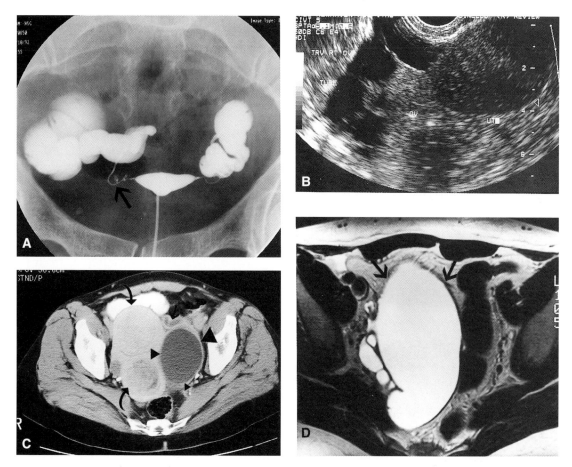

Figure 4 *Imaging of hydrosalpinx in four separate patients. (A) Hysterosalpingography demonstrates bilateral involvement. The left tube also displays evidence of salpingitis isthmica nodosa (arrow). (B) Ultrasound reveals a relative echogenic structure consistent with a dilated tube (OV, ovary; TUBE, fallopian tube; UT, uterus). (C) Pelvic computed tomography scan shows hydrosalpinx (small arrow) adjacent to an endometrioma in torsion (arrowheads). Also noted are uterine leiomyomas (curved arrow). (D) T_1-weighted axial magnetic resonance image of the pelvis displays a large midline cystic structure (arrows), proven at surgery to be hydrosalpinx of the right fallopian tube. This patient presented with a palpable mid-abdominal mass*

1887[36]. Although it is commonly associated with ectopic pregnancy and possibly infertility, the etiology and pathophysiology of salpingitis isthmica nodosa remain uncertain[37–42]. HSG continues to be the best modality for imaging of salpingitis isthmica nodosa.

The classic findings are multiple 1–2-mm outpouchings arising from the isthmic portion of the fallopian tube. These outpouchings give the appearance of diverticula, and can form complex-appearing contrast collections (Figures 3 and 4A)[2,38]. Histologically, the hallmark of salpingitis isthmica nodosa is the outpouching of tubal epithelium that

manifest as firm, nodular enlargements, ranging in diameter from 1–2 mm to 2 cm. The epithelium does not contain endometrial stroma, suggesting that salpingitis isthmica nodosa is not a form of tubal endometriosis. Usually, no inflammatory tissue is seen in association with salpingitis isthmica nodosa[38].

It is unknown whether the etiology of salpingitis isthmica nodosa is inflammatory, a form of adenomyosis, or a congenital condition that predisposes to infection[39,40]. Although the affected segment is usually not narrowed or obstructed, salpingitis isthmica nodosa is often seen in association with other

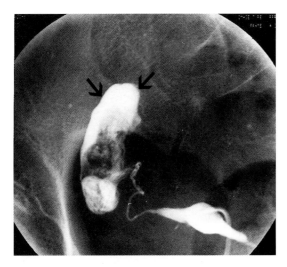

Figure 5 *Hysterosalpingogram of patient with peritubal adhesions. Contrast pools are evident immediately adjacent to the fimbriated portion of the right tube (arrows)*

obstructing tubal diseases, including hydro-salpinx (Figure 4A). As many as 50% of patients with salpingitis isthmica nodosa have tubal occlusion distal to the salpingitis isthmica nodosa-affected segment, and many have bilateral disease[33]. Histological studies have found salpingitis isthmica nodosa in 5% of control populations. Salpingitis isthmica nodosa is also well known as a risk factor for tubal pregnancy, with a reported incidence of up to 50% in tubes removed for ectopic pregnancy[40–42]. Salpingitis isthmica nodosa is also found in 7–25% of patients seeking treatment for proximal tubal obstruction. Thurmond and colleagues[40] have shown that salpingitis isthmica nodosa and associated tubal abnormalities were present on selective catheterization of the fallopian tube in 72% of patients studied. Moreover, these patients are well served by fallopian tube recanalization, as intrauterine pregnancies do occur via salpingitis isthmica nodosa-involved tubes.

Ectopic (tubal) pregnancy

Ectopic pregnancy is defined as the implantation and growth of products of conception anywhere outside the uterine cavity. Although the most common ectopic implantation site is within the fallopian tube, other sites of implantation include the cervix, ovary, or anywhere within the peritoneal cavity. Cervical implantation carries significant morbidity, as there is a risk of catastrophic hemorrhage as a result of the massive blood supply recruited by a placenta.

For the purposes of this chapter, emphasis is placed on imaging of the tubal pregnancy. The most common site within the fallopian tube for implantation is the ampullary segment. Of particular concern is the 'interstitial' (cornual) ectopic pregnancy, which is defined as implantation of products of conception within the mural portion of the fallopian tube. This phenomenon carries markedly higher morbidity and mortality than do other loci of tubal pregnancy, because it tends to present late, when placental blood supply is well established. Should tubal rupture occur, internal hemorrhage is severe. Although the classic clinical triad is pain, bleeding and an adnexal mass, rarely do patients exhibit all three at presentation.

Pelvic infection, a known contributor to the development of tubal obstruction, is suspected to increase the risk of tubal pregnancy. However, most patients presenting with tubal pregnancy (along with those presenting with tubal obstruction and infertility) have no clinical history of PID. Again, *Chlamydia* is thought to be the organism most commonly responsible for subclinical infection in patients with tubal pregnancy[43]. Approximately 8% of pregnancies after PID are ectopic, and approximately 50% of women undergoing surgery for ectopic pregnancy have pathological evidence of PID[43–45]. Previous abdominal surgery, including surgery for tubal pregnancy, has also been suggested as a risk factor for tubal pregnancy; however, this is controversial[32]. Advanced age is thought to be a relative risk factor due to decreased ciliary motion within the fallopian tubes.

Patients with a history of ectopic pregnancy are thought to have decreased fertility potential[46]. However if pregnancy develops, these patients should be evaluated early, even if they are asymptomatic. Early evaluation is also suggested when pregnancy is diagnosed in any patient at risk for pre-existing tubal disease, prior tubal surgery, assisted fertilization or indwelling intrauterine device[47].

The incidence of ectopic pregnancy has increased dramatically over the last few decades, however, the mortality rate has markedly decreased. This is thought to be due in large part to better methods of early detection[47,48]. Currently, the modality most associated with early detection of ectopic pregnancy is high-resolution transvaginal sonography (TVS). When used in combination with the serum measurement of the beta subunit of human chorionic gonadotropin (β-hCG), both transabdominal sonography and TVS are essential for the diagnosis of ectopic pregnancy[49–54], although TVS is the more sensitive and specific test[54–57]. Many patients can be treated before they become symptomatic, and before tubal rupture[58].

Many criteria for establishment of the diagnosis of ectopic pregnancy have been described with the use of transabdominal sonography and/or TVS, including: the empty uterus plus adnexal mass; an extrauterine gestational sac with or without a viable fetus; pseudodecidual reaction; adnexal ring; the 'halo' sign; decidual cysts within the endometrium; and the presence of echogenic extrauterine fluid[46,56,57,59–63]. With TVS, the criterion with the highest specificity (100%) is the identification of an extrauterine gestational sac. A detectable living fetus may or may not be present; however, these are rarely detected, and this sign has the lowest sensitivity (15–20%). A slightly less specific, but more sensitive (21–84%) criterion is the absence of an intrauterine pregnancy and a complex adnexal mass in a patient with a positive pregnancy test. This criterion has a specificity of 93–99.5% (Figure 6)[46,62,64]. Although the risk of simultaneous intrauterine and extrauterine heterologous pregnancies is low (1/7000–1/30 000 pregnancies), the likelihood is increased in patients undergoing assisted reproduction[46].

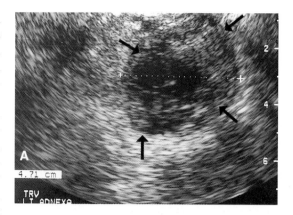

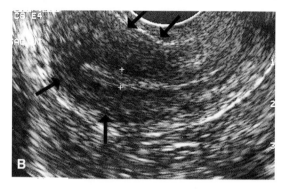

Figure 6 *The finding of a complex adnexal mass and a positive pregnancy test has a high specificity for ectopic pregnancy. (A) Complex adnexal mass with a relatively anechoic center (arrows). (B) Sagittal image of the uterus (arrows) in the same patient displays no evidence of an intrauterine gestational sac. Measurement cursors are on the endometrial stripe*

Transvaginal pulsed and color Doppler flow studies have recently been suggested for evaluation of ectopic pregnancy. Early data suggest that the presence, velocity and resistance index (RI) of blood flow may improve the diagnosis in a suspicious adnexal mass[65–69]. Both a corpus luteum cyst of pregnancy and an ectopic pregnancy adjacent to the ovary are highly vascular sonographically complex masses in the adnexa. Kurjak and colleagues[66] have described differences in RI between the corpus luteum cyst and the adnexal mass of tubal pregnancy. These differences, however, remain controversial, as the RIs of tubal pregnancy and the corpus luteum can vary widely, and overlap

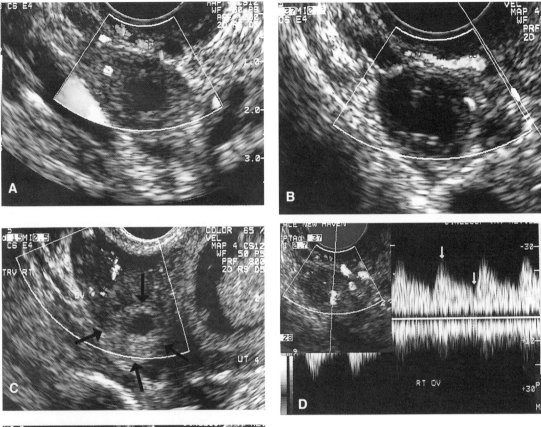

Figure 7 *The corpus luteum should be within the ovarian parenchyma, as seen here in sagittal (A) and transverse (B) images. A tubal pregnancy (arrows) is typically found between the ovary and uterine cornua. This distinction may be difficult (OV, ovary; UT, uterus) (C) and Doppler findings are variable and overlap significantly. In this example, the corpus luteum shows characteristic high-velocity, low-impedance flow (D), whereas the ectopic gestation is relatively avascular and probable non-viable (arrows on ectopic gestation, arrowheads on corpus luteum) (E)*

significantly[46,67]. Gray-scale imaging criteria to distinguish the adnexal mass from the ovary remain the standard for differentiating a corpus luteum cyst from a tubal pregnancy[67]. On the ultrasound image, a corpus luteum cyst is surrounded on all sides in three dimensions by ovarian tissue. A tubal pregnancy can be separated from the ovary, although the search can be technically challenging (Figure 7). The usefulness of Doppler in the evaluation of tubal pregnancy remains to be seen with further comparative studies.

MRI and CT have only a limited role in the imaging of tubal pregnancy, but can be helpful in locating ectopic pregnancy elsewhere in the pelvis or abdomen. In the past, HSG was used for diagnosing tubal pregnancy. Typical findings included obstruction by a filling defect caused by the gestational sac. HSG is no longer recommended, except in patients being treated by local uterine or tubal injection of drugs such as methotrexate[70,71]. In patients receiving systemic drugs for treatment (oral methotrexate, etc.), TVS is the optimal imaging modality for follow-up[72]. HSG can be used once the products of conception have been resorbed, to assess patency of the affected tube[73,74].

FALLOPIAN TUBE INTERVENTION

Fallopian tube recanalization (tuboplasty)

Since its first description in 1985 by Platia and Krudy[75], transcervical selective fallopian tube recanalization (FTR) under fluoroscopic guidance has been studied as an alternative to laparoscopic and microsurgical management of proximal tubal obstruction[10,12,13,75–85]. Many devices have been used to dilate the tube, including angioplasty balloons, coaxial catheter and guidewire combinations, and a guidewire alone[8,9,75,86–88].

In 1990, Thurmond and Rosch[10] published their results in the first 100 patients undergoing FTR with their coaxial wire/catheter system. The procedure was successful in opening one or both tubes in 86 patients. All patients had proximal obstruction of one or both tubes documented by HSG. The overall pregnancy rate was 26%. However, in a subset of 20 selected patients with bilateral proximal tubal obstruction and no other tubal disease, FTR was successful in one or more tubes in 19 patients (95%). Of these, nine conceived without further therapy (47%) with an average procedure to conception time of 4 months. All pregnancies were intrauterine[10]. In a review article published in 1991[80], Thurmond reported no clinically significant complications in 200 patients studied in an updated series. The estimated reocclusion rate of one or more tubes following FTR was 30%. Hovsepian and colleagues[89] performed 42 FTRs in 37 women. Their total number of pregnancies was 14 (33%), nine of them in diseased tubes (i.e. salpingitis isthmica nodosa or peritubal adhesions). Three of the 14 were tubal pregnancies. The authors concluded that FTR results can be favorable, even in

patients with intrinsic tubal disease. In our institution, we have performed FTR on over 100 patients. The current pregnancy rate is 40%.

In their study using a balloon catheter through a coaxial system, Confino and colleagues[90] reported successful cannulation in 71 of 77 patients, and a pregnancy rate approaching 34%, with one ectopic pregnancy and five spontaneous abortions. Gleicher and others[91] achieved an 82% recanalization rate using a system they called the Haus cervical balloon tuboplasty coaxial catheter. Pregnancies occurred in 35% of their population. On long-term follow-up, 70% of patients had either conceived or at least maintained unilateral tubal patency.

In a collective review by Darcy and coworkers[81], the overall pregnancy rate in nine studies ranged from 6 to 54% in series of 2–100 patients (total 361 patients). The rate of ectopic pregnancies ranged from 0 to 27% in a total of 14 patients out of 361. The tubal perforation rate ranged from 0–11%. These and other studies have established transcervical fluoroscopically guided tuboplasty as an essential treatment for selected patients with proximal tubal disease.

The usual etiology of proximal tubal obstruction is thought to be debris forming a 'plug' at the uterotubal junction. Most of the success of FTR is believed to result from dislodging this plug during catheterization and injection of the tube. The procedure is most useful for proximal tubal obstruction. Obstruction in the isthmic or ampullary portions are more difficult to recanalize, owing to the probable presence of adhesions and the frequent tortuosity of the tube. Therefore, patients with distal obstruction are not good candidates for this procedure[92].

FTR has been shown to be effective in the treatment of patients in whom surgical reconstruction of the proximal fallopian tube has failed. In a report by Lang and Dunaway[93], 19 patients who had undergone tubal reconstruction (surgical tuboplasty in 12 and reversal of tubal ligation in seven) were treated with FTR. In patients with tubal fistulae, FTR failed in all cases. In tubal stenosis, FTR was successful in 13 of 15 patients. Three patients conceived spontaneously 1–16 months after FTR, and two achieved success-ful pregnancy by *in vitro* fertilization and embryo transfer. Reocclusion occurred in two out of ten patients re-examined with HSG 6–36 months after FTR.

Concerns over the radiation dose to the patient during FTR have been raised. Hedgepeth and colleagues[94] calculated the absorbed radiation dose to the ovaries in 29 patients undergoing FTR. The average dose was 8.5 ± 5.6 mGy (0.85 ± 0.56 rad). This is comparable to the dose from an excretory urogram (8 mGy), and is much less than a barium enema (35 mGy).

Fallopian tube recanalization technique

At our institution FTR is performed by the technique described by Rosch and co-workers[9], with a few modifications. After the procedure is discussed with the patient and informed consent obtained, an intravenous line is started. During the procedure intravenous analgesics and sedatives are administered, and vital signs are continuously monitored. The patient receives antibiotics, either orally beginning the day before the procedure or intravenously immediately prior to the procedure. Following FTR, the patient will remain on oral antibiotics for 3–5 days.

The procedure itself can be considered in three steps: cannulation of the cervix; engagement of the tubal ostium with a catheter; and advancement of a catheter into the fallopian tube.

A number of instruments and techniques are available for insertion of a cannula into the uterine lumen. We use a Thurmond-Rosch Hysterocath® (Cook, Bloomington, IN), which fixes the cervix with a suction device rather than a tenaculum. The device establishes a conduit to the uterine lumen wide enough to receive a variety of catheter sizes but capable of sealing the cervical os to permit contrast medium injections. Any instrument or set that serves these functions can be used.

Injection of contrast medium after insertion of the uterine cannula demonstrates the anatomy of the uterus and the fallopian tubes. Spot films are obtained during this injection. Manipulation of catheters and guidewires within the cervix is a somewhat painful experience, and the pain is magnified by anxiety. Tubal spasm may occur in this setting. The reassuring presence of a nurse and the relaxation induced by sedation may aid in relieving spasm. If not, compounds such as aminophylline or glucagon may be used. Occasionally, fallopian tubes that were obstructed on prior HSG are patent at the time of this injection. Although it is possible that mechanical obstruction of some sort was relieved in the interim between diagnosis of proximal tubal obstruction and the current injection, it is most likely that tubal spasm caused factitious obstruction during HSG.

Once proximal tubal obstruction is confirmed (Figure 8A), attention is directed to the degree of rotation or angulation of the uterus and the locations of the cornua. In most instances a catheter with a curve of approximately 45° 2 or 3 cm from its tip will readily engage the ostia of the fallopian tubes after insertion through the cervical cannula. However, in uteri with unusual degrees of angulation or rotation the curve on the catheter may need to be modified.

We use a 5.5 French polyethylene catheter (Cook®, Bloomington, IN) for tubal cannulation. Since the tip of the catheter is quite stiff, a 0.035-inch guidewire with a soft 3-mm J curve is advanced through the tip of the catheter. During all manipulations within the uterine lumen the guidewire extends beyond the tip of the catheter and in this way protects the uterine mucosa from injury.

The catheter is manipulated towards the fallopian tube with fluoroscopy used for guidance. As the catheter tip approaches the ostium the guidewire is removed and the catheter is advanced to engage the ostium. Contrast medium injected through the catheter demonstrates its position. If the catheter tip is directed at the ostium, a straight 0.035-inch guidewire is advanced

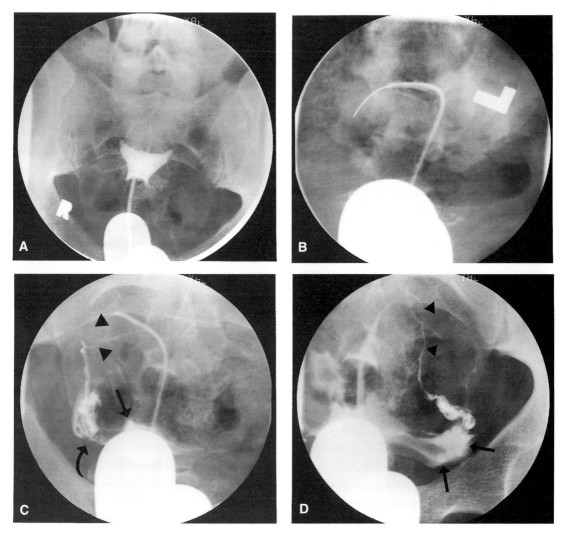

Figure 8 *Fallopian tube recanalization (FTR) in a patient with bilateral proximal obstruction. (A) Hysterosalpingography shows non-filling of both tubes proximally. (B) Through a 5.5 French catheter, a 0.018-inch guidewire is advanced into the right tubal orifice. (C) After FTR, contrast injection shows patent right tube (arrowheads) with spillage of contrast into the peritoneum (arrows). Overlying metallic artifact is due to vaginal speculum. (D) After FTR, contrast injection of the left tube reveals patency (arrowheads) and peritoneal spillage (arrows)*

through it to engage the fallopian tube, and the catheter is pushed to a wedged position. Contrast medium is then injected. In some instances the pressure of injection is sufficient to overcome the obstruction and opacify the fallopian tube. In these instances it seems likely that the obstruction was caused by cellular material within the tubal lumen.

If the tube remains obstructed, a 0.018-inch flexible tip guidewire fitted through a 3 French Teflon catheter (Cook, Bloomington,

IN) is advanced through the lumen of the 5.5 French catheter and carefully manipulated into the fallopian tube (Figure 8B). The guidewire is advanced into and through the obstruction. If this maneuver fails, a 0.018-inch wire with a hydrophilic coating (Glidewire®, Medi-tech, Watertown, MA) should be tried. After the wire has been advanced beyond the site of obstruction, the 3 French catheter is advanced over the wire to dilate the lumen. Confirmation of the anatomical result of the fallopian tube is then documented by selective injection (Figure 8C and D).

Inflatable angioplasty balloons have been used for dilatation of fallopian tube obstruction, as they have for obstructions and strictures of other tubular organs. Balloons exert axial force, which ought to be more effective than the longitudinal force produced by dilating with a catheter. However, dilatation balloons have the disadvantage that they require localization of the stricture and precise balloon placement. The precise location of a fallopian tube obstruction is seldom clear, since intraluminal debris may collect over an indeterminable length of the tube and obscure the actual site of obstruction.

Once the instruments are removed, the patient is observed until the effects of sedation are gone. The patient is given a prescription for oral antibiotics for 2 or 3 days. Vaginal spotting is likely for the next 2 or 3 days after the procedure, but severe bleeding has not occurred in our experience and has not been reported. Patients are instructed to avoid intercourse for 48 h.

Potential complications include infection and perforation of the fallopian tube. We have not seen clinically significant infection in our practice and attribute that to careful sterile technique during the procedure and antibiotic coverage. The wall of the fallopian tube is thin and offers little resistance to perforation. The flexible tip of the 0.018-inch guidewire is softer than the catheter. The catheter should never be advanced without the guidewire ahead of it. Within the fallopian tube the guidewire should always be advanced very gently and slowly, as should the catheter over the guidewire.

Perforation is particularly likely at points of sharp angulation or kinking. When any resistance is felt during advancement of the guidewire it should be removed from the catheter and contrast medium should be injected to demonstrate the course of the fallopian tube. Fluoroscopy with magnification should be used whenever possible, to improve visualization. Angulation or kinking

of the fallopian tube can occasionally be diminished in severity by moving the uterus. This can be accomplished by angling the cannula within the cervical canal contralaterally.

With frequent injections and judicious manipulation, perforation of the fallopian tube is avoidable in most cases. Occasionally, however, the obstruction will be so firm that, during attempts at passage, the tip of the guidewire will advance through the wall of the fallopian tube rather than through the obstruction. This is documented by injection and demonstration of extraluminal contrast medium. As long as the extravasation is small in volume and the perforation is no larger than the caliber of the guidewire, it seems to heal without sequelae. However, the physician must be alert to the possibility of perforation and check with contrast medium injections frequently when the guidewire does not pass freely, in order to ensure that any perforations that occur remain small and contained.

After successful tuboplasty, contrast medium passes freely from the fimbriae into the peritoneal cavity. Some investigators have suggested that injection of oily contrast medium (Ethiodol®, Savage Laboratories, Melville, NY) after HSG may improve fertility[15–19]. This hypothesis has not had rigorous scientific confirmation, but in the presence of patent tubes, it does no harm. We, therefore, inject a few milliliters of Ethiodol into the uterus just before removing the cannula at the end of successful procedures.

Hysteroscopy and laparoscopy

When tubal cannulation is carried out under hysteroscopy with concurrent laparoscopy, successful cannulation is reported in 88% of the patients, with a pregnancy rate of 52% and a 4% ectopic rate[95]. The advantages of the hysteroscopic approach include visualization of the uterine cavity and confirmation of tubal obstruction by chromotubation, along with the diagnosis and treatment of associated distal tubal disease or other pelvic pathology through the laparoscope.

Hysteroscopic gamete intra-fallopian transfer

Traditionally, tubal catheterization under hysteroscopic visualization has been used for contraceptive purposes or for recanalizing obstructed tubes[96]. More recently, successful hysteroscopic transfer of gametes into the fallopian tube has been reported[97–100]. Several techniques have been reported for transvaginal tubal cannulation and transfer of gametes into the fallopian tubes, with varying success rates. Hazout and colleagues[101] compared two techniques of tubal catheterization in a prospective randomized study in which the laparoscopic gamete intra-fallopian transfer (GIFT) procedure resulted in a 47% pregnancy rate as opposed to only 6% with the ultrasonically guided transcervical transfer. Jansen and Anderson[102], using ultrasound-guided transvaginal GIFT, reported a 20% pregnancy rate as compared with a 35% success rate with the laparoscopic GIFT procedure. However, in a prospective randomized comparison Serracchioli and colleagues[100] found that the pregnancy rate and implantation rate of hysteroscopic GIFT procedures (28.8% and 9%, respectively) were not significantly different from those obtained with laparoscopic GIFT (43.3% and 14%). Although these data are suggestive, they lack sufficient statistical power and any changes in practice should wait for larger controlled prospective trials.

FUTURE TRENDS IN FALLOPIAN TUBE IMAGING AND INTERVENTION

Among the near future advances likely to add simplicity to fallopian tube catheterization is the development of ultrasound for guidance. Currently, cannulation of a fallopian tube requires exposure of the patient and physician to ionizing radiation. Although the risk from radiation in this setting is small, ultrasound guidance will make direct tubal access incrementally safer. Although this is feasible with today's equipment[103,104], the current resolution of the ultrasound image of the uterine lumen is significantly inferior to that of fluoroscopy. Widespread use of ultrasound guidance awaits improved anatomical resolution and the development of reflective catheters[105].

The tools for fallopian tube catheterization will continue to be refined and simplified, but the technology is established and widely available. New applications will continue to evolve. The next two applications are likely to be intratubal treatment of ectopic pregnancy and fallopian tube closure for sterilization.

In patients with elevated hCG levels, direct catheter access to the fallopian tubes offers the opportunity for definitive localization of ectopic pregnancy and immediate treatment. Drugs injected into a fallopian tube are more likely to reach the target and less likely to cause side-effects than the same drugs injected systemically or even into the uterus. In a small clinical trial, intratubal injection of methotrexate successfully treated 87% of 31 patients[70]. Although the results are promising, the numbers in this study alone are not conclusive. However, they point the way towards a more definitive trial and suggest the power of the technique. When the optimal agent, its dose and its limits of efficacy are established, the direct access technique, because of its safety and simplicity, will find its way into the diagnostic workup and treatment of this increasingly common problem.

Direct catheter access to the fallopian tubes offers the likelihood of producing tubal sterilization with a less invasive procedure than laparoscopy. Several investigative attempts have been made to close fallopian tubes by introduction of mechanical occlusive devices. Mechanical obstruction requires a material small enough to be inserted via a catheter yet capable of enlarging to plug the lumen of the fallopian tube. It requires a material that gives rise to little or no tissue reaction, but can reliably maintain its position. A removable material is a theoretic goal but one that at present seems unachievable.

Two mechanical obstructive materials currently under investigation include a hydrogel, which is injected in liquid phase but which polymerizes in the fallopian tube to form a solid plug, and a metal mesh spindle, which is injected in a collapsed state but springs open when released from the catheter[106-108]. Other possible approaches include application of chemical cytotoxins or tissue-damaging energy in the form of heat, cold or electricity directly to the tubal lumen. Clinical application of a new sterilization technique, however, will require demonstration of safety and clinical effectiveness comparable to current surgical options.

These exciting therapeutic innovations that employ imaging have moved across the horizon and are slowly cruising towards clinical application. These are procedures over which obstetricians and radiologists will inevitably dispute territory, like many other interventions in many organ systems over the past 20 years, but they will be best resolved by a joint approach. Since interventional radiology began in the 1960s, the specialists who in the past had limited their practice to interpreting images have become more and more involved in direct patient care. This is only fair, since obstetrician/gynecologists have simultaneously become imagers and in many centers and many practices are the principal ultrasonographers.

Although the two medical specialties overlap at their peripheries, each brings a different point of view and a different craft. Whether procedures are performed jointly in a given center or practice or whether their responsibilities for procedures are separate, the patient will be better served if both specialties are involved. No organization of responsibilities can be suggested here, since the training, interest, experience and expertise of the individuals in each institution will govern who does what and in what proportion. Perhaps the larger challenge is to persuade the bureaucracies that pay the bills to recognize that collaboration among specialists achieves optimum patient care, which, in the long term, is the most cost-effective patient care.

References

1. Smith, T. W. (1849). New method of treating sterility by the removal of obstructions of the fallopian tube. *Lancet*, **1**, 603–5
2. Winfield, A. C. and Wentz, A. C. (eds.) (1992). *Diagnostic Imaging in Infertility*, 2nd edn, Hysterosalpingography of the Fallopian tube. pp. 167–91. (Baltimore: Williams and Wilkins)
3. Beyth, Y. and Kopolovic, J. (1982). Accessory tubes: a possible contributing factor in infertility. *Fertil. Steril.*, **38**, 382–3
4. Doyle, M. B. (1992). Magnetic resonance imaging in mullerian fusion defects. *J. Reprod. Med.*, **37**, 33–8
5. Letterie, G. S. and Sakas, E. L. (1991). Histology of proximal tubal obstruction in cases of unsuccessful tubal canalization. *Fertil. Steril.*, **56**, 831–5
6. Sulak, P. J., Letterie, G. S., Coddington, C. C. *et al.* (1987). Histology of proximal tubal occlusion. *Fertil. Steril.*, **48**, 437–40
7. Wadin, K., Lonnemark, M., Rasmussen, C. *et al.* (1994). Frequency of proximal tubal obstruction in patients undergoing infertility evaluation. *Acta Radiol.*, **35**, 357–60
8. Thurmond, A. S. and Rosch, J. (1990). Fallopian tubes: improved technique for catheterization. *Radiology*, **174**, 572
9. Rosch, J., Thurmond, A. S., Uchida, B. T. *et al.* (1988). Selective transcervical fallopian tube catheterization: technique update. *Radiology*, **168**, 1
10. Thurmond, A. S. and Rosch, J. (1990). Non-surgical fallopian tube recanalization for treatment of infertility. *Radiology*, **174**, 371
11. Thurmond, A. S. and Rosch, J. (1990). Device for hysterosalpingography and fallopian tube catheterization. *Radiology*, **174**, 571
12. Thurmond, A. S., Rosch, J., Patton, P. E. *et al.* (1988). Fluoroscopic transcervical fallopian tube catheterization for diagnosis and treatment of female infertility caused by tubal obstruction. *Radiographics*, **8**, 621
13. Lang, E. K., Dunaway, H. E. and Roniger, W. E. (1990). Selective osteal salpingography and transvaginal catheter dilatation in the diagnosis and treatment of fallopian tube obstruction. *Am. J. Roentgenol.*, **154**, 735
14. Thurmond, A. S., Hedgepeth, P. L. and Scanlan, R. M. (1991). Selective injection of

contrast media: inflammatory effects on rabbit fallopian tubes. *Radiology*, **180**, 97

15. Palmer, A. (1960). Ethiodol hysterosalpingography for the treatment of infertility. *Fertil. Steril.*, **11**, 311

16. Gillespie, H. W. (1965). The therapeutic aspect of hysterosalpingography. *Br. J. Radiol.*, **38**, 301

17. Makey, R. A., Glass, R. H., Olson, L. E. *et al.* (1971). Pregnancy following hysterosalpingography with oil and water soluble dye. *Fertil. Steril.*, **22**, 504

18. Horbach, J. G., Maathuis, J. B. and van Hall, E. V. (1973). Factors influencing the pregnancy rate following hysterosalpingography and their prognostic significance. *Fertil. Steril.*, **24**, 15

19. DeCherney, A. H., Kort, H., Barney, J. B. *et al.* (1980). Increased pregnancy rate with oil-soluble hysterosalpingography dye. *Fertil. Steril.*, **33**, 407

20. Balen, F. G., Allen, C. M., Siddle, N. C. *et al.* (1993). Ultrasound contrast hysterosalpingography – evaluation as an outpatient procedure. *Br. J. Radiol.*, **66**, 592

21. Yarali, H., Gurgan, T., Erdan, A. *et al.* (1994). Colour Doppler hysterosalpingography: a simple and potentially useful method to evaluate fallopian tube patency. *Hum. Reprod.*, **9**, 64

22. Gomel, V. (1977). Laparoscopy prior to reconstructive tubal surgery for infertility. *J. Reprod. Med.*, **18**, 251

23. Whitelaw, M. J. (1977). Use of nitroglycerin in hysterosalpingography. *Fertil. Steril.*, **28**, 327

24. Winfield, A. C., Pittaway, D., Maxon, W. *et al.* (1982). Apparent cornual occlusion in hysterosalpingography: reversal with glucagon. *Am. J. Roentgenol.*, **139**, 525

25. Green, D. F., Glickman, M. G. and Weiss, R. M. (1987). Preliminary results with aminophylline as smooth-muscle relaxant in percutaneous renal surgery. *J. Endourol.*, **1**, 243

26. Fortier, K. J. and Haney, A. F. (1985). The pathologic spectrum of uterotubal junction obstruction. *Obstet. Gynecol.*, **65**, 93

27. David, M. P., Ben-Zwi, D. and Langer, L. (1981). Tubal intramural polyps and their relationship to infertility. *Fertil. Steril.*, **35l**, 526

28. Glazener, C. M., Loveden, L. M., Richardson, S. J. *et al.* (1987). Tubo-cornual polyps: their relevance in subfertility. *Hum. Reprod.*, **2**, 59

29. Urman, B., Gomel, V., McComb, P. *et al.* (1992). Midtubal occlusion: etiology, management, and outcome. *Fertil. Steril.*, **57**, 747

30. Rosenfield, D. L., Seidman, S. M., Bronsen, R. A. and Scholl, G. M. (1983). Unsuspected chronic pelvic inflammatory disease in the infertile female. *Fertil. Steril.*, **39**, 44

31. Nakamura, K., Ishimaru, T., Kurata, S. *et al.* (1992). Association between chlamydial infections and pelvic lesions. *Asia-Oceania J. Obstet. Gynecol.*, **18**, 239

32. Markham, S. (1991). Cervico-utero-tubal factors in infertility. *Curr. Opin. Obstet. Gynecol.*, **3**, 191

33. Gomel, V. (1980). Microsurgical reversal of female sterilization: reappraisal. *Fertil. Steril.*, **33**, 587

34. Karasick, S. and Ehrlich, S. (1989). The value of hysterosalpingography before reversal of sterilization procedure involving the fallopian tube. *Am. J. Roentgenol.*, **153**, 1247

35. Karasick, S. (1991). Hysterosalpingography. *Urol. Radiol.*, **13**, 67

36. Chiari, H. (1987). Zur pathologischen Anatomie des Eileitercatarrhs. *Z. Heilkunde*, **8**, 457

37. Creasy, J. L., Clark, R. L., Cuttino, J. T. *et al.* (1985). Salpingitis isthmica nodosa: radiologic and clinical correlates. *Radiology*, **154**, 597

38. Jenkins, C. S., Williams, S. R. and Schmidt, G. E. (1993). Salpingitis isthmica nodosa: a review of the literature, discussion of clinical significance, and consideration of patient management. *Fertil. Steril.*, **60**, 599

39. Saracoglu, F. O., Mungan, T. and Tanzer, F. (1992). Salpingitis isthmica nodosa in infertility and ectopic pregnancy. *Gynecol. Obstet. Invest.*, **34**, 202

40. Thurmond, A. S., Burry, K. A. and Novy, M. J. (1995). Salpingitis isthmica nodosa: results of transcervical fluoroscopic catheter recanalization. *Fertil. Steril.*, **63**, 715

41. Green, L. K. and Kott, M. L. (1989). Histopathologic findings in ectopic tubal pregnancy. *Int. J. Gynecol. Pathol.*, **8**, 255

42. Majmudar, B., Henderson, P. H. and Semple, E. (1983). Salpingitis isthmica nodosa: a high-risk factor for tubal pregnancy. *Obstet. Gynecol.*, **62**, 73

43. Brunham, R. C., Peeling, R., Maclean, I. *et al.* (1992). *Chlamydia trachomatis* – associated ectopic pregnancy: serologic and histologic correlates. *J. Infect. Dis.*, **165**, 1076–81

44. Westrom, L., Bengtsson, L. P. H. and Mardh, P. A. (1981). Incidence, trends and risks of ectopic pregnancy in a population of women. *Br. J. Med.*, **282**, 15–18

45. Chow, W. H., Daling, J. R., Cates, W. *et al.* (1987). Epidemiology of ectopic pregnancy. *Epidemiol. Rev.*, **9**, 70–94

46. Maymon, R., Shulman, A., Maymon, B. B. *et al.* (1992). Ectopic pregnancy, the new gynecological epidemic disease: review of the modern work-up and the nonsurgical treatment option. *Int. J. Fertil.*, **37**, 146

47. Frates, M. C. and Laing, F. C. (1995). Sonographic evaluation of ectopic pregnancy: an update. *Am. J. Roentgenol.*, **165**, 251

48. Churgay, C. A. and Apgar, B. S. (1993). Ectopic pregnancy. An update on technologic advances in diagnosis and treatment. *Prim. Care*, **20**, 629

49. Batzer, F. R., Weiner, S. W., Corson, S. L. *et al.* (1983). Landmarks during the first forty-two days of gestation demonstrated by the β-subunit of human chorionic gonadotropin and ultrasound. *Am. J. Obstet. Gynecol.*, **146**, 973

50. Shapiro, B. S., Cullen, M., Taylor, K. J. W. *et al.* (1988). Transvaginal ultrasonography for the diagnosis of ectopic pregnancy. *Fertil. Steril.*, **50**, 425

51. Chambers, S. E., Muir, B. B. and Haddad, N. G. (1990). Ultrasound evaluation of ectopic pregnancy including correlation with human chorionic gonadotropin levels. *Br. J. Radiol.*, **63**, 246

52. Penzias, A. S. and Huang, P. L. (1992). Imaging in ectopic pregnancy. *J. Reprod. Med.*, **37**, 47

53. Braffman, B. H., Coleman, B. G., Ramchandani, P. *et al.* (1994). Emergency department screening for ectopic pregnancy: a prospective US study. *Radiology*, **190**, 797

54. Barnhart, K., Mennuti, M. T., Benjamin, I. *et al.* (1994). Prompt diagnosis of ectopic pregnancy in an emergency department setting. *Obstet. Gynecol.*, **84**, 1010

55. Cacciatore, B., Stenman, U. H. and Ylostalo, P. (1989). Comparison of abdominal and vaginal sonography in suspected ectopic pregnancy. *Obstet. Gynecol.*, **73**, 770

56. Timor-Tritch, I. E., Yeh, M. N., Peisner, D. B. *et al.* (1989). The use of transvaginal sonography in the diagnosis of ectopic pregnancy. *Am. J. Obstet. Gynecol.*, **161**, 157

57. Thorsen, M. K., Lawson, T. L., Aiman, E. J. *et al.* (1990). Diagnosis of ectopic pregnancy: endovaginal vs. transabdominal sonography. *Am. J. Roentgenol.*, **155**, 307

58. Burry, K. A., Thurmond, A. S., Suby-Long, T. D. *et al.* (1993). Transvaginal ultrasonographic findings in surgically verified ectopic pregnancy. *Am. J. Obstet. Gynecol.*, **168**, 1796

59. Stiller, R. J., Haynes de Regt, R. and Blair, E. (1989). Transvaginal ultrasonography in patients at risk for ectopic pregnancy. *Am. J. Obstet. Gynecol.*, **161**, 930

60. Fleischer, A. C., Pennell, R. G., McKee, M. S. *et al.* (1990). Ectopic pregnancy: features at transvaginal sonography. *Radiology*, **174**, 375

61. Taylor, K. J. and Meyer, W. R. (1991). New techniques in the diagnosis of ectopic pregnancy. *Obstet. Gynecol. Clin. North Am.*, **18**, 39

62. Nyberg, D. A., Hughes, M. P., Mack, L. A. *et al.* (1991). Extrauterine findings of ectopic pregnancy of transvaginal US: importance of echogenic fluid. *Radiology*, **178**, 823

63. Ackerman, T. E., Levi, C. S., Lyons, E. A. *et al.* (1993). Decidual cyst: endovaginal sonographic sign of ectopic pregnancy. *Radiology*, **189**, 727

64. Brown, D. L. and Doubilet, P. M. (1994). Transvaginal sonography for diagnosing ectopic pregnancy: positivity criteria and performance characteristics. *J. Ultrasound Med.*, **13**, 259

65. Taylor, K. J. W., Ramos, I. M., Feylock, A. L. *et al.* (1989). Ectopic pregnancy: duplex Doppler evaluation. *Radiology*, **173**, 93

66. Kurjak, A., Zalud, I. and Schulman, H. (1991). Ectopic pregnancy: transvaginal color Doppler of trophoblastic flow in questionable adnexa. *J. Ultrasound Med.*, **10**, 685

67. Pellerito, J. S., Taylor, K. J. W., Quedens-Case, C. *et al.* (1992). Ectopic pregnancy: evaluation with endovaginal color flow imaging. *Radiology*, **183**, 407

68. Emerson, D. S., Cartier, M. S., Altieri, L. A. *et al.* (1992). Diagnostic efficacy of endovaginal color Doppler flow imaging in an ectopic pregnancy screening program. *Radiology*, **183**, 413

69. Tekay, A. and Jouppila, P. (1992). Color Doppler flow as an indicator of trophoblastic activity in tubal pregnancies detected by transvaginal ultrasound. *Obstet. Gynecol.*, **80**, 995

70. Risquez, F., Foreman, R., Maleika, F. *et al.* (1992). Transcervical cannulation of the fallopian tube for the management of ectopic pregnancy: prospective multicenter study. *Fertil. Steril.*, **58**, 1131

71. Confino, E., Binor, A., Molo, M. W. *et al.* (1994). Selective salpingography for the diagnosis and treatment of early ectopic pregnancy. *Fertil. Steril.*, **62**, 286

72. Brown, D. L., Felker, R. E., Stovall, T. G. *et al.* (1991). Serial endovaginal sonography of ectopic pregnancies treated with methotrexate. *Obstet. Gynecol.*, **77**, 406

73. Ory, S. J. (1992). New options for diagnosis and treatment of ectopic pregnancy. *J. Am. Med. Assoc.*, **267**, 534

74. Carson, S. A. and Buster, J. E. (1993). Ectopic pregnancy. *N. Engl. J. Med.*, **329**, 1174

75. Platia, M. D. and Krudy, A. G. (1985). Transcervical fluoroscopic recanalization of a proximally occluded oviduct. *Fertil. Steril.*, **44**, 704

76. Thurmond, A. S., Novy, M., Uchida, B. T. and Rosch, J. (1987). Fallopian tube obstruction: selective salpingography and recanalization. Work in progress. *Radiology*, **163**, 511

77. Winfield, A. C., Moore, D., Segars, J. *et al.* (1990). Selective fallopian tube canalization (abstr.). *Am. J. Roentgenol.*, **154**, 195

78. Amendola, M. A., Banner, M. P., Pollack, H. M. *et al.* (1990). Preliminary experience with fluoroscopic transcervical fallopian tube recanalization (abstr.). *Am. J. Roentgenol.*, **154**, 196

79. Kumpe, D. A., Zwerdinger, S. C., Rothbarth, L. J. *et al.* (1990). Proximal fallopian tube occlusion: diagnosis and treatment with transcervical fallopian tube catheterization. *Radiology*, **177**, 183

80. Thurmond, A. S. (1991). Selective salpingography and fallopian tube recanalization. *Am. J. Roentgenol.*, **156**, 33

81. Darcy, M. D., McClennan, B. L., Picus, D. *et al.* (1991). Transcervical salpingoplasty: current techniques and results. *Urol. Radiol.*, **13**, 74–9

82. Isaacson, K. B., Amendola, M., Banner, *et al.* (1992). Transcervical fallopian tube recanalization: a safe and effective therapy for patients with proximal tubal obstruction. *Int. J. Fertil.*, **37**, 106–10

83. Risquez, F. and Confino, E. (1993). Transcervical tubal cannulation: past, present and future. *Fertil. Steril.*, **60**, 211

84. Martensson, O., Nilsson, B., Ekelund, L. *et al.* (1993). Selective salpingography and fluoroscopic transcervical salpingoplasty for diagnosis and treatment of proximal fallopian tube occlusions. *Acta Obstet. Gynecol. Scand.*, **72**, 458–64

85. Hercz, P., Vine, S. J. and Walker, S. M. (1994). Experience with transcervical fallopian tube catheterization. *Fertil. Steril.*, **61**, 551–3

86. Fernando, C. C. and Fraser, H. H. (1992). Technical report: fallopian tube recanalization facilitated by a hydrophilic guidewire. *Australas. Radiol.*, **36**, 323

87. Eckstein, N., Orron, D. E., Vagman, I. *et al.* (1993). Combined transvaginal tubal catheterization and adhesiolysis of filmy uterine synechiae performed with a newly developed device under the guidance of digital road mapping fluoroscopy. *Fertil. Steril.*, **59**, 1325–8

88. Millward, S. F., Claman, P., Leader, A. *et al.* (1994). Technical report: Fallopian tube recanalization – a simplified technique. *Clin. Radiol.*, **49**, 496–7

89. Hovsepian, D. M., Bonn, J., Eschelman, D. J. *et al.* (1994). Fallopian tube recanalization in an unrestricted patient population. *Radiology*, **190**, 137

90. Confino, E., Tur-Kaspa, I., DeCherney, A. *et al.* (1990). Transcervical balloon tuboplasty. A multicenter study. *J. Am. Med. Assoc.*, **264**, 2079

91. Gleicher, N., Confino, E., Corfman, R. *et al.* (1993). The multicentre transcervical balloon tuboplasty study: conclusions and comparison to alternative technologies. *Hum. Reprod.*, **8**, 1264

92. Hayashi, N., Kimoto, T., Sakai *et al.* (1994). Fallopian tube disease: limited value of treatment with fallopian tube catheterization. *Radiology*, **190**, 141

93. Lang, E. K. and Dunaway, H. H. (1994). Transcervical recanalization of strictures in the postoperative fallopian tube. *Radiology*, **191**, 507–12

94. Hedgepeth, P. L., Thurmond, A. S., Fry, R. *et al.* (1991). Radiographic fallopian tube recanalization: absorbed ovarian radiation dose. *Radiology*, **180**, 121

95. Das, K., Nagel, T. C. and Malo, J. W. (1995). Hysteroscopic cannulation for proximal tubal obstruction: a change for the better? *Fertil. Steril.*, **63**, 1009

96. Seigler, A. M., Hulka, J. and Pevetz, A. (1985). Reversibility of female sterilization. *Fertil. Steril.*, **43**, 499

97. Wurfel, W., Steck, T., Spingler, H., Krusmann, G., Hirsch, P. *et al.* (1990). Hysteroscopy for gamete intrafallopian transfer (GIFT). *Acta Eur. Fertil.*, **21**, 133–7

98. Posati, G., Seracchioli, R., Melega, C., Pareschi, A., Maccolini, A. and Flamigni, C. (1991). Gamete intrafallopian transfer by hysteroscopy as an alternative treatment for fertility. *Fertil. Steril.*, **56**, 496–9

99. Serracchioli, R., Porcu, E., Maccolini, A., Ciotti, P., Cattoli, M. and Fabri, R. (1993). A new approach to gamete intrafallopian transfer via hysteroscopy. *Hum. Reprod.*, **12**, 2093–5

100. Serracchioli, R., Fabri, R., Porcu, E., Colombi, C., Ciotti, P. and Flamigni, C. (1995). Gamete intrafallopian transfer: prospective randomized comparison between hysteroscopic and laparoscopic transfer techniques. *Fertil. Steril.*, **64**, 355–9

101. Hazout, A., Glissant, A. and Frydman, R. (1989). Transvaginal ultrasound guided GIFT. Proceedings of the *VI World Congress of IVF and Alternate Assisted Reproduction*, p. 30. Jerusalem, Israel

102. Jansen, R. P. S. and Anderson, J. C. (1989). Transvaginal gamete and embryo transfer to the fallopian tubes. In Capitanio, G. L., Asch, R. H. and DeCecco (eds.) *GIFT: from Basics to Clinics*, vol. 63, pp. 383–9. (New York: Raven Press)

103. Stern, J. J., Peters, A. J. and Coulam, C. B. (1991). Transcervical tuboplasty under ultrasonographic guidance: a pilot study. *Fertil. Steril.*, **56**, 359–61

104. Thurmond, A. S., Patton, P. E., Hector, D. M. *et al.* (1991). US-guided fallopian tube catheterization. *Radiology*, **180**, 571

105. Confino, E., Tur-Kaspa, I. and Gleicher, N. (1992). Sonographic transcervical balloon tuboplasty. *Hum. Reprod.*, **7**, 1271–3

106. Schmitz-Rode, T., Ross, P. L., Timmermans, H., Thurmond, A. S., Gunther, R. W. and Rosch, J. (1994). Experimental nonsurgical

female sterilization: transcervical implantation of microspindles in Fallopian tubes. Genitourinary intervention and fertility. *JVIR*, **5**, 905–10

107. Maubon, A. J., Thurmond, A. S., Laurent, A., Honiger, J. E., Scanlan, R. M. and Rouanet, J. P. (1994). Selective tubal sterilization in rabbits: experience with a hydrogel combined with a sclerosing agent. *Radiology*, **193**, 721–3

108. Brundin, J. (1991). Transcervical sterilization in the human female by hysteroscopic application of hydrogelic occlusive devices into the intramural parts of the Fallopian tubes: 10 years experience of the P-block. *Eur. J. Obstet. Gynecol. Reprod. Biol.*, **39**, 41–9

Imaging of the uterus in reproductive failure

6

J. P. Heneghan and R. N. Troiano

MORPHOLOGIC ABNORMALITIES OF THE UTERUS

The true incidence of congenital uterovaginal anomalies remains unknown, as approximately 75% are asymptomatic and hence not usually diagnosed. However, it is estimated that they occur in 2–3% of the population and are associated with infertility in 25% of those affected[1]. Embryologically, these defects are the sequelae of failure of formation of the two Müllerian ducts, resulting in uterine agenesis if complete, and unicornuate if incomplete; failure of fusion of the ducts, resulting in didelphys or a bicornuate uterus; or failure of resorption of the medial walls following fusion, resulting in a complete or partial septum.

The original Buttram and Gibbons classification[2] and the subsequent American Fertility Society (AFS) classification system for Müllerian duct anomalies attempt to group the structural changes into distinct classes based on the stage of failure of normal embryogenesis, as well as similar clinical findings and treatment (Figure 1). Unfortunately, it is difficult to ascribe many congenital anomalies to a single class, as failure of development can occur at any point along a continuum, resulting in overlapping configurations. One case in point is the mixed bicornuate–septal configuration. Attempts to differentiate septate from bicornuate uteri have been based on the external uterine contour, as well as on the histological component of the internal division. Convexity of the fundus with a fibrous internal division has been ascribed to septate uteri, whereas concavity of the fundal contour with myometrium in the internal division has been attributed to the bicornuate uterus. Recent advances in magnetic resonance imaging (MRI) have shown this classification to be somewhat

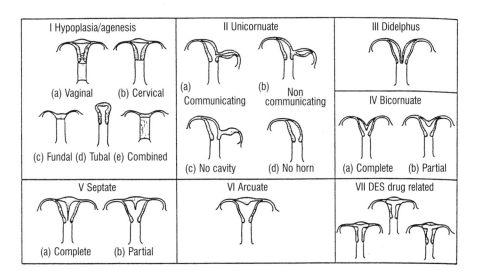

Figure 1 *Classification system of Müllerian anomalies developed by the American Fertility Society. DES, diethylstilbestrol*

arbitrary. There is often significant overlap in both fundal contour and histology of the internal division, precluding simple designation as septate or bicornuate.

Investigation for uterine anomaly should be initiated in patients presenting with two consecutive first-trimester losses, and in those presenting with premature labor or an apparent normal pregnancy loss in the second trimester.

The correct diagnosis of Müllerian duct anomalies is important, as the surgical approaches to treatment vary. The goal of imaging is to provide a detailed description of the anomaly that can be correlated with the clinical manifestation of infertility. When these are considered together, the need and type of necessary surgical intervention can be determined.

Hysterosalpingography (HSG) has traditionally been used as the primary imaging modality for evaluating congenital uterine anomalies. Performed in the mid-follicular phase, HSG relies on the angle of divergence of the uterine horns in differentiating septate from bicornuate uteri[3]. HSG is most useful if the angle of divergence is less than 75°, indicative of a septate uterus (Figure 2). However, angles greater than 75° could not definitively differentiate the two anomalies. A diagnostic accuracy of only 55% was reported on HSG alone, with the most common error being misdiagnosis of a septate as a bicornuate uterus[3] (Figure 3). HSG is additionally limited by its inability to define the external uterine contour. Supplementing HSG by ultrasound reportedly increased the accuracy to 90% in differentiating septate from bicornuate configurations[3]. Further limitations of HSG are found in evaluating and differentiating more complex anomalies: a unicornuate uterus may have a similar radiographic appearance to a bicornuate or didelphic uterus with an associated obstructed vaginal septum.

HSG can accurately assess the hypoplastic changes of the uterus in patients with a history of diethylstilbestrol (DES) exposure. DES exposure carries a risk of up to 50% for

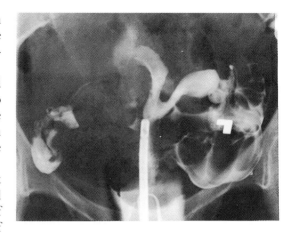

Figure 2 *Septate uterus. Hysterosalpingogram demonstrates an angle of divergence of less than 75°*

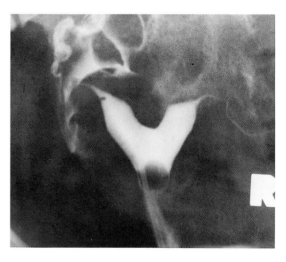

Figure 3 *Bicornuate uterus. Hysterosalpingogram is indeterminate in differentiating bicornuate from septate in this example*

structural abnormalities of the cervix, and up to 66% for abnormalities of the endometrial cavity[4,5]. The endometrial cavity is classically 'T-shaped' with associated constriction bands.

Identification of uterine anomalies with ultrasound is optimally performed during the midluteal phase of the menstrual cycle, when the endometrium is thickest. Sonography can not only demonstrate separate echogenic endometrial cavities, but also delineate external uterine contour (Figure 4). These features are best appreciated with an endovaginal technique, allowing increased resolution, as compared to the transabdominal approach. Endovaginal ultrasound alone has been shown to have an accuracy of 92% in correctly diagnosing duplication anomalies[6]. Limitations to sonographic diagnosis include associated distorting leiomyomas and/or adnexal masses which can obscure fine detail and lead to misinterpretations.

Sonographic evaluation of the DES-exposed uterus is somewhat difficult. Findings on ultrasound have demonstrated a small uterus with loss of the normal fundal bulbous expansion[7].

Sonohysterography performed while infusing sterile saline as a contrast medium during sonographic examination has also been advocated for detecting duplication anomalies. Infusion of saline distends the endometrial cavity, producing more dramatic interfaces and resolution. Although this technique is less commonly employed, sensitivities and specificities between 98% and 100% have been reported[8].

MRI has proven to be the modality of choice in the evaluation of uterine anomalies, with a reported accuracy of 100%[6–11]. Its multiplanar imaging ability and unsurpassed soft tissue resolution provides exquisite anatomical detail without being invasive or requiring exposure to ionizing radiation. In one study, MRI was not only 100% diagnostically accurate, but additionally detected coincidental gynecological disease in one-third of the patients imaged, and altered patient management in 24%[9]. T_2-weighted images are extremely accurate in defining uterine architecture. Zonal anatomy of the uterine corpus on these sequences is depicted as a central stripe of high signal intensity corresponding to the endometrium. This is surrounded by a layer of intermediate signal corresponding to the junctional zone, and a more superficial layer representing the outer myometrium. The uterine cervix also demonstrates a central high-signal stripe corresponding to the endocervical canal,

which is surrounded by a low-signal fibrous stroma.

Uterine agenesis can be documented by inability to visualize the organ discretely, or by visualization of a small ill-defined remnant. Hypoplasia is manifested as a uterus small for the patient's age, with poor zonal differention and decrease in the width of the endometrium and myometrium[9] (Figure 5).

Unicornuate uteri have a 'banana-shaped' contour with a normal width of the endometrium and myometrium (Figure 6).

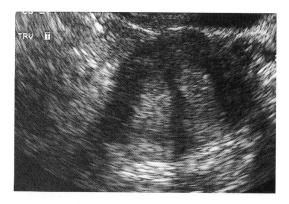

Figure 4 *Septate uterus. Sonogram demonstrates separate endometrial cavities with an intervening septum and a convex uterine contour*

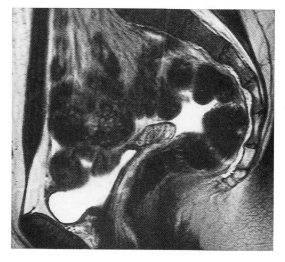

Figure 5 *Uterine hypoplasia. Sagittal magnetic resonance fast spin echo T_2-weighted image demonstrates a hypoplastic uterus*

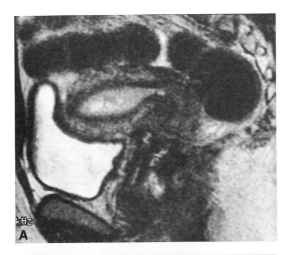

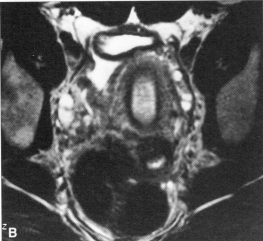

Figure 6 *Unicornuate uterus. Sagittal (A) and axial (B) fast spin echo T$_2$-weighted magnetic resonance images demonstrate loss of normal bulbous expansion of the fundus*

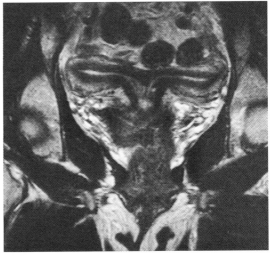

Figure 7 *Bicornuate uterus. Coronal fast spin echo T$_2$-weighted magnetic resonance image demonstrates wide divergence of the uterine horns*

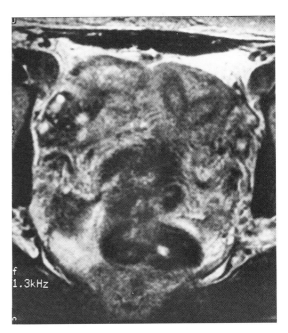

Figure 8 *Septate uterus. Axial fast spin echo T$_2$-weighted magnetic resonance image demonstrates the upper myometrial portion of the septum, the lower fibrous portion and the convex fundal contour*

Rudimentary horns can be identified as small low-signal masses extending from the level of the cervix[9].

Didelphic uteri demonstrate a duplicated uterine corpus, cervix and upper vagina. Bicornuate uteri exhibit two distinct uterine horns with a widened intercornual distance (Figure 7). Septate uteri have a normal inter-cornual distance with the endometrial cavity reduced in volume[9] (Figure 8). T$_1$-weighted images obtained parallel to the long axis of the uterus are of value in delineating the external uterine contour. MRI additionally provides information regarding the composi-tion of the internal division, differentiating myometrium from fibrous tissue. Myometrium is of intermediate signal intensity on T$_2$-weighted images, whereas fibrous tissue is of uniform very low signal intensity. This provides useful information, especially in mixed septate–bicornuate anomalies. More complex anomalies, such as duplications with obstructed vaginal septums, are also well defined by MRI (Figure 9).

In DES-exposed patients, MRI demonstrates hypoplasia of the endometrial cavity, uterine corpus and cervix. The classic 'T-shaped' endometrial cavity and constriction bands, as well as thickening of the junctional zone, are visualized[12]. Intrauterine synechiae result in a variable degree of obliteration of the endometrial cavity and endocervical canal. Although the majority of cases of intrauterine synechiae appear to result from curettage after either birth or abortion, infection, such as tuberculosis, may also result in adhesions[14]. The condition may result in infertility, fetal loss or menstrual abnormalities, including amenorrhea. The AFS classifies intrauterine adhesions according to the extent of the cavity involved (less than one-third, one-third to two-thirds or more than two-thirds), the type of adhesions and the menstrual pattern. Treatment is by hysteroscopic division of adhesions performed in the early proliferative phase of the cycle. Restoration of menses occurs in the majority of cases.

HSG has been the standard method of investigation[14]. Synechiae appear as irregular, angular, well-defined filling defects within the endometrial cavity, with a variable degree of cavity obliteration (Figure 10). Unfortunately, HSG is limited when cannulation of the endocervical canal cannot be performed. Differential considerations include complete endometrial obliteration, an obstructive synechia at the lower uterine body, or cervical stenosis. Synechiae have been sonographically described as echogenic, serpiginous endometrial bridges which are asymmetrically located in the endometrial cavity[15]. Endovaginal sonography is more useful than transabdominal ultrasound because of its increased spatial resolution.

MRI can also demonstrate synechiae, with the extent of disease accurately defined. MRI not only can differentiate complete endo-

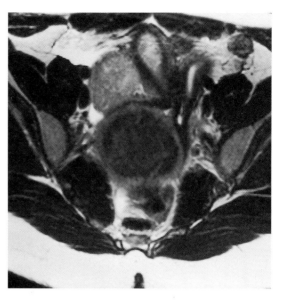

Figure 9 *Didelphic uterus with obstructed vaginal septum. Axial fast spin echo T$_2$-weighted magnetic resonance image. Incidental note is made of a right-sided dysgerminoma lying anterior to the obstructed vagina*

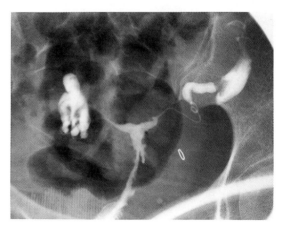

Figure 10 *Intrauterine synechiae. Hysterosalpingogram demonstrates multiple irregular filling defects within the endometrial cavity*

metrial obliteration from obstructive lower uterine body adhesions, but can also delineate the extent of the remaining endometrial tissue (Figure 11). Reports have been published in which the MRI findings were more accurate and clinically relevant than the findings at HSG[16].

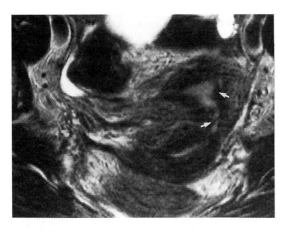

Figure 11 *Intrauterine synechiae. Oblique fast spin echo T₂-weighted magnetic resonance image demonstrates low signal fibrous bands with adhesions (arrows)*

Cervical incompetence is painless dilatation of the cervix, associated with recurrent second-trimester pregnancy loss. It is a diagnosis of exclusion, as it is not associated with congenital uterine anomalies or with immunological, endocrine, infective or other abnormalities. A prior history of cervical trauma is noted in a majority of cases. The diagnosis is usually made following careful history taking and physical examination; however, an unsuspected cervical dilatation may be noted during a routine second-trimester ultrasound examination and should always be considered when a relevant history is obtained. On ultrasound scanning, cervical incompetence is manifested as shortening of the cervix to < 3.0 cm in length with dilatation of the internal os and ballooning of membranes[17–19].

On MRI, this is demonstrated as shortening of the cervical canal (< 3 cm), widening of the internal os (> 3.5 cm) and absence of the normal low signal intensity cervical stroma. These features may occur in isolation or in combination[20].

Uterine leiomyomas are tumors of smooth muscle origin and occur in up to 40% of women of reproductive age. As they are an infrequent cause of infertility, a search for an alternative etiology should be undertaken before leiomyomas are designated as the cause for infertility. Leiomyomas are thought to be associated with infertility secondary to mass effect and alteration of uterine vascularity. Mechanical compression by submucosal or intramural myomas may obstruct the cornua, preventing migration of the embryo. Diminished vascularity with attenuation of the overlying endometrium may interfere with implantation or normal growth. Secondary uterine irritability may result in spontaneous abortion or premature labor.

Imaging is an important tool for defining the number and location of myomas, especially in surgical planning for myomectomy, as the type of surgical intervention will vary with location of the myoma within the myometrium. Small submucosal leiomyomas can be removed via hysteroscopy, whereas larger intramural myomas necessitate transabdominal surgery.

Ultrasound is the modality of choice in screening and for initial evaluation of leiomyomas. Transvaginal scanning is optimal; however, transabdominal imaging may be necessary to increase the field of view in patients with markedly enlarged uteri. Leiomyomatous uteri exhibit lobulation of the serosal contour if the leiomyomas are subserosal or are large in an intramural location. These cause changes in the echogenicity of the myometrium. Leiomyomas are usually hypoechoic and well defined. However, small tumors may be isoechoic with myometrium and therefore not apparent as discrete lesions. Ultrasound can differentiate between submucosal, intramural and subserosal leiomyomas in many cases (Figure 12), but this differentiation is not always reliable, but is improved with the addition of saline infusion sonohysterography. Identification of a uterine flow pattern using color flow and Doppler interrogation aids in differentiating a pedunculated myoma from an adnexal mass when a discrete pedicle is not appreciated. Sonography may be hindered in cases of retroverted or displaced uteri, because of limitations in the resolution and field of view[21–24].

MRI is a highly accurate method for evaluating leiomyomas. This is particularly

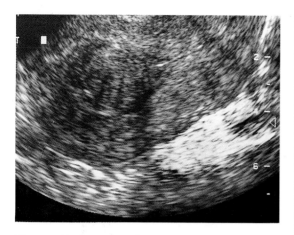

Figure 12 *Sagittal endovaginal sonogram demonstrating a well-defined submucosal leiomyoma*

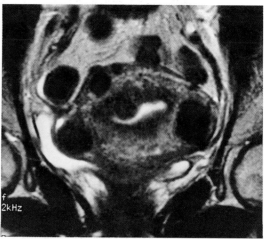

Figure 13 *Coronal fast spin echo T_2-weighted magnetic resonance image demonstrates multiple leiomyomas in submucosal, intramural and subserosal locations*

relevant for preoperative assessment as the exact number, size, location and morphologic changes can be ascertained (Figure 13). Studies have demonstrated that MRI is more accurate than ultrasound in the localization of leiomyomas[25–28]. Leiomyomas are well defined and are of medium signal intensity on T_1-weighted images, similar to the signal of myometrium. On T_2-weighted images, they are generally of low signal intensity, although 'cellular' leiomyomas may often appear as intermediate to high in signal intensity. Degenerating leiomyomas demonstrate a range of signal intensities varying from high to low, depending on the degree of hemorrhage, infarction, fatty degeneration or myomatous degeneration[29]. MRI is also useful in monitoring the response to therapy in patients undergoing conservative medical management with gonadotropin releasing hormone (GnRH) analogs. Precise volumes of individual myomas as well as overall uterine volumes may be sequentially measured.

Adenomyosis is characterized by the presence of endometrial glands and stroma within the myometrium, and has a reported incidence in hysterectomy specimens of 15–30%. The incidence is higher in multiparous women. Symptoms include menorrhagia and dysmenorrhea. The uterus is often tense, globular and enlarged on examination. Although this usually involves a diffuse process, it may be focal, forming an adenomyoma that includes smooth muscle[30].

On ultrasound examination, the uterus is typically enlarged with a thickened myometrium, which has poorly defined hypoechoic and heterogeneous areas. Small myometrial cysts ranging from 2 mm to 7 mm are noted in approximately half of the patients. The absence or thickening of the endometrial halo does not correlate with the presence of disease. Adenomyomas may present as more well-defined hypoechoic masses[31–35]. Ultrasound has been shown to be comparable to MRI in accuracy of diagnosis of adenomyosis; however, it is operator dependent and requires meticulous imaging technique[33].

MRI is a highly accurate modality for diagnosing adenomyosis[36]. Uterine enlargement with focal or diffuse thickening of the junctional zone of > 12 mm is best appreciated on T_2-weighted images. High signal foci may be identified within the myometrium and correspond to glandular and/or hemorrhagic changes (Figure 14). Adenomyomas are demonstrated as oval masses of low signal intensity with poorly defined borders[33] (Figure 15).

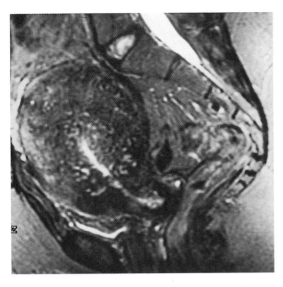

Figure 14 *Adenomyosis. Sagittal fast spin echo T_2-weighted magnetic resonance image demonstrates a globular uterus, diffuse thickening of the junctional zone and punctate foci of high signal intensity*

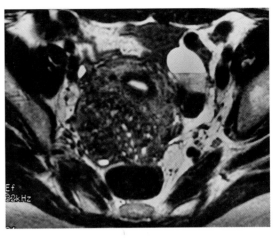

Figure 15 *Axial fast spin echo T_2-weighted magnetic resonance image demonstrates a well-demarcated adenomyoma extending from the posterior uterine body*

Differentiation from leiomyomas has important clinical repercussions, as therapeutic approaches are often different between the two. MRI is highly accurate in making this distinction, as leiomyomas appear as spherical low signal masses that are well defined and smooth in contour[37,38].

LUTEAL PHASE EVALUATION

The functional layer of the endometrium is influenced by the levels of circulating estrogen and progesterone throughout the menstrual cycle, and the glandular, mucous and water composition of the layer varies with the phase of the cycle. The sonographic appearances of the endometrium during the menstrual cycle have been well documented. During menses, the endometrial layer is thin and echogenic. During the proliferative phase, the endometrium becomes thicker and is made up of alternating hypoechoic and hyperechoic layers. At ovulation, the hypoechoic component is most obvious. During the secretory phase, the endometrium becomes increasingly echogenic, with the previously noted alternating layers becoming

obliterated into a single layer, measuring up to 14 mm. Mucous and water content during the late luteal phase is high, and acoustic enhancement is noted[39].

Luteal phase defect results in insufficient progesterone production secondary to abnormal function of the corpus luteum. It is associated with infertility, recurrent abortion and an increased incidence in ectopic pregnancy[40]. Characterization of the endometrium is best achieved by transvaginal ultrasonography, which guides therapeutic options. If the endometrium is abnormally thin, then hormonal analysis and luteal phase endometrial biopsy are generally recommended. Work has been carried out to investigate the uterine and ovarian artery flow characteristics of women with luteal phase defects in comparison with controls[41,42]. Women with luteal phase defects demonstrated high resistance indices in the ovarian arteries during the follicular phase. One study demonstrated poor endometrial flow in 48% of infertile patients[43]. Following hormonal therapy, uterine perfusion improved, and there was a concomitant rise in the pregnancy rate.

ABNORMALITIES OF EARLY GESTATION

Ultrasound remains the method of choice for the imaging of pregnancy. In the first trimester, an endovaginal approach should be employed.

Ninety-five per cent of ectopic pregnancies are tubal in location, but the remainder occur in a variety of locations including the ovary, cervix and peritoneal cavity. An additional 2–3% of ectopic pregnancies occur in the uterine cornua and are designated as interstitial ectopic pregnancies. These pregnancies are associated with a mortality rate that is more than twice that of tubal pregnancy secondary to life-threatening hemorrhage from late rupture. Diagnosing interstitial ectopic pregnancies can be very difficult. The gestational sac is generally eccentrically located, and is associated with an incomplete myometrial mantle[44,45] (Figure 16). However, other studies demonstrated that these findings could not be reliably and consistently identified. An 'interstitial line' sign has been described, referring to a thin echogenic line that extends to the gestational sac or cornual mass, and is felt to represent the endometrial cavity or the interstitial portion of the fallopian tube itself[46].

Ectopic pregnancies are rarely located within the cervix, and the reported rate is between 1 : 9500 and 1 : 16 000. Prior curettage is a recognized risk factor. Sonographic findings are of a gestational sac located in the cervix, without the clinical findings that accompany a spontaneous abortion. As surgical intervention is often accompanied by massive hemorrhage, conservative treatment with methotrexate has been alternatively advocated[47–49].

In the first trimester, endovaginal ultrasound examination is usually performed to assess accurate gestational dating, fetal viability and normal progression of pregnancy. Non-visualization of a discrete gestational sac raises several differential diagnostic considerations. The intrauterine pregnancy may be of less than 4 weeks, and thus not yet visible, or other considerations might include spontaneous abortion or

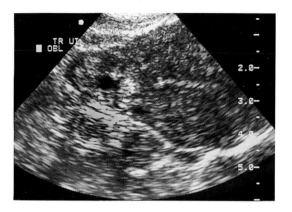

Figure 16 *Interstitial (cornual) ectopic pregnancy. Transverse endovaginal sonogram demonstrates an eccentrically located gestational sac within the right cornua. Note the thin endometrial stripe*

ectopic pregnancy. Clinical and laboratory correlation with serum β-human chorionic gonadotropin (β-hCG) levels as well as ultrasound follow-up will clarify the findings.

Visualization of an early gestational sac yields important information with regard to fetal viability. A gestational sac that is either enlarged or abnormally small may be associated with early fetal loss (Figure 17). A mean sac diameter of > 8 mm on endovaginal ultrasound is abnormal if an associated yolk sac is not visualized[50]. If the mean sac diameter is 18 mm and is without a fetal pole or cardiac activity, the findings are consistent with fetal demise[51].

Correlation of the mean sac diameter with reference to the crown–rump length has also been investigated. A gestational sac is abnormal if the mean sac diameter is < 5 mm larger than the crown–rump length (Figure 18). This was associated with a 94% spontaneous abortion rate, despite documentation of fetal cardiac activity at the time of the scan[52]. Alternatively, when the amniotic cavity is large relative to the crown–rump length and chorionic cavity, the findings also speak for a poor outcome. At 5–6 weeks' gestation, the normal difference in the crown–rump length from the diameter of the amniotic cavity was 0.11 cm (± 0.20 cm), whereas with abnormal embryos a difference

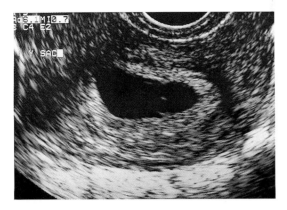

Figure 17 *Large gestational sac, with evidence of a yolk sac, but not of a fetal pole*

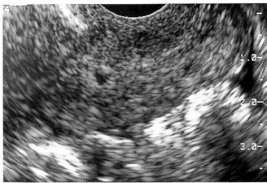

Figure 19 *Abnormal location of gestational sac. A small irregular gestational sac is located in the lower uterine segment, just above the internal os*

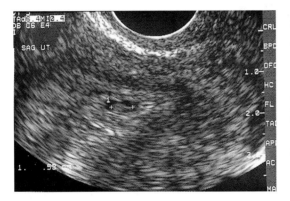

Figure 18 *Discordance of crown–rump length (5.3 mm) and mean sac diameter. The gestational sac is abnormally small*

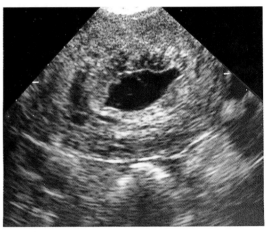

Figure 20 *Abnormal, irregular contour of gestational sac. Fetal parts are not identified*

of 0.86 cm ($\pm$ 0.38 cm) was noted[53]. A guarded prognosis must also be considered when cardiac activity cannot be documented in embryos with a crown–rump length of < 4 mm[54].

Location and shape of the gestational sac within the uterus also have important prognostic implications. A low-lying sac is often associated with impending spontaneous abortion[55] (Figure 19), and an irregularly shaped sac is associated with a poor outcome (Figure 20). However, in pregnancies resulting from *in vitro* fertilization, there appears to be a high incidence of apparent morphological abnormalities of the gesta-

tional sac without necessarily a poor fetal outcome. Abnormality of the gestational sac is found in up to 40% of *in vitro* fertilization patients in comparison to 7% of controls. In *in vitro* fertilization, abnormalities of the sac contents, such as the yolk sac, were much more relevant than sac morphology in predicting prognosis. Only 29% of these patients with abnormal sac contents gave birth to a live infant, whereas 90% of those with an abnormal appearance of the sac itself delivered a live infant[56].

Also of clinical importance is the morphological appearance of the yolk sac. A yolk sac diameter of 0.56 mm at less than 10 weeks' gestation is not associated with a normal outcome[57]. Embryonic demise is also associated with a calcified yolk sac[58] (Figure 21).

Evaluation of embryonic cardiac activity also carries prognostic implications. Absence of cardiac motion in an embryo larger than 5 mm is associated with demise. Bradycardia in the first trimester also implies poor outcome. In embryos with heart rates less than 70 beats/min at 8 weeks' gestation, eventual demise was noted in all cases[59].

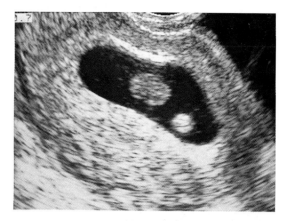

Figure 21 *Calcified yolk sac noted, associated with an abnormal fetal pole*

References

1. Golan, A., Langer, R., Bukovsky, L. *et al.* (1979). Congenital anomalies of the Mullerian system. *Fertil. Steril.*, **32**, 40–6

2. Buttram, V. C. and Gibbons, W. E. (1979). Mullerian anomalies: a proposed classification (an analysis of 144 cases). *Fertil. Steril.*, **32**, 40–6

3. Reuter, K. L., Daly, D. C. and Cohen, S. M. (1989). Septate versus bicornuate uteri: errors in imaging diagnosis. *Radiology*, **172**, 749–52

4. Kaufman, R. H., Adam, E., Noller, K. *et al.* (1986). Upper genital tract changes and infertility in diethylstilbestrol exposed women. *Am. J. Obstet. Gynecol.*, **154**, 1312

5. Kaufman, R. H., Noller, K., Adam, E. *et al.* (1984). Upper genital tract abnormalities and pregnancy outcome in diethylstilbestrol-exposed progency. *Am. J. Obstet. Gynecol.*, **148**, 973

6. Pellerito, J. S., McCarthy, S. M., Doyle, M. B. *et al.* (1992). Diagnosis of uterine anomalies: relative accuracy of MR imaging, endovaginal sonography, and hysterosalpingography. *Radiology*, **183**, 795–800

7. Viscomi, G. N., Gonzales, R. and Taylor, K. J. W. (1987). Ultrasound detection of uterine anomalies after diethylstilbestrol (DES) exposure. *Radiology*, **136**, 733–5

8. Randolph, J. R., Ying, Y. K., Maier, D. B. *et al.* (1986). Comparison of real-time ultrasonography, hysterosalpingography, and laparotomy/ hysteroscopy in the evaluation of uterine abnormalities and tubal patency. *Fertil. Steril.*, **46**, 828–32

9. Carrington, B. M., Hricak, H., Nuruddin, R. N. *et al.* (1990). Mullerian duct anomalies: MR imaging evaluation. *Radiology*, **176**, 715–20

10. Mintz, M. C., Thickman, D. I., Gussman, D. *et al.* (1987). MR evaluation of uterine anomalies. *Am. J. Roentgenol.*, **148**, 287–90

11. Fedele, L., Dorta, M., Brioschi, D. *et al.* (1989). Magnetic resonance evaluation of double uteri. *Obstet. Gynecol.*, **74**, 844–7

12. Van Gils, A. P., Tham, R. T., Falke, T. H. *et al.* (1989). Abnormalities of the uterus and cervix after diethylstilbestrol exposure: correlation of findings on MR and hysterosalpingography. *Am. J. Roentgenol.*, **153**, 1235–8

13. Krysiewicz, S. (1992). Infertility in women: diagnostic evaluation with hysterosalpingography and other imaging techniques. *Am. J. Roentgenol.*, **159**, 253–61

14. Taylor, P. J., Cumming, D. C. and Hill, P. J. (1981). Significance of intrauterine adhesions detected hysteroscopically in eumenorrheic infertile women and role of antecedent curettage in their formation. *Am. J. Obstet. Gynecol.*, 139–239

15. Confino, E., Friberg, J., Griglia, R. V. *et al.* (1985). Sonographic imaging of intrauterine adhesions. *Obstet. Gynecol.*, **66**, 596–8

16. Letterie, G. S. and Haggerty, M. F. (1994). Magnetic resonance imaging of intrauterine synechiae. *Gynecol. Obstet. Invest.*, **37**, 66–8

17. Andersen, H. F. (1991). Transvaginal and transabdominal ultrasonography of the uterine cervix during pregnancy. *J. Clin. Ultrasound*, **19**, 77–83

18. Podobnik, M., Bulic, M., Smiljanis, N. *et al.* (1988). Ultrasonography in the detection of cervical incompetence. *J. Clin. Ultrasound*, **13**, 383–91

19. Michaels, W. H., Montgomery, C., Karo, J. *et al.* (1986). Ultrasound differentiation of the competent from the incompetent cervix: prevention of preterm delivery. *Am. J. Obstet. Gynecol.*, **154**, 537–46

20. Hricak, H., Chang, Y. C. F., Cann, C. E. *et al.* (1990). Cervical incompetence: preliminary evaluation with MR imaging. *Radiology*, **174**, 821–6

21. O'Brien, W. F., Buck, D. R. and Nash, J. D. (1984). Evaluation of sonography in the initial assessment of the gynecologic patient. *Gynecology*, **149**, 598–602

22. Fleischer, A. C., Gordon, A. N. and Entman, S. S. (1989). Transabdominal and transvaginal sonography of pelvic masses. *Ultrasound Med. Biol.*, **15**, 529

23. Gross, B. H., Silver, T. M. and Jaffe, M. H. (1983). Sonographic features in uterine leiomyomas. *JIUM*, **2**, 401–6

24. Baltarowich, O. H., Kurtz, A. B., Pennel, R. *et al.* (1988). Pitfalls in the sonographic diagnosis of uterine fibroids. *Am. J. Roentgenol.*, **154**, 725–8

25. Dudiak, C. M., Turner, D. A. A., Patel, S. K. *et al.* (1988). Uterine leiomyomas in the infertile patient: preoperative localization with MR imaging versus US and hysterosalpingography. *Radiology*, **167**, 627–30

26. Hamlin, D. J., Petersson, H., Fitzsimmons, J. *et al.* (1985). MR imaging of uterine leiomyomas and their complications. *J. Comput. Assis. Tomogra.*, **9**, 902–7

27. Hricak, H., Tscholakoff, D., Heinrichs, L. *et al.* (1986). Uterine leiomyoma correlation by magnetic resonance imaging: clinical symptoms and histopathology. *Radiology*, **158**, 385–91

28. Zawin, M., McCarthy, S., Scoutt, I. *et al.* (1990). High field in MRI and US evaluation of the pelvis in women with leiomyomas. *Magn. Res. Imaging*, **8**, 371–6

29. Hricak, H., Finck, S., Honda, G. *et al.* (1992). MR imaging in the evaluation of benign uterine masses: value of gadolinium dimeglumine-enhanced T_1-weighted images. *Am. J. Roentgenol.*, **158**, 1043–250

30. Tiltman, A. J. (1980). Adenomatoid tumours of the uterus. *Histopathology*, **4**, 437

31. Reinhold, C., Atri, M., Mehio, A. *et al.* (1995). Diffuse uterine adenomyosis: morhologic criteria and diagnostic accuracy of endovaginal sonography. *Radiology*, **197**, 609–14

32. Mitchell, D. G., Scholholz, L., Hilpert, P. L. *et al.* (1990). Zones of the uterus: discrepancy between US and MR images. *Radiology*, **174**, 827–31

33. Reinhold, C., McCarthy, S., Bret, P. *et al.* (1996). Diffuse adenomyosis: comparison of endovaginal US and MR imaging with histopathological correlation. *Radiology*, **199**, 151–8

34. Federle, L., Bianchi, S., Dorta, M. *et al.* (1992). Transvaginal ultrasonography in the differential diagnosis of adenomyoma versus leiomyoma. *Am. J. Obstet. Gynecol.*, **167**, 603–6

35. Walsh, J. W., Taylor, K. J. W. and Rosenfield, A. T. (1979). Gray scale ultrasonography in the diagnosis of endometriosis and adenomyosis. *Am. J. Roentgenol.*, **132**, 87–90

36. Togashi, K., Nishimura, K., Itoh, K. *et al.* (1988). Adenomyosis: diagnosis with MR imaging. *Radiology*, **166**, 111–14

37. Mark, A. S., Hricak, H., Heinrichs, L. W. *et al.* (1987). Adenomyosis and leiomyoma: differential diagnosis with MR imaging. *Radiology*, **163**, 527–9

38. Ascher, S. M., Arnold, L. L., Patt, R. H. *et al.* (1994). Adenomyosis: prospective comparison with MR imaging and transvaginal sonography. *Radiology*, **190**, 803–6

39. Bakos, O., Lundkvist, O. and Bergh, T. (1993). Transvaginal sonographic evaluation of endometrial growth and texture in spontaneous ovulatory cycles – a descriptive study. *Hum. Reprod.*, **8**, 799–806

40. Guillame, A. J., Benjamin, F., Sicuranza, B. *et al.* (1995). Luteal phase defects and ectopic pregnancy. *Fertil. Steril.*, **63**, 30–3

41. Tinkanen, H., Kujansuu, E. and Laippala, P. (1994). Vascular resistence in uterine and ovarian arteries: its association with infertility and the prognosis of infertility. *Eur. J. Obstet. Gynecol. Reprod. Med.*, **57**, 111–15

42. Glock, J. L. and Brumsted, J. R. (1995). Color flow pulsed Doppler ultrasound in diagnosing luteal phase defects. *Fertil. Steril.*, **64**, 500–4

43. Goswamy, R. K. and Steptoe, P. C. (1988). Doppler ultrasound studies of the uterine artery in spontaneous ovarian cycles. *Hum. Reprod.*, **3**, 721–6

44. Fleischer, A. C., Pennell, R. G., McKee, M. S. *et al.* (1990). Ectopic pregnancy: features at transvaginal sonography. *Radiology*, **174**, 375–8

45. Graham, M. and Cooperberg, P. L. (1979). Ultrasound diagnosis of interstitial pregnancy: findings and pitfalls. *J. Clin. Ultrasound*, **7**, 433–7

46. Ackerman, T. E., Levi, C. S., Dashefsky, S. M. *et al.* (1993). Interstitial line: sonographic finding in interstitial (cornual) ectopic pregnancy. *Radiology*, **189**, 83–7

47. Hoffmann, H. N., Urdl, W., Hoffler, H. *et al.* (1987). Cervical pregnancy: case reports and current concepts in diagnosis and treatment. *Arch. Gynecol. Obstet.*, **241**, 63–9

48. Yankowitz, J., Leake, J., Huggins, G. *et al.* (1990). Cervical ectopic pregnancy: review of the literature and report and a case treated by single-dose methotraxate therapy. *Obstet. Gynecol. Surv.*, **45**, 405–14

49. Palti, Z., Rosenn, B., Goshen, R. *et al.* (1989). Successful treatment of a viable cervical pregnancy with methotrexate. *Am. J. Obstet. Gynecol.*, **161**, 1147–8

50. Levi, C. S., Lyons, E. A. and Lindsay, D. J. (1988). Early diagnosis of nonviable pregnancy with endovaginal ultrasound. *Radiology*, **167**, 383–5

51. Rempen, A. (1990). Diagnosis of viability in early pregnancy with vaginal sonography. *J. Ultrasound Med.*, **9**, 711–16

52. Bromley, B., Harlow, B. L., Laboda, L. V. *et al.* (1991). Small sac size in the first trimester: a predictor of poor fetal outcome, *Radiology*, **178**, 375–7

53. Horrow, M. H. (1992). Enlarged amniotic cavity: a new sonographic sign of early embryonic death. *Am. J. Roentgenol.*, **158**, 359–62

54. Levi, C. S., Lyons, E. A., Zheng, X. H. *et al.* (1990). Endovaginal US: demonstration of cardiac activity in embryos of less than 5.0 mm in crown rump length. *Radiology*, **176**, 71–4

55. Nyberg, D. A., Laing, F. C. and Filly, R. A. (1986). Threatened abortion: sonographic distinction of normal and abnormal gestational sacs. *Radiology*, **158**, 397–400

56. Wax, M. R., Frates, M., Benson, C. B. *et al.* (1992). First trimester findings in pregnancies after *in vitro* fertilization. *J. Ultrasound Med.*, **11**, 321–5

57. Lindsay, D. J., Lovett, I. S., Lyons, E. A. *et al.* (1992). Yolk sac diameter and shape at endovaginal US: predictors of pregnancy outcome in the first trimester. *Radiology*, **183**, 115–18

58. Harris, R. D., Vincent, L. M. and Askin, F. B. (1988). Yolk sac calcification: a sonographic finding associated with intrauterine demise in the first trimester. *Radiology*, **166**, 109–10

59. Benson, C. B. and Douibilet, P. M. (1994). Slow embryonic heart rate in early first trimester: indicator of poor pregnancy outcome. *Radiology*, **192**, 343–4

Hysteroscopic fluid distension media and their complications

7

D. L. Olive

As an imaging technique, hysteroscopy has only recently found its niche within the armamentarium of the gynecologist. The procedure was initially termed 'a technique in search of an indication'. Today, however, its role in diagnosing and treating abnormal uterine bleeding and specific Müllerian anomalies is without question. Among those specializing in infertility, too, this procedure has proved to be of value. Structural abnormalities of the uterus are identified hysteroscopically, and surgical correction can often follow. The hysteroscope also provides a means of access to the proximal fallopian tube for a variety of diagnostic and interventional procedures.

To achieve this level of capability with hysteroscopy, it is imperative that adequate visualization of the uterine cavity be achieved. This generally requires a high-quality hysteroscope (either rod–lens or fiberoptic), appropriate lighting and the use of a video camera and monitor. However, at least as critical to the achievement of such visualization is the use of an appropriate method to distend the uterine cavity.

Two types of distension methods can be used. Gaseous distension is popular for a variety of reasons, including cost, ease of administration and storage ability. Liquid media are also employed; this area is highly variable in type of media and consequences of use. This chapter reviews hysteroscopic distension media, their assets and complications.

GAS DISTENSION: CARBON DIOXIDE

The most commonly used gaseous distension medium is carbon dioxide. The popularity of

this approach stems from the ease of use and safety, since the gas is rapidly absorbed into the blood and readily released as the patient is ventilated[1]. No other gas can or should be used for hysteroscopic uterine distension.

Carbon dioxide is useful for diagnostic hysteroscopy, but its use in operative procedures is problematic. Blood from the operative site can quickly obscure the view of the hysteroscopist. Furthermore, gas is less than ideal even for diagnosis: bubbles created by infusion of the gas can distort and obscure visibility.

The primary complication associated with carbon dioxide is intravasation. Little potential risk exists from this factor if a maximum pressure of 100 mmHg and a maximum flow rate of 100 ml/min are not exceeded[2]. The rate of intravasation clearly increases in direct proportion to infusion pressure, and some intravasation has been noted in 52% of women undergoing hysteroscopy[3].

When significant gas extravasation occurs, results can be catastrophic. Metabolic changes due to increased intravascular carbon dioxide include an increase in partial pressure of carbon dioxide and a decrease in partial pressure of oxygen. The resulting metabolic profile is one of metabolic acidosis and this can cause cardiac irregularity[4]. Small amounts of carbon dioxide intravascularly can cause embolization, but in limited volumes this is not dangerous. However, large amounts of undissolved carbon dioxide can accumulate in the right heart and prove fatal.

Treatment of carbon dioxide intravasation consists of cessation of hysteroscopy, patient ventilation and vascular supportive measures. Placing the patient on her left side may also be helpful if a carbon dioxide embolus resides in the right heart.

Occasional reports point out odd and unique complications resulting from the use of carbon dioxide as a distension medium. One adverse reaction can be rupture of a blocked fallopian tube[5]. Generally, however, excessive infusion pressure is required.

LIQUID DISTENSION

High-viscosity media: dextran 70

Hyskon is a solution of 32% dextran 70 in 10% glucose. Dextrans are glucose polymers produced by bacteria. Dextran 70 is a mixture of dextrans of varying sizes, but whose mean molecular weight is 70 000. These molecules were originally used as plasma expanders, but as the solution's clarity and immiscibility with blood were noted it was promoted as an endoscopic distension medium for surgical procedures. Their benefit as to intravascular expansion is a direct result of their increasing of the plasma oncotic pressure and their slow rate of elimination from the body. The latter effect is due to the size of the molecules: while molecules of 50 000 molecular weight or less can be eliminated by filtration through the kidney, larger molecules require metabolism by the reticuloendothelial system[6] and have a half-life in the circulation of up to 4 days. These properties, however, are problematic when Hyskon is used for uterine distension.

A major complication associated with absorption of excessive amounts of Hyskon is pulmonary edema. This effect is probably due to an increase in intravascular volume. As previously stated, dextrans have been used clinically as plasma expanders. With dextrans of high molecular weight, their presence in the intravascular space results in an increase in oncotic pressure and intravascular volume. Fluid and electrolytes are drawn into the intravascular compartment, with each gram of dextran 70 capable of drawing 20 to 27 ml of water into the circulation[7,8]. Thus, absorption of 100 ml of Hyskon intravascularly will expand the intravascular space an additional 860 ml[9]. Importantly, there is no resulting electrolyte imbalance, as both fluid and electrolytes are drawn into the intravascular space.

Treatment of volume overload secondary to excessive dextran absorption includes supportive measures, such as ventilatory assistance. Diuresis may be considered, but only with mild use under careful observation, as this technique will not remove the underlying cause and could result in intracellular fluid depletion. In cases of intractable pulmonary edema, plasmapheresis may be considered. Dialysis is not effective in removing dextrans.

A second complication noted with Hyskon is anaphylactic shock. It is theorized that in most cases prior sensitization may have occurred to naturally occurring antigens, such as in sugar beets, or bacterial antigens. The rate of such a response has been estimated at 1/10 000[10]. At present there does not seem to be any reliable method to predict anaphylaxis when using dextran, including the use of skin testing[11]. When anaphylaxis occurs, the dextran infusion should immediately be stopped. Resuscitation with epinephrine (adrenaline) and hydrocortisone may be necessary, and administration of antihistamines seems reasonable.

Dextran 70 has been associated with coagulation disorders, ranging from mild abnormalities in the coagulation profile to disseminated intravascular coagulation. The antithrombotic effect is thought to be due to decreased platelet adhesiveness to the endothelium, a result of both surfaces being coated with dextrans. In addition, the structure of fibrin clots is altered, making them more susceptible to lysis[6]. Further, numerous coagulation factors are reduced in concentration; this is compounded by dilution of such factors due to increased circulating plasma volume[12].

Intravascular dextran absorption has also been associated with oliguria and renal failure. Such changes may be transient or more severe, and are due to both a change in hydrostatic pressure gradients in the glomeruli and precipitation of dextrans of low molecular weight in the renal tubules. Dextrans may also cause factitious laboratory results, such as spuriously elevated glucose levels, abnormal bilirubin assays and faulty blood cross-matching[6].

Prevention of Hyskon side-effects is best accomplished by minimizing absorption. This is accomplished by keeping the maximum infusion pressure under 150 mmHg and utilizing less than 500 ml per procedure. When these recommendations are exceeded, the frequency of pulmonary edema is 1.1% and the rate of disseminated intravascular coagulation is 0.5%[13].

Low-viscosity media

A variety of low-viscosity fluids have been utilized for uterine distension, and their use has increased dramatically with the introduction of the continuous-flow hysteroscope. These fluids require large volumes with rapid circulation through the system, as blood and debris are fully miscible with each. As a result, the potential for substantial absorption of these fluids exists.

Two categories of low-viscosity media can be used: electrolyte-free or electrolyte-balanced. The latter, although useful for diagnostic procedures, in mechanical interventions and with the use of the Nd : YAG laser, cannot be utilized with electrosurgical instrumentation; in such instances, the electrical current is dissipated away from the electrode, rendering it ineffective. With the widespread use of hysteroscopic electrosurgery, the popularity of low-viscosity electrolyte-free solutions has therefore expanded.

Electrolyte-balanced solutions

The use of normal saline or Ringer's lactate solutions for uterine distension obviate any concern about electrolyte imbalance with excessive fluid absorption. However, pulmonary edema is still a potential problem with these media. Rates of fluid overload with myoma resection are reportedly as high as 1.1%[14]. Treatment for such overload is diuresis, generally with furosemide.

Electrolyte-free solutions: glycine

The most commonly used electrolyte-free distension medium is glycine, a 1.5% simple amino acid solution in water. Its osmolarity is approximately 200 mOsm/l. Intravascular absorption of this solution may cause water intoxication with hypervolemia and hyponatremia. Patients present with bradycardia and hypertension followed by hypotension, nausea, vomiting, headache, visual disturbances, agitation, confusion and lethargy[15]. If this is untreated, seizures, coma, cardiovascular collapse and death may result. This is the post-TURP syndrome, a condition encountered by urologists in up to 2% of surgical cystoscopies in which glycine is used.

Glycine accesses the vascular space when uterine vessels are transected during surgery. Fluid under pressure in the distended uterine cavity rapidly passes into the vasculature. As this fluid enters the circulation, sodium concentration in the serum decreases. Osmolarity is initially maintained as glycine molecules fill the osmolar gap. However, these molecules have a half-life of 85 min in the circulation; with removal of the glycine, a surplus of free water remains in the vascular tree. Hypo-osmolar hyponatremia is the resulting condition. This can result in cerebral edema, injuring the brain owing to the bony confines of the skull (Figure 1). In addition, increased intracranial pressure can lead to decreased cerebral blood flow and hypoxia. Finally, an increase in intracranial volume of 5% may lead to herniation. Additionally, hyponatremia itself can cause central nervous system depression, with lethargy, convulsions and coma[15].

Treatment of hypo-osmolar hyponatremia involves the removal of the excess free water and correction of the serum sodium level. It is important to correct these abnormalities even in the asymptomatic patient, as rapid deterioration can occur.

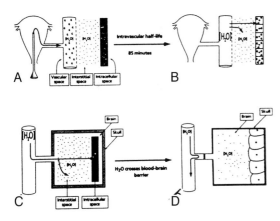

Figure 1 (A) *Intravascular osmolarity is initially maintained by glycine molecules (G) contained in the intravascular space. (B) When glycine moves from the intravascular space into the cell, intravascular osmolarity falls. The concentration of water ([H_2O]) is greater in the intravascular space than in the interstitial space. As a result, water moves from the vascular space into the interstitial and intracellular spaces (arrows). (C) Because of the intravascular hypo-osmolar state, water moves across the blood–brain barrier into the interstitial and intracellular spaces. (D) Cerebral edema develops with compression of the brain against the skull. Water will continue to move into the brain until the hydrostatic pressure of the brain offsets the osmotic force. From reference 15*

The length of time the patient has been hyponatremic is critical to determining the speed and method of correction. If the patient is found to be profoundly hyponatremic in the operating room (minutes), complete correction can be rapidly performed. This can be achieved by the infusion of normal saline and the administration of either furosemide or mannitol. There is no need to use hypertonic saline, as this solution is potentially dangerous and correction will occur with sufficient rapidity using the aforementioned treatment combination.

When hypo-osmolar hyponatremia is noted hours or days after surgery, however, care must be taken in correcting the abnormalities. The reason for this is that too rapid correction can result in an obscure brain injury called central pontine myelinolysis (CPM)[16]. This disorder occurs as a result of the brain's ability to compensate for osmolarity abnormalities. In the hyponatremic patient, water is osmotically drawn into the central circulation, potentially resulting in cerebral edema. Unlike other tissues, however, the brain attempts to compensate for this hypo-osmolarity by the extrusion of small molecules. Initially, potassium leaves the cells. Over the following days there is loss of cytoplasmic organic osmolytes such as taurine, phosphocreatinine, myoinositol, glutamine and glutamate[17]. It is the extrusion of these molecules that allows the brain cells to maintain their integrity in the face of osmolar variation.

Unfortunately, the compensated brain cells are highly vulnerable to rapid correction of hyponatremia. Because the brain decreases its solute concentration to decrease swelling as it reaches equilibrium with the plasma, it becomes vulnerable to dehydration if serum osmolarity increases rapidly (Figure 2). The resulting clinical presentation is one of neurological deterioration, with paresis, mutism, pseudobulbar palsy, behavioral changes and movement disorders.

Therefore, the strategy for correction of

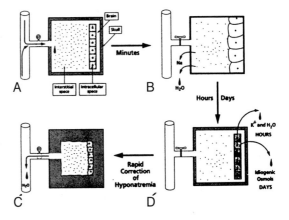

Figure 2 (A) *As a result of intravascular hypo-osmolarity, water moves into the brain. The brain swells and is compressed against the skull. (B) Within minutes, sodium and water are extruded from the extracellular space into the cerebrospinal fluid and ultimately into the vasculature. (C) To decrease swelling, the brain cells release potassium and 'idiogenic osmols'. The brain now has decreased the number of osmotically active particles. This response takes up to several days. (D) A rapid increase in plasma osmolarity (as with rapid correction of hyponatremia) leads to movement of water out of the brain and into the vascular space, causing desiccation of the brain. From reference 15*

hyponatremia is dependent upon the degree of chronicity. If the disorder is recognized several hours after surgery, but within the first 24 h, correction of serum sodium should occur at a rate of 1–2 mEq/l per hour, with no more than a 12-mEq/l increase in sodium in the first 24 h. If, however, the hyponatremia is not recognized for more than 24 h, a slow correction of 0.6 mEq/l per hour is recommended[18,19].

In addition to the above disorders, glycine can produce other adverse effects. The metabolic products of glycine may cause postoperative complications. Oxalate crystals may form in the urine. Hyperammonemia may develop, with resulting encephalopathic symptoms. Finally, glycine may alter neurotransmitter function to produce a transient decrease in visual acuity.

Sorbitol and mannitol

Two other solutes used in solution for uterine distension are sorbitol and mannitol, either alone or in combination. A solution of 3% sorbitol has been used extensively, owing to its excellent visual characteristics. One distinct characteristic of sorbitol is the much shorter half-life in the circulation. Therefore, development of hypo-osmolarity should be more rapid than with glycine. Unfortunately, comparative studies do not exist for these two solutions.

Mannitol can be used in either a 3% or a 5% solution. Only a small portion of intravascular mannitol is metabolized; the remainder (90+%) is freely filtered by the kidney and excreted in the urine. The half-life in the circulation is only 15 min, thus allowing mannitol to act as an osmotic diuretic. Hyponatremia should still be a concern, but the risk of hypo-osmolar problems should be severely diminished. No data exist to confirm any advantages or disadvantages of these solutions compared to glycine.

Sorbitol and mannitol are also used in combination (Cytal, Abbot laboratories), with the commercially available solutions containing 2.7% sorbitol and 0.54% mannitol.

Again, data do not exist on the relative merits of these solutions.

Prevention of complications of low-viscosity fluids

There are several important precautions that can be taken to prevent adverse effects of low-viscosity fluids[20]. First, it is imperative that the operating room team keep meticulous track of the amount of fluid absorbed, and this calculation should be made and recorded no less often than every 10 min during an operation. The use of a multichannel continuous flow instrument is essential. Preoperative medical preparation of the endometrium will help decrease vascularity and duration of surgery. Chilling the distension medium may also decrease fluid absorption by initiating blood vessel constriction.

All patients should undergo preoperative electrolyte assessment to establish the baseline values. If, during the course of the procedure, there is a 500-ml deficit noted, stat serum electrolytes should be sent to the laboratory. If a 1000-ml deficit is observed, electrolytes should again be determined and the operation halted until the results are returned. Furosemide may be administered empirically at a dose of 20 mg intravenously (Figure 3). The same protocol is used at a 1500-ml deficit. If a 2-l deficit is observed, or if the serum sodium level is less than

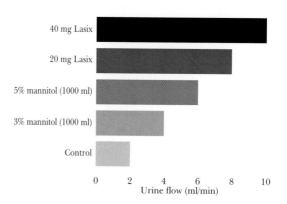

Figure 3 *Diuretic effect of various treatment modalities. Lasix (furosemide)*

120 mEq/l, the operation should be immediately discontinued.

In utilizing this protocol for the past 4 years, we have been successful at minimizing instances of hyponatremia and other adverse effects. However, such an approach is not a panacea, and diligent monitoring as well as prompt recognition and response is the best defense against complications arising from use of these fluids.

References

1. Salat-Baroux, J., Hamou, J. E., Maillard, G. *et al.* (1984). Complications from microhysteroscopy In Siegler, A. M. and Lindemann, H. J. (eds.) *Hysteroscopy: Principles in Practice*, pp. 112–17. (Philadelphia: JB Lippincott)
2. Loffer, F. D. (1995). Complications of hysteroscopy – their cause, prevention, and correction. *J. Am. Assoc. Gynecol. Laparosc.*, **3**, 11–26
3. Rythen-Alder, E., Brundin, J., Notini-Gudmarsson, A. *et al.* (1992). Detection of carbon dioxide embolism during hysteroscopy. *Gynaecol. Endosc.*, **1**, 207–10
4. Lindemann, H. J. and Mohr, J. (1976). CO_2 hysteroscopy: diagnosis and treatment. *Am. J. Obstet. Gynecol.*, **124**, 129–33
5. Siegler, A. M., Valle, R. F., Lindemann, H. J. *et al.* (1990). *Therapeutic Hysteroscopy: Indications and Techniques*, pp. 53–61. (St Louis: CV Mosby)
6. Data, J. L. and Nies, A. S. (1974). Dextran 40. *Ann. Intern. Med.*, **81**, 500–4
7. Ljungstrom, K. G. (1990). Safety of dextran 70 for hysteroscopy [letter]. *Am. J. Obstet. Gynecol.*, **163**, 2029–30
8. Lukascko, P. (1985). Noncardiogenic pulmonary edema secondary to intrauterine instillation of 32% dextran 70 [letter]. *Fertil. Steril.*, **44**, 560–1
9. Mangar, D., Gerson, J. I., Constantine, R. M. and Lenzi, V. (1989). Pulmonary edema and coagulopathy due to Hyskon (32% dextran 70) administration. *Anesth. Analg.*, **68**, 686–7
10. Jedeikin, R. and Olsfanger, D. (1990). Disseminated intravascular coagulopathy and adult respiratory distress syndrome: life-threatening complications of hysteroscopy. *Am. J. Obstet. Gynecol.*, **162**, 44–5
11. Ahmed, N., Falcone, T., Tulandi, T. and Houle, G. (1991). Anaphylactic reaction because of intrauterine 32% dextran-70 instillation. *Fertil. Steril.*, **55**, 1014–16
12. Cronberg, S., Robertson, B., Nilsson, I. M. and Nilehn J. E. (1966). Suppressive effect of dextran on platelet adhesiveness. *Thromb. Diath. Haemorrh.*, **16**, 384–92
13. Ruiz, J. M. and Neuwirth, R. S. (1992). The incidence of complications associated with the use of Hyskon during hysteroscopy: experience in 1783 consecutive patients. *J. Gynecol. Surg.*, **8**, 219
14. Loffer, F. D. (1994). Removing intrauterine lesions: myomectomy and polypectomy. In Biever, E. J. and Loffer, F. D. (eds.) *The Gynecologic Resectoscope*, pp. 168–94. (Cambridge MA: Blackwell)
15. Witz, C. A., Silverberg, K. M., Burns, W. N., Schenken, R. S. and Olive, D. L. (1993). Complications associated with the absorption of hysteroscopic fluid media. *Fertil. Steril.*, **60**, 745–56
16. Ayus, J. C., Krothapalli, R. K. and Arieff, A. I. (1987). Treatment of symptomatic hyponatremia and its relation to brain damage. *N. Engl. J. Med.*, **5**, 1190–5
17. Sterns, R. H. (1990). The management of symptomatic hyponatremia. *Semin. Nephrol.*, **10**, 3–14
18. Arieff, A. I. and Ayus, J. C. (1991). Treatment of symptomatic hyponatremia: neither haste nor waste. *Crit. Care Med.*, **19**, 748–51
19. Stern, R. H. (1990). The treatment of hyponatremia: first, do no harm. *Am. J. Med.*, **88**, 557–60
20. Kim, A. H., Keltz, M. D., Arici, A., Rosenberg, M. and Olive, D. L. (1995). Dilutional hyponatremia during hysteroscopic myomectomy with sorbitol–mannitol distension medium. *J. Am. Assoc. Gynecol. Laparasc.*, **2**, 237–42

Normal anatomy of the male genital system

8

J. Mulhall and S. C. Honig

INTRODUCTION

The male genital system can be divided by function into organs involved with sperm production, sperm maturation and sperm transport. Sperm production occurs in the testis and may be affected by intra- and para-testicular factors. Sperm maturation occurs in the epididymis. Sperm transport starts in the epididymis, continues through the vas deferens and may be affected by its communication with the seminal vesicles and prostate. Sperm-containing semen travels into the prostatic urethra via the ejaculatory duct, and is propelled in an antegrade fashion by perineal muscular contractions resulting in the production of a forceful ejaculation.

The purpose of this chapter is to delineate the normal anatomy of the male reproductive tract, which is important in the diagnosis and treatment of male infertility. We outline the 'gold standards', minimally invasive diagnostic tests and 'state-of-the-art' approaches to imaging of the male genital tract. The modalities that are most helpful in defining the anatomic detail of these structures are ultrasonography, magnetic resonance imaging (MRI) and contrast studies of the venous system and vas deferens.

SPERM PRODUCTION

Testis

The imaging modalities used most frequently in the evaluation of the testis are gray-scale ultrasonography, color-flow Doppler ultrasonography and magnetic resonance imaging (MRI). The scrotum is best imaged ultrasono-graphically using a high frequency probe (7.5–12.5 MHz) which provides minimal attenuation and maximal resolution of intra-scrotal structures.

The testis has a dual function. More than two-thirds of the normal testicular parenchyma is composed of seminiferous tubules which house spermatogenic tissue. The remainder of the testis comprises interstitial tissue composed of Leydig cells which produce testosterone.

The normal testis measures approximately 3–5 cm in length, 2–3 cm in width and 2–3 cm in anteroposterior depth with a normal volume of approximately 20 cc by physical examination. The normal testis demonstrates a uniform, homogeneous texture of low to moderate echogenicity[1] (Figure 1). The echotexture of the two testes should be similar. The mediastinum of the testis is that portion of the tunica albuginea that folds in upon itself protruding into the testicular parenchyma posteriorly as a septum. This mediastinum appears on ultrasonography as a highly echogenic band, but this band must not be used as a reference for testicular orientation as the testes are highly mobile[2]. Testicular volume has been estimated by several methods including manual palpation with comparison to testis models[3–5], use of an orchidometer[6], calipers[7] and ultrasonography[8–11]. Ultrasonography, while operator-dependent, has been shown to have good correlation with true volume measurement[8,10]. The most commonly utilized formula for the estimation of testicular volume by ultrasonography is:

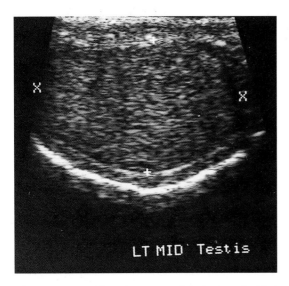

Figure 1 *Normal testis: gray-scale ultrasound. Note homogeneous echotexture throughout the parenchyma of the testis. Cursors show size measurement of testis. (From Honig SC: Use of ultrasonography in the evaluation of the infertile male.* World J Urol *1993;11:102–7)*

$$V = L \times W \times D \times \pi/6$$

where V is volume, L is length, W is width, D is anteroposterior depth and $\pi/6 = 0.52$. As little difference exists between W and D, some authors use the formula $V = L \times W^2 \times 0.52$. Since most of the testis consists of sperm producing cells, if the volume is significantly below 20 cc impairment of sperm production is likely.

Normal arterial supply to the testis is a major prerequisite for normal function. Interference with the blood supply may reduce fertility. The duplex and color flow Doppler (CFD) characteristics of the testicular blood supply have been previously outlined[12]. The testicular and capsular (circumferential) arteries travel in the periphery of the testis with the capsular artery giving rise to intra-testicular branches that course toward the mediastinum of the testis (Color plate K). Capsular and centripetal arteries should be detectable on CFD in the normal testis. MRI may be a useful modality in the evaluation of the scrotal contents[13–18]. MRI has certain advantages over ultrasonography, although it is more expensive and less accessible. Its advantages include high sensitivity for intrascrotal pathologies, high contrast and spatial resolution and simultaneous assessment of the right and left hemiscrotum and inguinal regions. Furthermore, it has been demonstrated that MRI has no deleterious effects on spermatogenesis[19]. At the present time, indications for scrotal MRI for diagnosis of male fertility-related disorders are limited to situations where scrotal ultrasonography is equivocal.

The normal testis on MRI is well demarcated by the low signal tunica albuginea. Most importantly, the normal testicular parenchyma has a homogeneous signal on all imaging sequences. On T_1-weighted images the signal is of medium signal intensity, brighter than water and darker than fat. It has a homogeneous high signal intensity on T_2-weighted images and often the low signal mediastinum testis can be identified (Figure 2). If there is fluid within the tunica vaginalis, i.e. hydrocele, this can be used as an internal standard to detect any changes in the testicular signal. Thin 5 mm slices are standard and the use of a surface coil is recommended for optimal imaging[15–18,20,21].

Paratesticular structures

The normal venous anatomy of the testis is depicted ultrasonographically by venous channels less than 2 mm in diameter that do not usually demonstrate reversal of flow with the Valsalva maneuver. This is the standard diagnostic imaging modality used to identify a varicocele. The normal venous anatomy may also be identified on venography, however this is usually reserved for patients undergoing therapeutic intervention for a varicocele using embolotherapy. Normal venography shows a competent valve in the internal spermatic vein, as demonstrated in Figure 3.

Ultrasonography cannot differentiate between the various layers of the spermatic cord nor delineate the two layers of the tunica vaginalis unless a hydrocele is present. The tunica vaginalis is indistinguishable from the tunica albuginea. The tunica vaginalis does

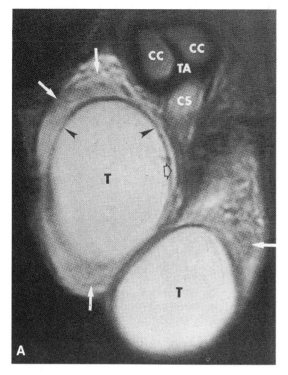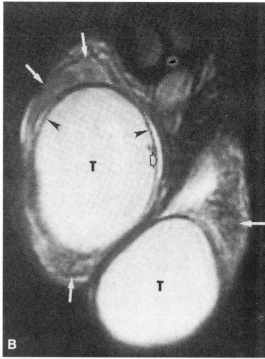

Figure 2 *Normal testis; magnetic resonance images in the coronal plane. There is a homogeneous pattern on T_1 (A) and T_2 (B) weighted images. T, normal testis; white arrows, epididymis; arrowheads, tunica albuginea of testis; CC, corpus cavernosum; CS, corpus spongiosum; TA, tunica albuginea of penis; open arrow, small hydrocele. (From Baker et al. MR Imaging of the scrotum: Normal anatomy.* Radiology *1987;163:89–92)*

not invest the entire testis but leaves a bare area posteriorly where the tunica albuginea invaginates as the low-signal mediastinum of the testis.

SPERM MATURATION

Epididymis

The epididymis, which is in close association with the testis on its posterolateral aspect, is involved in both the storage and maturation of sperm. Careful examination of the epididymis is important in a male infertility evaluation. Both real-time and CFD scanning are helpful, but in different situations. The normal epididymis measures 7.7 mm in thickness by ultrasonography which is helpful in the detection of epididymal thickening[22]. In general, the head of the epididymis (caput) is larger in width than the body (corpus) or

tail (cauda). The echogenicity of the epididymis is similar to, or just a little greater than, that of the testis[2] (Figure 4). On CFD scanning, the normal epididymis rarely exhibits an active blood flow pattern but in certain pathological states, such as epididymitis, increased blood flow may be seen on CFD imaging.

On MRI, the epididymis has a heterogeneous signal on T_1 which is less pronounced on the T_2-weighted images. The head and tail are generally well seen but the body is difficult to distinguish from the scrotal wall (Figure 2). Tortuous tubular structures lying above the epididymal head represent the pampiniform venous plexus.

SPERM TRANSPORT

Great interest has arisen recently in the use of minimally-invasive imaging modalities in the

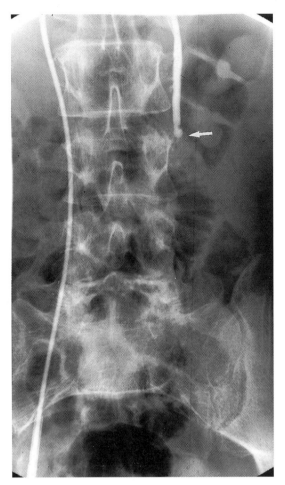

Figure 3 *Normal venogram. White arrow depicts level of competent left internal spermatic valve preventing reflux down towards the testis. (Courtesy Robert White MD)*

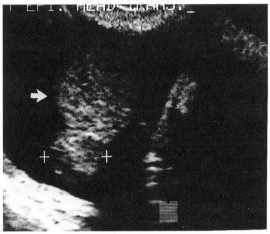

Figure 4 *Normal epididymis (cursor) on gray-scale ultrasound with the same echotexture as the adjacent testis (white arrow). The cursor is measuring the size of the epididymal head. (From Honig SC: Use of ultrasonography in the evaluation of the infertile male. World J Urol 1993;11:102–7)*

evaluation of the distal genital ductal system. The distal genital duct system includes the seminal vesicles, vasa deferentia, vasal ampullae, prostate and urethra. Transrectal ultrasongraphy (TRUS) and MRI have come to the forefront in this respect and have supplanted vasography as the imaging modality of choice. Scrotal vasography is still considered the gold standard, however it is invasive and may result in obstruction from scarring. Transrectal ultrasonography allows for precise anatomic delineation of the vasal ampullae, prostate, seminal vesicles and ejaculatory ducts in a minimally invasive fashion. The experience with MRI is growing

and its multiplanar capabilities coupled with its sensitivity allow for differentiation of tissue elements. When transrectal ultrasonography is non-diagnostic or contraindicated, MRI is a secondary choice for the evaluation of this anatomic area in the management of the infertile male.

Seminal vesicles

The seminal vesicles are androgen-dependent accessory organs that function in the production and storage of seminal fluid, which is essential to male fertility. The seminal vesicles are best studied ultrasonographically using a multiplanar high-frequency (7.5–10 MHz) probe. An 'end-firing' probe has the advantage over an axial probe of being able to examine the superior parts of the seminal vesicles. Transaxial imaging is useful in determining seminal vesicle size, volume, symmetry and echotexture.

Normal seminal vesicles are seen as flat, paired structures that lie cephalad to the prostate behind the bladder with a 'bow-tie' appearance on transverse imaging[23–27]. They are seen as symmetric, well-defined, saccular, elongated organs (Figure 5). In its normal collapsed state the center of the gland is homogeneous, with areas of increased echogenicity corresponding to the folds of secretory epithelium. Caudally, the seminal vesicles diverge laterally into the perivesical fat.

The dimensions of the seminal vesicles vary with age but not with the ejaculatory state[28]. On transrectal ultrasonography, their dimensions have been estimated at 30 ± 5 mm in length and 15 ± 4 mm in width with a mean estimated volume of 13.7 ± 3.7 cc[28]. The age of the patient and the degree of prostate enlargement have been shown to cause variations in the size of the seminal vesicles[29,30] (Figure 6).

Magnetic resonance imaging may also be helpful in delineating the normal anatomy of the seminal vesicles. Using MRI, the signal intensity of the seminal vesicles can be compared to those of the matter surrounding

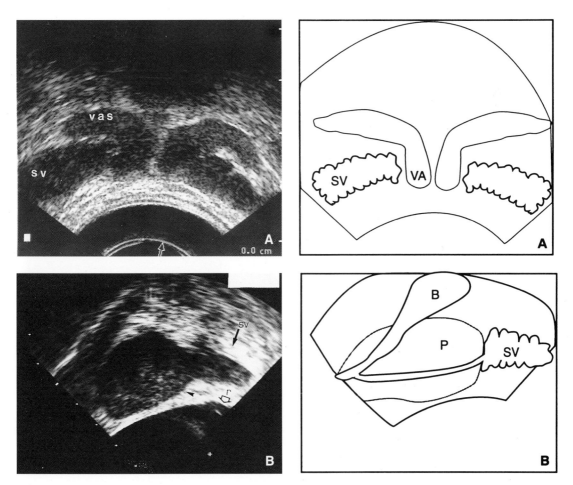

Figure 5 *Normal pelvic anatomy on transrectal ultrasound (TRUS), with accompanying schematic representation. (A), transverse plane. sv, normal seminal vesicle; vas, normal vasal ampulla; arrow, rectum. Note 'bow-tie' appearance of seminal vesicles. (Courtesy Brian Ginsberg MD, Keith Jarvi MD, Mount Sinai Hospital, Toronto, Canada). (B), sagittal plane. SV, normal seminal vesicle; arrowhead, normal prostate; r, rectum. (from Honig SC: Use of ultrasonography in the evaluation of the infertile male.* World J Urol 1993;11:102–7). *Schematic of normal pelvic anatomy. (A) transverse plane: SV, normal seminal vesicle; VA, normal vasal ampulla. (B) sagittal plane: SV, normal seminal vesicle; P, normal prostate; B, bladder*

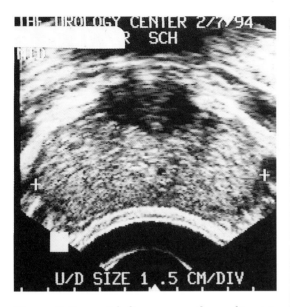

Figure 6 *Transrectal ultrasonogram of normal prostate in transverse plane. Note no evidence of ejaculatory duct abnormalities and no calcifications. There are no hypoechoic lesions in the peripheral zone to suggest prostate cancer*

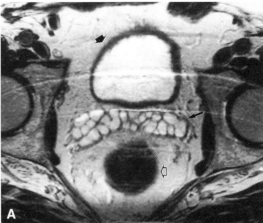

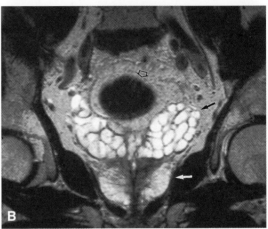

Figure 7 *Magnetic resonance image of normal male pelvis with sequential fast T_2 coronal views showing (A) seminal vesicles (narrow black arrow), bladder (wide black arrow) and rectum (open arrow); and (B) seminal vesicles (narrow black arrow), prostate (white arrow) and rectum (open arrow). (By permission of Shirley McCarthy, MD, PhD)*

them, that is skeletal muscle, fat and urine. The signal intensity on T_1-weighted images of normal seminal vesicles in adult males is similar to, or slightly higher than, that of skeletal muscle and always greater than that of urine[20,31,32]. On T_2-weighted images the signal intensity is variable, but the internal signal of these saccular structures is usually of high intensity (Figure 7). Prepubertally, and in men over 70 years of age (androgen-deprived males) the signal intensity is generally lower than that of skeletal muscle or urine. Convolutions of the seminal vesicles are best seen on T_2-weighted images or on T_1-weighted images with the use of intravenous contrast agents such as gadolinium-diethylene trianine pentacetic acid (gadolinium-DTPA)[32] (Figure 7B). Whether using an endorectal coil will be helpful in better defining anatomic detail is unclear at present[33].

A paucity of literature exists on the use of computed tomography (CT) scanning in the evaluation of this anatomic area[33-35]. In general, CT is not as useful as ultrasonography or MRI in demonstrating the anatomy of the distal genital tract.

Vas deferens/vasal ampullae

The vas deferens acts as a conduit carrying sperm between the epididymis and the ejaculatory ducts. The vasal ampullae pass medial to the seminal vesicles and are best seen on transaxial transrectal ultrasonography views (Figure 5A). Imaging of the vasa and seminal vesicles by injection of contrast materials is an established modality for the evaluation of the male with infertility, particularly azoospermia. Indeed, the first attempts at vaso-seminal vesiculography took place in the early part of this century[36,37]. The normal seminal vesiculogram has been previously outlined[38].

From a technical standpoint, contrast study of the vasa and seminal vesicles can be performed optimally at the time of scrotal exploration by performance of a microsurgical hemivasotomy and cannulation of the vasal lumen with a 24 French (Fr) angiographic catheter using a 50/50 mixture of renograffin and indigo carmine[39–41] (Figure 8) (compare to Figures 14 and 16 in Chapter 9). Intraoperative vasal fluid sampling is an essential part of this procedure. The gross quality of the exuding fluid from the vas should be noted and the fluid should be examined microscopically for the presence or absence of sperm. Data are not available on the fluid quality in the normal unobstructed vas deferens; however, generally a small amount of fluid and a few sperm are usually present. This is significantly different from the obstructed state. Imaging studies are not necessary if low vasal irrigation pressure is present (subjective) when flushing the vas towards the prostate with a 24 Fr cannula. This is confirmation of the non-obstructed normal state. Alternatively, vasal flushing with indigo carmine followed by urethral catheterization will show the return of bluish-green urine in the normal or minimally obstructed state.

Recently, contrast imaging of the seminal vesicles has been attempted via both the transperineal route[42,43] and the transrectal route with transrectal ultrasonographic guidance (Figure 9)[44]. A normal vaso-seminovesiculogram shows contrast in the scrotal and inguinal vas deferens, contrast in non-distended vasal ampullae, seminal vesicle and ejaculatory duct with free flow of contrast into the bladder.

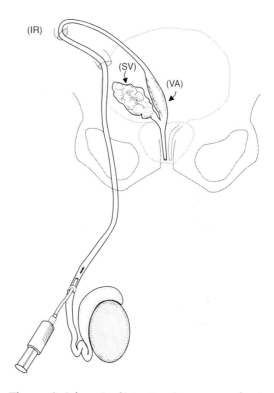

Figure 8 *Schematic of intraoperative vasogram showing normal anatomy of vas deferens traversing through internal ring (IR), seminal vesicle (SV), ejaculatory duct and vasal ampulla (VA). Compare to Figure 9 in this chapter and Figures 14 and 16 in Chapter 9*

Ejaculatory ducts/prostate

The seminal vesicles and vasal ampullae join together to form the ejaculatory duct. The ejaculatory duct travels through the prostate and enters the urethra at the level of the verumontanum. The junction between the seminal vesicle and the ejaculatory duct lies within the prostate and in the normal unobstructed system is not seen on imaging studies. Small echodense areas are frequently seen at the junction of the ejaculatory ducts and the verumontanum in the urethra. These provide useful landmarks and are felt to represent concretions within the periurethral glands surrounding the verumontanum[45]. The prostate is a homogeneous structure that is nicely imaged on transrectal ultrasonography. The normal prostate on transrectal ultrasonography shows minimal hyperechoic calcification, no evidence of dilated ejaculatory ducts and no hypoechoic lesions in the posterior zone (Figure 6).

Urethra/penis

The urethra is the final conduit for semen to pass through in the body. During normal ejaculation, seminal emission results in semen deposition in the prostatic urethra. Retrograde ejaculation is prevented by normal closure of the bladder neck. The normal urethra is smooth and capacious allowing

expulsion of semen during antegrade ejaculation[46]. Abnormalities that narrow the urethra or affect bladder neck closure can be identified by either a retrograde urethrogram (RUG), voiding cystourethrogram (VCUG) or ultrasonography or cystoscopy. On ultrasonography, the normal urethra measures 4 mm, has smooth echogenic walls and is identified travelling through the corpus spongiosum[47]. The urethra is best imaged by retrograde urethrography (Figure 10). The normal urethrogram shows a uniform caliber tubular structure up to the external sphincter where normal tightening may be seen. Some contrast is usually seen in the bladder.

Successful coitus is a prerequisite for semen deposition in the vagina and a full and sustained erection is necessary for vaginal penetration. Some patients may have problems with erectile dysfunction that results in coital factor infertility. Radiological evaluation of this problem is beyond the scope of this chapter. However, associated penile problems such as penile curvature (Peyronie's disease) and hypospadias may preclude successful semen deposition near the cervix. Peyronie's disease is usually diagnosed

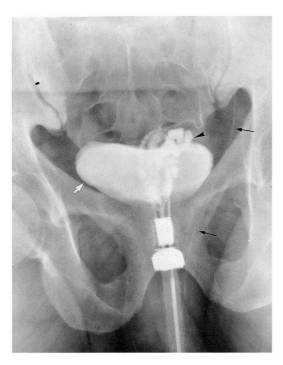

Figure 9 *Normal vasoseminovesiculogram. Note normal outline of left vasal ampulla, seminal vesicle (arrowhead) and scrotal vas deferens (two black arrows) with contrast filling the bladder (white arrow). Using a transrectal ultrasonography-guided needle, the seminal vesicle was injected with renograffin to delineate this anatomy. (From Riedendlau E, Buch JP, Jarow JP. Diagnosis of vasal obstruction with seminal vesiculography: an alternative to vasography in select patients. (Fertil Steril 1995;64(6):1224–7)*

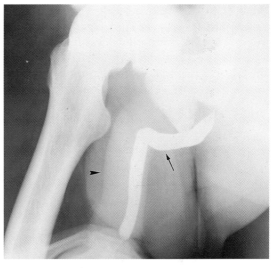

Figure 10 *Normal retrograde urethrogram. Note normal contour of urethra (black arrow) with no evidence of scar or stricture and outline of penis (arrowhead). (Courtesy Morton Glickman MD)*

clinically; however, sometimes ultrasonography or MRI is helpful in delineating the size and extent of plaque formation in the penis responsible for the curvature. Figure 11 shows a normal MRI of the flaccid penis. This can be compared to Figure 18 in the following chapter showing scar tissue of the penis resulting in severe penile curvature and coital factor infertility.

SUMMARY

A complete understanding of the anatomy of the male reproductive system radiologically is a prerequisite to identification of abnormalities that may result in male factor infertility. Ultrasonography, magnetic resonance imaging and contrast studies are the imaging modalities most useful for this purpose. The normal radiographs in this chapter should be helpful as a reference guide for the following chapter which shows anatomic abnormalities responsible for male factor infertility.

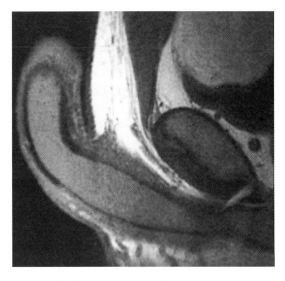

Figure 11 *Normal penis: sagittal magnetic resonance T₁ image. The corpus cavernosum is homogeneous without evidence of curvature, scar tissue or inflammation. (Courtesy Robert Smith MD)*

References

1. O'Mara, E. M. and Rifkin, M. D. (1991). Scrotum and contents. In Resnick, M. I. and Rifkin, M. D. (eds.) *Ultrasonography of the Urinary Tract*, 3rd edn. pp. 386–435 (Baltimore: Williams & Wilkins)

2. Feld, R. and Middleton, W. D. (1992). Recent advances in sonography of the testis and scrotum. *Radiol. Clin. North Am.*, **30**, 1033–51

3. Schonfeld, W. A. and Beebe, G. N. (1942). Normal growth and variation in male genitalia from birth to maturity. *J. Urol.*, **48**, 759–77

4. Nakamura, R. (1961). Normal growth and maturation in male genitalia of the Japanese. *Jap. J. Urol.*, **52**, 172–88

5. Prader, A. (1966). Testicular size: assessment and clinical importance. *Testes*, **7**, 240–3

6. Takihara, H., Sakatoku, J., Fujii, M., Nasu, T., Cosentino, M. J. and Cockett, A. T. K. (1983). Significance of testicular size measurement in andrology I: A new orchidometer and its clinical application. *Fertil. Steril.*, **39**, 836–40

7. Lambert, B. (1951). The frequency of mumps and of mumps orchitis and the consequences for sexuality and fertility. *Acta Gen. Stat. Media*, **2** (Suppl. 1), 68–9

8. Fuse, H., Takahara, M., Ishii, H., Sumiya, H. and Shimakazi, J. (1990). Measurement of testicular volume by ultrasonography. *Int. J. Androl.*, **13**, 267–72

9. Lomeo, A. M. and Giambersio, A. M. (1991). Measurement of testicular volume. *Int. J. Androl.*, **14**, 241–2

10. Behre, H. M., Nashan, D. and Nieschlag, E. (1989). Objective measurement of testicular volume by ultrasonography: evaluation of the technique and comparison with orchidometer estimates. *Int. J. Androl.*, **12**, 395–403

11. Costabile, R. A., Skoog, S. and Radowich, M. (1992). Testicular volume assessment in the adolescent with a varicocele. *J. Urol.*, **147**, 1348–50

12. Middleton, W. D., Thorne, D. A. and Melson,

G. L. (1989). Color Doppler ultrasound of the normal testis. *Am. J. Radiology,*, **152**, 293–7

13. Fritzsche, P. J. (1988). MRI of the scrotum. *Urol. Radiol.,* **10**, 52–7

14. Mattrey, R. F. (1991). Magnetic resonance imaging of the scrotum. *Semin. Ultrasound Comput. Tomogr. Magn. Reson.,* **12**, 95–108

15. Baker, L. L., Hajek, P. C., Burkhard, T. K. *et al.* (1987). MR imaging of the scrotum: normal anatomy. *Radiology,* **163**, 89–92

16. Rholl, K. S., Lee, J. K. T., Ling, D., Heiken, J. P. and Glazer, H. S. (1987). MR imaging of the scrotum with a high resolution surface coil. *Radiology,* **163**, 99–103

17. Thurner, S., Hricak, H., Carroll, P. R., Filly, R. A. and Pobiel, R. (1988). Imaging the testis: comparison between MR imaging and ultrasound. *Radiology,* **167**, 631–6

18. Sohn, M., Neuerburg, J., Bohndorf, K., Sikora, R. and Daus, H. J. (1989). The value of magnetic resonance imaging at 1.5T in the evaluation of the scrotal content. *Urol. Int.,* **44**, 284–91

19. Withers, H. R., Mason, K. A. and Davis, C. A. (1985). MR effect on murine spermatogenesis. *Radiology,* **156**, 741–2

20. Hricak, H. and Carrington, B. M. (1991). *MRI of the Pelvis: A Text Atlas,* pp. 313–53. (Norwalk, CT: Appleton and Lange)

21. Costabile, R. A., Choyke, P. L., Frank, J. A. *et al.* (1993). Dynamic enhanced magnetic resonance imaging of testicular perfusion in the rat. *J. Urol.,* **149**, 1195–7

22. Nashan, D., Behre, H. M., Grunert, J. H. *et al.* (1990). Diagnostic value of scrotal sonography in infertile men: report on 658 cases. *Andrologia,* **22**, 387–95

23. Carter, S. S. C., Shinohara, K. and Lipshultz, L. I. (1989). Transrectal ultrasonography in disorders of the seminal vesicles and ejaculatory ducts. *Urol. Clin. North Am.,* **16**, 787–99

24. Braeckman, J. and Denis, L. (1983). The practice and pitfalls of ultrasonography in the lower urinary tract. *Eur. Urol.,* **9**, 193

25. Colpi, G. M., Ballerini, G., Zanollo, A. *et al.* (1985). Ultrasonography of seminal vesicles in infertility. In Bollack, C. and Calvert, A. (eds.) *Seminal Vesicles and Fertility: Biology and Pathology,* pp. 124–42. (Basel: S. Karger)

26. Honig, S. C. (1994). New diagnostic techniques in the evaluation of anatomic abnormalities of the infertile male. *Urol. Clin. North Am.,* **21**, 417–32

27. Lee, F., Torp-Pedersen, S. T., Siders, D. B. *et al.* (1989). Transrectal ultrasound in the diagnosis and staging of prostatic carcinoma. *Radiology,* **170**, 609–11

28. Hernandez, A. D., Urry, R. L. and Smith J. A. (1990). Ultrasonographic characteristics of the seminal vesicles after ejaculation. *J. Urol.,* **144**, 1380–2

29. Littrup, P. J., Lee, F. and McLeary, R. D. (1985). Transrectal ultrasound of the seminal vesicles and ejaculatory ducts: clinical correlation. *Radiology,* **168**, 625–8

30. Grayhack, J. T. (1961). Changes with ageing in human seminal vesicle fluid fructose concentration and seminal vesicle weight. *J. Urol.,* **86**, 142–3

31. Nilsson, S. (1962). The human seminal vesicle. *Acta. Chir. Scand.* (Suppl.) **296**, 3–13

32. Secaf, E., Nuruddin, R. N., Hricak, H., McClure, R. D. and Demas, B. (1991). MR imaging of the seminal vesicles. *Am. J. Radiology,* **156**, 989–94

33. Ramchandani, P., Banner, M. P. and Pollack, H. M. (1993). Imaging of the seminal vesicles. *Semin. Roentgenol.,* **1**, 83–91

34. Silverman, P. M., Dunnick, N. R. and Ford, K. K. (1985). Computed tomography of the normal seminal vesicles. *Comput. Radiol.,* **9**, 379–85

35. Korobkin, M., Callen, P. W. and Fisch, A. E. (1979). Computed tomography of the pelvis and retroperitoneun. *Radiol. Clin. North Am.,* **17**, 301–19

36. Belfield, W. T. (1913). Vasotomyoradiography of the seminal duct. *J. Am. Med. Assoc.,* **61**, 1867–9

37. Belfield, W. T. (1926). Vesiculography by means of iodized oils. *J. Urol.,* **16**, 73–84

38. Banner, M. P. and Hassler, R. (1978). The normal seminal vesiculogram. *Radiology,* **128**, 339–44

39. Al-Omari, H., Girgis, S. M. and Hanna, A. Z. (1985). Diagnostic value of seminal vesiculography. *Arch. Androl.,* **15**, 187–92

40. Devasia, A. and Gopalakrishnan, G. (1993). Atraumatic cannulation of the vas for perioperative vasography. *Br. J. Urol.,* **72**, 989–90

41. Feldman, A., Lanigan, D. and Choa, R. G. (1993). Simple technique for vasography. *Br. J. Urol.,* **72**, 390

42. Castineiras, J., Lopez, A., Parra, R. *et al.* (1993). Vesiculography with echo-guided transperineal puncture: a complement to intracavitary transrectal echography. *Acta. Urol. Esp.,* **17**, 268–74

43. Ospedale, S. and Giovanni, B. (1992). Trans.perineal vesiculodeferentography under ultrasound control: first experiences. *Arch. Ital. Urol. Nefrol. Androl.,* **64**, 133–6

44. Jarow, J. P. (1994). Seminal vesicle aspiration in the management of patients with ejaculatory duct obstruction. *J. Urol.,* **152**, 899–901

45. Sanders, R. C. (1984). Normal ultrasonic anatomy of the genitourinary system. In Resnick, M. I. (eds.) *Ultrasound in Urology.* (Baltimore: Williams & Wilkins)

46. Pollack, H. M. (1990). Retrograde urethrography. In Pollack, H. M. (ed.) *Clinical Urography.* (Philadelphia: W. B. Sanders), 895

47. McAninch, J. W., Laing, F. C. and Jeffrey, R. B. (1988). Sonourethrography in the evaluation of urethral strictures: a preliminary report. *J. Urol.,* **139**, 294–7

Abnormal anatomy of the male genital system

9

J. Mulhall and S. C. Honig

The previous chapter summarized the normal anatomical structures important in the diagnosis and treatment of male fertility-related disorders. This chapter emphasizes the anatomical detail of male genital system abnormalities that result in treatable male fertility disorders. We again divide this review into categories of pathology that affect sperm production, sperm maturation and sperm transport. Please use the figures showing normal structures in the previous chapter to help identify the abnormalities shown here.

SPERM PRODUCTION

Testis

Imaging modalities are helpful in delineating abnormalities in the testis parenchyma. Specifically, tumor identification and measurement of testicular size for atrophy or retarded growth may account for problems with sperm production. Abnormalities of the testis are best studied radiographically with real-time ultrasonography.

Testicular tumors are most common in the same age group in which fertility disorders of the male are most prevalent. Testicular tumors on physical examination have been identified in patients presenting with infertility, with semen analyses revealing mild or severe oligoasthenospermia or azoospermia[1]. A heterogeneous pattern within the parenchyma with localized hypoechoic areas are ultrasonographic findings consistent with a testicular tumor, specifically a seminoma

(Figure 1). Cystic degeneration, focal hemorrhage and necrosis will appear ultrasonographically with a more heterogeneous architecture and tend to be associated with non-seminomatous germ cell tumors. The epididymis is almost always of normal size. Magnetic resonance imaging (MRI) of the testis may be helpful in situations in which ultrasound scanning of the testis is equivocal. Classically, testicular neoplasms have a low signal intensity on T_2-weighted imaging (Figure 2) in association with a heterogeneous pattern[2–8]. This can usually be compared to a normal homogeneous high signal intensity in the contralateral testis or the non-affected

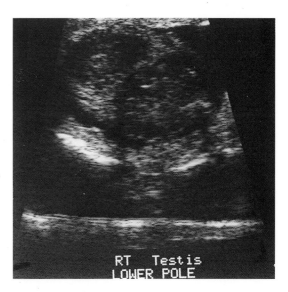

Figure 1 *Testis tumor: gray-scale ultrasound scan. Note heterogeneity of parenchyma of testis with mass effect. From reference 49, with permission*

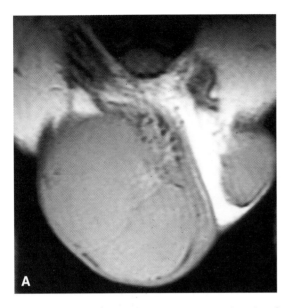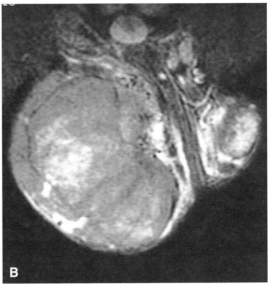

Figure 2 *Testis tumor: magnetic resonance imaging fast stir T_1-weighted (A) and T_2-weighted (B) images. T_1-weighted image appears to show homogeneous testis; however, with T_2-weighted images the heterogeneous nature of testis parenchyma is evident. Usually, comparison can be made with normal-appearing contralateral testis (see Figure 2, Chapter 8). In this case, a benign tumor was noted in an atrophic contralateral testis; note the heterogeneous pattern. (Courtesy Robert Smith MD)*

testis parenchyma in the same testis. The signal intensity on MRI is dependent on the histological nature of the tumor, seminomas usually appearing as a homogeneous low signal mass, whereas non-seminomatous testicular tumors have a heterogeneous low signal intensity[4]. MRI may be specifically helpful in situations in which there is a suspicion that a bilateral process is present or when a diffuse infiltrative disease, e.g. lymphoma, is suspected[8].

The fertility status of the young male patient should always be considered in the diagnosis and treatment of any process affecting the testes, paratesticular structures or genital ducts. In cases of acute testicular pain, real-time gray-scale ultrasonography will not be helpful in differentiating testicular torsion from acute epididymo-orchitis. Color flow Doppler imaging is very helpful in this situation. In testicular torsion, intratesticular color flow is completely absent. Comparison is made with the contralateral testis showing normal intratesticular flow (see Color plate K). In cases of epididymo-orchitis, increased epididymal and intratesticular blood flow are depicted by increased color and brightness[9,10]. Severe epididymitis may result in compression of the testicular vessels, resulting in testicular ischemia or infarction, mimicking torsion. This clinical entity, if identified on color flow Doppler, could be relieved by a relaxing incision in the tunica of the epididymis without entering an epididymal tubule. Witherington reported that, with this approach, the testicular salvage rate was 86%[11]. The long-term salvage effects on fertility are unclear, but certainly identification by color flow Doppler imaging and treatment of this ischemic insult[12] seem likely to be beneficial.

Ultrasonography is being used with increasing frequency to assess testicular size when progressive atrophy or retarded growth of the testicle would change the approach to therapy in a patient with a varicocele. Kass observed that the best way to assess testicular size in an adolescent is to compare size differences between testicles[13]. Use of semi-annual ultrasound examinations repeated by the same operator is sensitive in assessing progressive atrophy. This is indicated in the adolescent with a varicocele or the adult male with a varicocele and associated normal semen parameters who is not currently trying to achieve a pregnancy.

Benign intratesticular pathology that may be noted on scrotal ultrasound examination includes intratesticular cysts, testiculiths, microlithiasis and old hematoma[14]. Small intratesticular cysts are hypoechoic and may represent cysts of the rete testis. On MRI, these cysts are sharply outlined, demonstrate low signal intensity on T_1-weighted images and an increase in signal intensity on T_2-weighted images[8]. However, the relationship to the fertility status of the patient is unclear. Mixed echogenicity from a hematoma resulting from significant trauma is very difficult to differentiate from a testicular tumor. A history of trauma suggests a hematoma, but very often surgical exploration is necessary to rule out a testicular tumor.

Paratesticular structures: varicoceles and hydroceles

The mainstay of diagnosis of a varicocele is physical examination in a warm room. Active cremasteric muscles can sometimes mimic the venous augmentation seen on the Valsalva maneuver, and therefore confirmatory imaging tests are sometimes necessary. Ultrasonography, nuclear scintigraphy, thermography and venography have been used to confirm the presence of a suspected varicocele. We review several of the modalities that are currently used in the diagnosis and treatment of a varicocele.

Historically, the imaging modality used most often as the 'gold standard' for radiographic diagnosis of a varicocele was venography. Early studies comparing physical exmination with venography for the presence of a varicocele showed that physical examination had a 23% false-negative rate[15]. In another study, 33% of patients without clinical varicoceles had radiological evidence of reflux by venography. In patients with a clinically palpable varicocele, reflux was noted in 58% of patients[16]. Thus, venography cannot be relied upon to be the absolute gold standard. The procedure is extremely operator- and experience-dependent. However, most would agree that, despite its invasive nature, it is probably the most accurate method for diagnosing a radiographic varicocele.

Because venography is relatively invasive compared to other diagnostic modalities, its role has become somewhat limited in clinical practice. Indications for venography at present are:

(1) Identification of reflux channels prior to therapeutic radiological embolization of a varicocele;

(2) Confirmation of recurrent or persistent varicocele after surgical repair; and

(3) Contradictory findings on physical and ultrasound examinations.

A venogram showing free reflux into the left spermatic vein is shown in Figure 3. Very often, collateral vessels will run along with the main internal spermatic veins. Important collaterals include high communications such as proximal renal hilar veins, capsular renal veins and left colic veins, and lower communications such as external spermatic veins and possibly gubernacular veins[17].

When a varicocele is identified on venography, radiographic occlusive procedures may be performed. This has been reported using different materials such as sclerosing agents, detachable balloons and stainless steel coils[17]. The success rates with radiographic occlusion of varicoceles approaches that with surgical repair. Good randomized studies have not been performed to date. Complications and recurrence rates are low; however, theoretical major risks of balloon migration and lack of operator experience have limited its widespread use.

The mainstay of radiological identification of a varicocele using current technology is ultrasonography. Ultrasonographic techniques are non-invasive and include a Doppler stethoscope, real-time ultrasound and color flow Doppler imaging. In any radiological examination for a varicocele, the patient

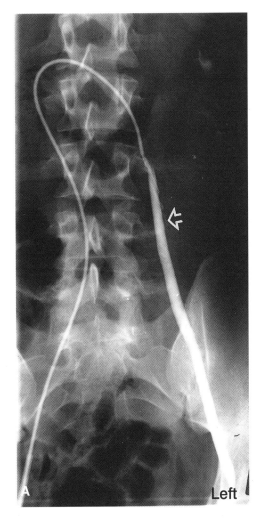

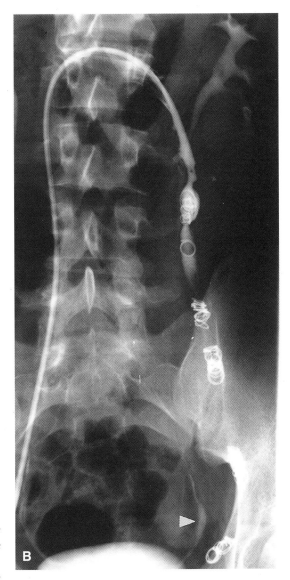

should be scanned in both the supine and the upright position with and without the Valsalva maneuver.

The Doppler stethoscope confirms the presence of a varicocele when a prolonged venous flow augmentation or reflux is detectable, usually as a venous rush during the Valsalva maneuver. This must be differentiated from the mild and transient flow augmentation seen with the Valsalva meneuver in some normal individuals. In addition, active cremastic musculature can make it difficult to obtain exact placement of the ultrasound probe on venous structures.

Because of these shortcomings, real-time ultrasound has been used more reliably to identify varicoceles. Since penetration depth

Figure 3 *Varicocele: internal spermatic venography. (A) Catheter inserted via right femoral vein with tip into left spermatic vein (open arrow) identifies patency of system without valves. Commonly there are some collateral channels in the retroperitoneum that are identified as well. (B) Venogram after placement of coils in the left spermatic vein. Note good embolization (no contrast) of left spermatic vein. Contrast is also being excreted into the kidney (pyelogram) and left distal ureter (arrowhead). From reference 17, with permission*

is short, the use of a high-frequency, 7–10-mHz ultrasound probe is optimal for highest resolution. A varicocele is defined ultrasonographically as a hollow, tubular structure that increases in size on the Valsalva maneuver (Figure 4). Different authors have used different criteria for an ultrasonographic varicocele. McClure and colleagues[18] have defined a varicocele as being present if three veins are present, with one of them at least 3 mm in diameter at rest or an increase in venous diameter with the Valsalva maneuver (Figure 4). However, several other investigators[19,20] have used 2–3 mm as the cut-off value. Variable definitions have created difficulty in comparing results of diagnostic modalities and treatment. However, there appears to be a good correlation between real-time ultrasound and venography[19].

Confirmation of the presence of a varicocele has most recently been described by color flow Doppler imaging. This modality combines real-time ultrasound with pulsed Doppler in one non-invasive scan using color identification of blood flow superimposed on the gray-scale image. Prolonged flow augmentation seen as lightened hues within a colored flow area depicted on real-time imaging confirms the reversal of flow characteristic of a varicocele (Color plate L). As with most ultrasound studies, color flow Doppler imaging is very operator-dependent.

Excellent correlation is seen between venography and color flow Doppler imaging in the diagnosis of varicoceles. Petros and co-workers[21] identified more varicoceles with this method than with routine physical examination when venography was used as the gold standard. Eskew and colleagues[22] noted that color flow Doppler was very sensitive (85%) in identifying subclinical varicoceles when venography was used as the gold standard. Recently, Meacham and associates[23] evaluated 34 asymptomatic young men in the general population by physical examination, gray-scale ultrasound and color flow Doppler ultrasound and noted the incidence of varicoceles to be 15%, 18% and 35%, respectively. It appears that color-coded reversal of venous flow is identifying more subclinical varicoceles. The importance of these 'color Doppler reversal of flow' varicoceles to the infertility status of the couple is unclear at present.

Ligation of a clinical (palpable) varicocele is generally accepted as a reasonable treatment for improvement of semen quality and pregnancy rates in infertile men. However, the management of the radiologically identified (non-palpable) subclinical varicocele is controversial. In their report on 150 men with a varicocele and infertility, Dubin and Amelar[24] concluded that the size of the varicocele did not correlate with the degree of impairment of spermatogenesis. Therefore, a small varicocele detected only by radiological

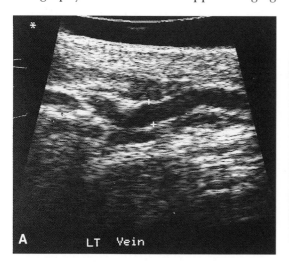
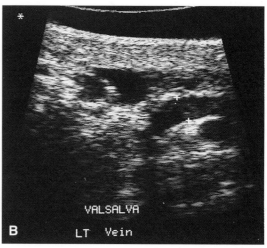

Figure 4 *Varicocele: gray-scale ultrasound scans. Tubular structure (cursors) shows dilated vein (A) that increases in size with the Valsalva maneuver (B). From reference 49, with permission*

assessment may have a profound effect on spermatogenesis. The incidence of the subclinical varicocele in the infertile population ranges from 21 to 80%. Table 1 summarizes the most recent studies[18,20,25–28] evaluating the treatment of subclinical varicoceles.

Overall, there appears to be an improvement in semen quality after varicocelectomy in patients with a subclinical varicocele. However, none of these studies contained a control observation arm. Different techniques and criteria were used by different authors to define a subclinical varicocele, making it difficult to compare data from different groups. A prospective, randomized study using the same detection technique, with cross-over of the non-treatment group at 1 year, would answer this question, but has not been performed to date. We do not recommend routine repair of a subclinical varicocele and therefore do not scan all infertile males for such an entity. However, we do use real-time ultrasound to confirm a varicocele (at least one vein of ≥ 3 mm) suspected on physical examination.

A hydrocele is another clinical entity that can be identified radiographically. The tunica vaginalis is visualized on ultrasound only if a fluid interface is present. A hydrocele is characterized ultrasonographically by a hypoechoic image anterior to and laterally surrounding the testis (Figure 5). Although this entity has been identified by MRI, MRI for this purpose is limited to situations with equivocal findings on ultrasound. Hydroceles may be communicating or non-communicating, but this cannot be identified by ultrasound. Sometimes if a hydrocele is present, testicular and epididymal appendages may be visualized. If the hydrocele is loculated, there may be streaks of hyperechoic lines running within the anechoic-appearing sac. This suggests bleeding or infection. The presence of a hydrocele in the infertile male requires careful examination of the testis for the presence of ultrasonographic abnormalities consistent with a testis tumor. Most testicular tumors will have an associated small

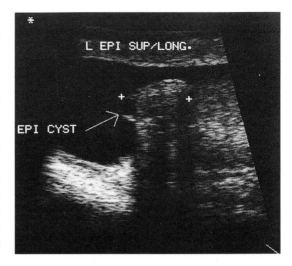

Figure 5 *Epididymal cyst, hydrocele: gray-scale ultrasound scan. Normal epididymis is identified by cursors; adjacent cyst has no internal echoes (arrow). Hydrocele is also present. From reference 49, with permission*

hydrocele. Fluid movement within a hydrocele may be confused with a varicocele on color flow Doppler imaging, because moving fluid of any type will be identified by color[9]. Correlation with the real-time image is necessary for differentiation.

SPERM MATURATION

Epididymis

Careful examination of the epididymis is important in a male infertility evaluation. Real-time and color flow Doppler scanning of the epididymis are helpful, but in different situations.

Patients presenting to a male infertility clinic may have infection or inflammation of the epididymis as a clinical finding. Although acute epididymitis is a clinical diagnosis, ultrasonographic findings include an enlarged, heterogeneous epididymis with decreased echogenicity. Chronic inflammation usually results in an enlarged, indurated epididymis with mixed echogenicity, sometimes with hyperechoic calcification (Figure 6). In a comparison of epididymal size, Nashan and

Table 1 Summary of subclinical varicocele data. From reference 48

Year	Authors	Detection method	Definition of varicocele	No. of patients	Method of treatment	% improved	Improved parameter	Follow-up (months)
1992	Dhabuwala et al.[28]	Doppler	⊕ reflux	16	surgery	81	concentration; morphology	12
1991	McClure et al.[18]	real-time	> 3 mm diameter	18	surgery	N/A	motility ($p < 0.09$)	12
1989	Yarborough et al.[26]	venography	retrograde flow	13	embolization	N/A	concentration	6
1988	Bsat and Masabni[27]	Doppler	⊕ reflux	15	surgery	27	concentration; motility	12
1987	Gonda et al.[20]	real-time scintigraphy	> 2 mm diameter	19	surgery	94	concentration; motility	?
1985	Marsman[25]	venography	retrograde flow	24	embolization	55	concentration; motility	> 6

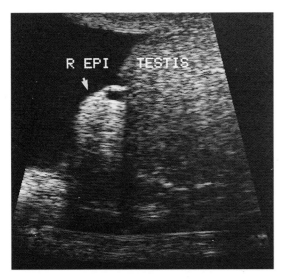

Figure 6 *Chronic epididymitis: gray-scale ultrasound scan. Note the hyperechoic epididymis (arrow) suggestive of scarring and possible epididymal obstruction. Normal testis on right. From reference 49, with permission*

they may be loculated. Spermatoceles (containing sperm) and epididymal cysts (containing no sperm) have similar ultrasonographic patterns and are usually located at the head of the epididymis. Rarely, an epididymal cyst will compress the epididymal tubules and cause an epididymal obstruction. Epididymal obstruction can usually be confirmed on ultrasound by the increased size of the epididymis. However, this sign is not completely reliable. Most epididymal cysts do not cause obstruction. However, an epididymal cyst associated with severe oligoasthenospermia or azoospermia may be compressing the epididymis, causing obstruction. A formal scrotal exploration and possibly unroofing of the cyst may be helpful in improving semen quality. This should be approached very cautiously, however, in the non-azoospermic patient.

colleagues[29] confirmed their clinical suspicion of epididymal thickening by ultrasound. A thickened epididymis (mean 12.1 mm) on palpation was significantly different in size ($p < 0.5$) from the normal epididymis by palpation (mean 7 mm).

Color flow Doppler imaging has been helpful in differentiating acute epididymitis from testicular torsion. The normal epididymis rarely reveals an active blood flow pattern on this type of imaging. With acute epididymitis, increased vascularity cannot be identified on gray-scale real-time imaging, but will be noted on color flow Doppler[9]. Evaluation of intratesticular blood flow by color flow Doppler imaging is the key to differentiating torsion from epididymitis. Early aggressive treatment of epididymitis with antibiotics and anti-inflammatory medications may result in a decreased incidence of scarring and epididymal obstruction.

Spermatoceles and epididymal cysts palpated on physical examination may be confirmed by ultrasound. Cysts are hypoechoic masses with through transmission and posterior enhancement (Figure 5). Sometimes

SPERM TRANSPORT

In the previous chapter, we reviewed the normal anatomy of the distal genital ductal system. Herein, we discuss the evolving role of transrectal ultrasound (TRUS), MRI, intraoperative and TRUS-guided vasoseminovesiculography, and intraoperative diagnostic maneuvers in the diagnosis and treatment of anatomical abnormalities of the distal genital ductal system.

Seminal vesicles

The anatomical abnormalities of the seminal vesicles are best imaged by TRUS or MRI. Extrinsic compression by a large seminal vesicle (Wolffian duct) cyst can result in ejaculatory duct obstruction. This is a congenital anomaly which results from an ectopic ureter[30,31] inserting into the seminal vesicle or ejaculatory duct, associated with a hypoplastic kidney. TRUS will reveal a laterally positioned, cystic, anechoic mass where the seminal vesicle should be.

MRI will also identify seminal vesicle cysts that obstruct the ejaculatory ducts. Signal intensity on T_1- and T_2-weighted images depends on the fluid content in the seminal vesicles[32]. Classically, however, seminal vesicle cysts are of low signal on T_1- and high signal on T_2-weighted images, suggesting that they are fluid filled[33]. Such cysts may obstruct the ejaculatory duct and may be treated by drainage, transrectally[34]. However, they may recur.

Distal ejaculatory duct obstruction may result in dilatation of the seminal vesicles as seen on TRUS and MRI. In this situation, the seminal vesicles lose their internal echo pattern and appear as hypoechoic saccules on TRUS (Figures 7A and 8A). This situation is also nicely depicted in TRUS and MRI images in the transverse plane (see Figure 12). On MRI, the thickened walls of the seminal vesicles have very low signal intensity on T_2-weighted images consistent with chronic inflammation[35,36]. The MRI internal signal intensity pattern of dilated seminal vesicles has not been characterized to date.

Patients with bilateral congenital absence of the vas deferens received an embryological insult that affects the development of the mesonephric ductal system. In one study, most patients with this condition were shown by TRUS to have evidence of at least a unilateral seminal vesicle abnormality[37]. A total of 72 individual seminal vesicle units were examined, with 29% shown as normal, 17% as hypoplastic, 36% as atrophic and 18% as completely absent. Figures 7 and 8 show a spectrum of seminal vesicle abnormalities in bilateral congenital absence of the vas deferens. These may involve absent, atrophic or dilated seminal vesicles.

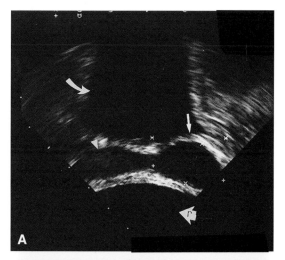

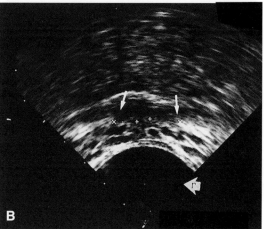

Figure 7 *Spectrum of seminal vesicle abnormalities: transverse transrectal ultrasound images. (A) Dilated right seminal vesicle (thin white arrow), normal left seminal vesicle (arrowhead), distended bladder (curved arrow) and rectum (broad white arrow, r). (B) Absent seminal vesicles in patient with congenital bilateral absence of the vas deferens. Arrows point to area where seminal vesicles should be (broad white arrow, r, rectum). From reference 49, with permission*

Ejaculatory ducts/prostate

Extrinsic or intrinsic processes may cause ejaculatory duct obstruction that is responsible for male factor infertility. Perineal pain, hematospermia or epididymitis may also be present. Although these patients usually have a low volume of ejaculate, a normal volume does not rule out ejaculatory duct obstruction[30,38]. Absence of seminal

fructose is not a reliable sign of obstruction, as partial obstruction accounting for subfertility may be present. It is clear that partial ejaculatory duct obstruction does occur, and therefore the indications for TRUS in the infertile male have been broadened. TRUS has replaced vasography as the first-line diagnostic modality of evaluation for ejaculatory duct obstruction. Indications for

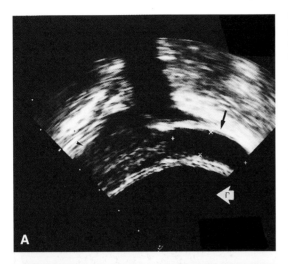

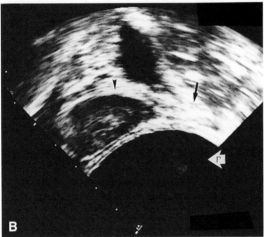

Figure 8 *Spectrum of seminal vesicle abnormalities: Sagittal transrectal ultrasound images. (A) Dilated seminal vesicle: black arrow (note hypoechoic nature), black arrowhead shows normal prostate; broad arrow, r, rectum. (B) Absent seminal vesicle: black arrow shows area where seminal vesicle is usually located; black arrowhead shows normal prostate; broad white arrow, r, rectum. From reference 49, with permission*

Table 2 *Indications for transrectal ultrasonography in the subfertile male. From reference 42*

Absolute indications

  Low-volume azoospermia, absence of severe testicular atrophy

  Low-volume severe oligospermia (concentration < 5 million/ml)

  Palpable abnormality on digital rectal examination

  Unexplained retrograde ejaculation

Relative indications

  Normal-volume oligospermia or azoospermia, absence of severe testicular atrophy

  Severe motility defects (motility less than 25% and/or sluggish forward progression)

  Severe sperm morphology defects

  Any ejaculatory abnormality (e.g. anejaculation, hematospermia, painful ejaculation)

  History suggestive of genital duct abnormalities (unilaterally non-functioning kidney, history of severe hypospadias)

  Elevated seminal leukocytes, history of prostatitis

TRUS in the infertile male are listed in Table 2. Meacham and co-workers[39] reported that patients with partial ejaculatory duct obstruction (i.e. not azoospermic) identified by TRUS showed improved semen quality after transurethral resection of the ejaculatory ducts (TURED) in 72% of cases with an overall pregnancy rate of 54%. However, more recent data with broadened indications for TURED based on TRUS findings have indicated lower success rates[38]. Patients with ejaculatory duct obstruction usually have normal-sized testes and a normal serum level of follicle stimulating hormone (FSH). Digital rectal examination rarely reveals any significant masses, but sometimes a palpable mass is present. Associated epididymal induration as a result of long-standing obstruction is not uncommon. A history of prior bladder neck surgery or other pelvic surgery may suggest an iatrogenically induced ejaculatory duct obstruction.

Ejaculatory duct cysts, ejaculatory duct calcification, dilated ejaculatory ducts and dilated seminal vesicles are findings consistent with obstruction (Figures 9–12). A Müllerian duct cyst (prostatic utricular cyst; see Figure 11) may be present under the base of the bladder, between the seminal vesicles, causing extrinsic compression of the ejaculatory duct[40,41]. A history of severe hypospadias and subsequent repair may alert the clinician to such an entity. A Wolffian duct cyst can be differentiated from a Müllerian duct cyst because of the presence of sperm in the former[40]. Any of these findings strongly

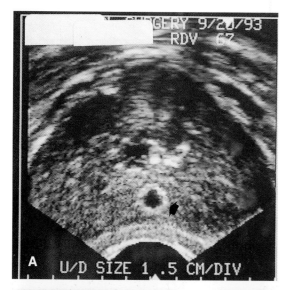

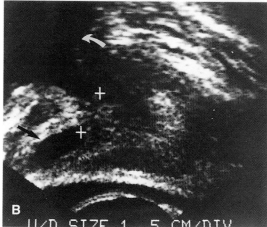

Figure 9 *Dilated ejaculatory duct: transrectal ultrasound scans. (A) Transverse view of dilated ejaculatory duct (black arrow) in prostate. (B) Sagittal view of dilated ejaculatory duct. Cursors measure distance from ejaculatory duct cyst (black arrow) to urethra; see bladder (curved white arrow) above. From reference 49, with permission*

suggest ejaculatory duct obstruction, which can be treated successfully in most cases with transurethral resection of the ejaculatory ducts (TURED).

MRI has been used to identify dilated ejaculatory ducts suspected from the patient's history and semen analysis[35,36]. MRI of the pelvis with and without an endorectal coil has been helpful in identifying dilated ejaculatory

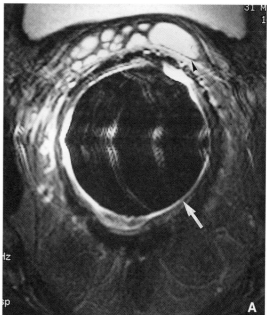

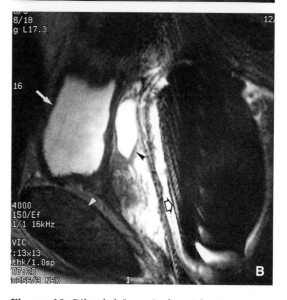

Figure 10 *Dilated left seminal vesicle: T₂-weighted magnetic resonance image using endorectal coil. (A) Transverse plane shows cross-sections of normal seminal vesicle on right and dilated seminal vesicle on left (arrowhead), rectum with coil (white arrow). (B) Sagittal view shows dilated seminal vesicle (black arrowhead), bladder (white arrow), endorectal coil (open black arrow) and pubic bone (white arrowhead)*

ducts. This has best been displayed on coronal and sagittal T₂-weighted spin echo imaging. Fluid in an obstructed ejaculatory duct or

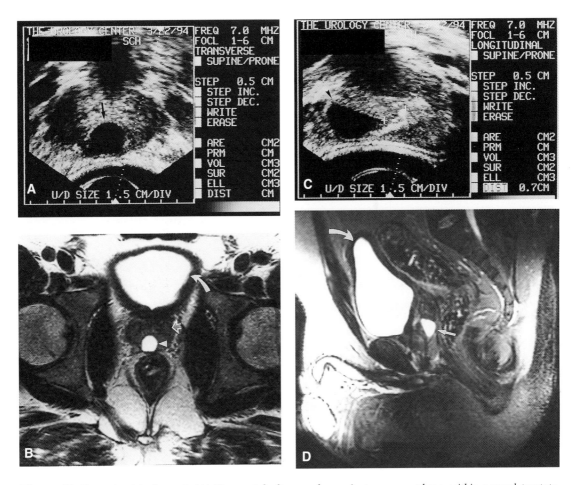

Figure 11 *Prostatic utricular cyst. (A) Transrectal ultrasound scan in transverse plane: within normal prostate, hypoechoic mass (black arrow) is shown obstructing seminal vesicle. (B) T_2-weighted magnetic resonance image in transverse plane. The same patient, with cyst (arrowhead) within prostate (open arrow); bladder above (curved arrow). (C) Transrectal ultrasound scan in sagittal plane. Same patient, with hypoechoic cyst (black arrowhead); cursors measure distance from urethra. (D) T_2-weighted magnetic resonance image in sagittal plane. The same patient, with prostatic cyst (white arrow); bladder (curved arrow)*

prostatic utricular cyst usually shows a high signal on T_2-weighted MRI imaging consistent with hemorrhage or high protein content (see Figure 11B and D).

In cases in which ejaculatory duct obstruction is suspected but TRUS or MRI is indeterminate, formal vasography can confirm ejaculatory duct obstruction. Vasography is still considered the 'gold standard' for identification of distal ejaculatory duct obstruction and obstruction of the vas deferens in areas proximal to the vasal ampulla. Lack of contrast in the bladder associated with a dilated seminal vesicle and ejaculatory duct

on vasography is pathognomonic of complete ejaculatory duct obstruction. This is confirmed by subjectively high injection pressure (vas irrigated with a 50 : 50 mixture of renograffin and indigo carmine) into the vas deferens and lack of indigo carmine-colored urine on bladder catheterization. Whereas TRUS identifies anatomical abnormalities, vasal injection pressure gives subjective physiological information about the ductal system.

Intraoperative examination of vasal fluid is an essential part of a vasal exploration[42]. The gross quality of the exuding fluid should be

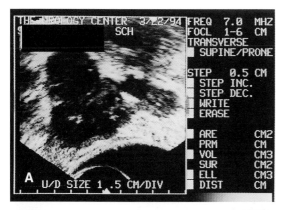

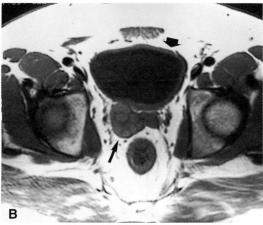

Figure 12 *Dilated right seminal vesicle from prostatic utricular cyst. (A) Transrectal ultrasound scan in transverse plane: hypoechoic, dilated and obstructed right seminal vesicle, resulting from prostatic utricular cyst, seen in Figure 11. (B) T₁-weighted magnetic resonance image in transverse plane. Thin arrow points to dilated right seminal vesicle obstructed by prostatic utricular cyst, seen in Figure 11. Broad arrow, bladder*

noted (i.e. clear, cloudy or inspissated), and then examined microscopically for the presence or absence of sperm. The presence of many sperm (motile or non-motile) confirms that obstruction is present distal to the vasotomy site. If sperm are absent, the system is either not obstructed, and there is an associated epididymal obstruction, or there is a problem with sperm production. In the contrary situation in which vasal exploration shows high injection pressure, sperm are not present in thick inspissated vasal fluid and the epididymal tubules are dilated, we usually

perform TURED and microscopic epididymal reconstruction at the same sitting. If the decision is made to perform TURED only, and postoperatively the seminal volume increases but the patient remains azoospermic, microscopic epididymal reconstruction may be performed subsequently.

Partial obstruction of the ejaculatory duct is characterized by high vasal injection pressure associated with dilated seminal vesicles and ejaculatory ducts and some contrast noted in the bladder on vasography (Figure 13). If high vasal injection pressure is noted subjectively and blue urine is noted on bladder catheterization, the diagnosis of partial obstruction is made. Usually, intra-operative vasal fluid sampling reveals motile sperm in the proximal vasal fluid.

Some have recommended a vasal exploration and formal vasography prior to all TURED procedures. This is helpful to determine whether the ejaculatory ducts have been opened by TURED. In this situation, once communication between the ejaculatory duct and urethra is established after TURED, indigo carmine (blue-black) is seen exuding from the ejaculatory duct. Confirmation of patency of an opened ejaculatory duct has been made by passing an 0.038 guidewire endoscopically through the newly opened ejaculatory duct (approximately 2–3 cm)[42].

Potential complications of vasal exploration include vasal stricture formation (from scar formation or loss of blood supply), bleeding, infection and sperm granuloma formation. For these reasons, vasal exploration is not recommended in straightforward cases of ejaculatory duct obstruction identified with TRUS prior to TURED.

Recently, some experience has been gained with TRUS-guided vasoseminovesiculo-graphy[43]. Under TRUS guidance, a dilated seminal vesicle may be aspirated and then injected with contrast to delineate the anatomy of the distal genital ductal system (Chapter 8, Figure 9). The aspirated fluid is examined microscopically for the presence of sperm. Normally, sperm are not present in the seminal vesicles. The presence of motile

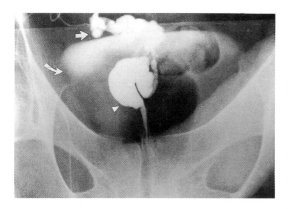

Figure 13 *Partial ejaculatory duct obstruction on vasography. Right vasogram shows dilated seminal vesicle (white arrow), dilated ejaculatory duct (arrowhead) and some contrast in bladder (curved arrow) consistent with partial ejaculatory duct obstruction. From reference 42, with permission*

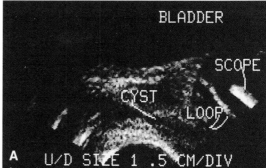

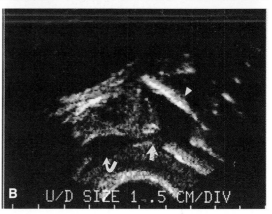

Figure 14 *(A) intraoperative ultrasound scan of ejaculatory duct cyst just prior to resection. (B) Ejaculatory duct cyst just after resection (resectoscope indicated by arrowhead). Note communication (arrow) between cyst (curved arrow) and urethra, not seen on (A). From reference 49, with permission*

or non-motile sperm, however, confirms obstruction of the seminal vesicles.

We have used intraoperative transrectal ultrasonography to identify the location of a small ejaculatory duct cyst in relationship to the urethra. This may be helpful in determining the depth of resection and may be re-checked intraoperatively after each step of endoscopic resection performed, if proximity to the anterior rectal wall is a concern. In Figure 14A, ultrasonographic evidence of an ejaculatory duct cyst is seen. After the resection, a communication between the ejaculatory duct cyst and the urethra is clearly visualized (Figure 14B). An 0.038 guidewire has been used to cannulate the ejaculatory ducts endoscopically, to document patency.

The prevalence of ejaculatory duct cysts in the infertile population and the elderly screened population has been reported[44]. Of the screening group, 5% (20/400) had evidence of cystic dilatation of the ejaculatory duct. In the infertile population, 17% (23/135) had similar findings. The difference in prevalence was statistically significant ($p < 0.01$). An infertility questionnaire was given to all patients in the older screened group. Of patients with normal ejaculatory ducts, 14% did not have children; however, of those with ejaculatory duct cysts, 35% did not have

children ($p < 0.01$). These patients were not age-matched control groups, and thorough infertility histories were not obtained. These data do suggest, however, that ejaculatory duct cysts may affect fertility status, and are relatively uncommon in the general population.

Vas deferens/vasal ampulla

The vasal ampullae are well visualized by TRUS in the transverse plane in the normal condition (Figure 5 in Chapter 8). In patients with bilateral congenital absence of the scrotal vas deferens, the vasal ampulla was absent in 64% of cases in a study using TRUS[37]. Sometimes when the spermatic cord is thickened, palpation of the vas deferens can be difficult. In this situation, the use of TRUS is recommended to determine whether a vasal ampulla is present. MRI using coronal sections may also be helpful in this regard. An acidic, low-volume ejaculate with azoospermia and absence of the vasal ampulla with associated seminal vesicle abnormalities confirms the diagnosis of bilateral congenital absence of the vas deferens. Appropriate counselling regarding treatment with microscopic epididymal sperm aspiration in conjunction with *in vitro* fertilization is instituted. These patients have a significantly higher risk of being a carrier of genes responsible for cystic fibrosis (Δ508 and others) and therefore must be counselled appropriately prior to any fertility-related procedures[45]. Bilateral congenital absence of the vas deferens has a spectrum of anomalies. A case of this is shown in the vasogram in Figure 15. This shows a patient with unilateral left congenital absence of the vas deferens, a palpable right contralateral scrotal vas deferens and azoospermia, where the palpable right vas deferens ends blindly in the retroperitoneum.

Because minimally invasive testing has been able to delineate male genital anatomical abnormalities quite well, the indications for vasal exploration and vasography have decreased significantly. Indications for formal vasography are:

(1) Suspected inguinal vasal obstruction;

(2) Indeterminate TRUS or MRI with clinical suggestion of ejaculatory duct obstruction; and

(3) Prior to transurethral resection of ejaculatory duct (only advocated by some).

When inguinal vasal obstruction is suspected, formal vasography should be performed, to determine the site of obstruction. If this is a result of a prior inguinal hernia repair, the obstruction is almost always at the level of the internal ring. On the vasogram in Figure 15, the large white arrow indicates the area where the vas will end abruptly in the case of an

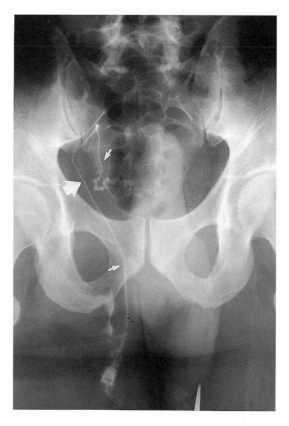

Figure 15 *Vas deferens: intraoperative scrotal vasogram. Note contrast in vas deferens (small arrows) which never reaches seminal vesicle or bladder, but ends blindly in retroperitoneum. Transrectal ultrasound showed very atrophic seminal vesicles. If inguinal vasal injury were present, contrast would stop at the level of the large arrow (compare to Chapter 8, Figure 9)*

inguinal vasal injury. Alternatively, a zero proline suture may be passed through the vasal lumen to determine the distance from the vasotomy to the site of obstruction. It should be emphasized that the vasal lumen on the testicular side should never be injected with contrast or fluid to document epididymal obstruction. This is likely to result in high epididymal pressure with subsequent epididymal blowout, scarring and obstruction.

More recently, attempts have been made to identify inguinal vasal obstruction using TRUS-guided vasoseminovesiculography[43]. If the scrotal vas deferens is identified, no inguinal obstruction is present. If the vas deferens fills to the level of the internal ring and stops abruptly, this is suggestive but not pathognomonic of inguinal vasal obstruction. If obstruction is present microscopic inguinal vasovasotomy would be performed to restore continuity to the sperm transport system.

Urethra/penis

The urethra is the final conduit through which the semen travels during ejaculation. Abnormalities of the urethra or bladder neck can result in partial or complete retrograde ejaculation[46]. Clinically, this presents as no antegrade ejaculation or low-volume ejaculation. The diagnosis can be made by examination of a post-ejaculate urine specimen for the presence of sperm. If retrograde ejaculation is present, the cause of the problem must be ascertained, since treatment may often restore strong and forceful antegrade ejaculation. A common cause of non-neurogenic retrograde ejaculation is the presence of a urethral stricture. A history of trauma, urethral instrumentation or sexually transmitted diseases suggest this. Patients may complain of decreased urinary stream or a spraying urinary stream. The diagnosis may be made with either cystoscopy or retrograde urethrography. Figure 16 shows a retrograde urethrogram with evidence of a mid-urethral stricture. Note the narrowing of the mid-portion of the urethra with contrast in urethral veins as a result of back pressure. A simple endoscopic incision of the narrowing will usually restore antegrade ejaculation and may allow a couple to achieve a pregnancy through natural timed intercourse. Bladder neck abnormalities such as a ureterocele affecting the bladder neck or previous surgical injury from Y–V plasty surgery of the bladder neck may result in retrograde ejaculation[46]. Transrectal ultrasound will identify an open bladder neck in these cases.

If antegrade ejaculation is present, deposition of semen in the vagina near the cervix is a prerequisite for achieving a pregnancy through natural intercourse. Peyronie's disease is a pathological deposition of collagen in the tunica albuginea of the

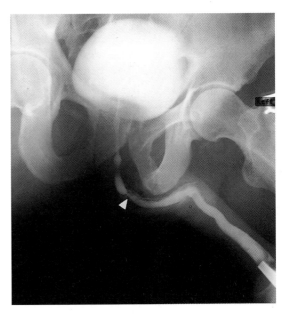

Figure 16 *Urethra: retrograde urethrogram. Arrowhead points to area of narrowing in the urethra with distal dilatation. Note retrograde filling of urethral veins from back pressure. This lesion could result in retrograde ejaculation. (Courtesy Morton Glickman MD)*

penis that results in penile curvature. This disease will sometimes preclude a couple's ability to have intercourse. In general, the diagnosis of Peyronie's disease is clinical; however, both ultrasound and MRI (Figure 17) have been used to identify scar formation in the penis. Penile straightening procedures may be performed to permit successful vaginal penetration and semen deposition.

Problems with erectile dysfunction may also result in coital factor infertility. Radiological studies such as duplex Doppler ultrasound examination of penile vasculature, dynamic cavernosometry or cavernosography may be helpful in determining the etiology of the problem[47]. However, review of these radiological tests is beyond the scope of this chapter.

CONCLUSION

New diagnostic imaging modalities have taken on a major role in the diagnosis and treatment of disease entities related to male infertility. When any disease process affects

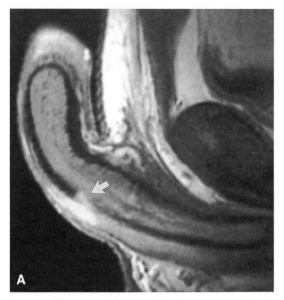 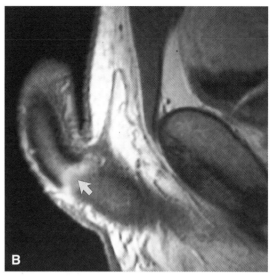

Figure 17 *Penis with Peyronie's disease: T_1-weighted magnetic resonance images with gadolinium; serial sagittal sections. Note the scar at the ventral aspect of mid-shaft of penis in (A) (arrow) and the circumferential scar in (B) (arrow), resulting in penile curvature. (Courtesy Robert Smith MD)*

the male in the reproductive or pre-reproductive years, potential repercussions on subsequent male factor fertility should always be addressed in the treatment plans of such patients.

Scrotal ultrasound examination is extremely helpful in identification of abnormalities of the testis parenchyma, paratesticular structures and blood flow in the region of the testes. TRUS has replaced the vasogram as the initial diagnostic test for evaluation of the prostate, ejaculatory duct and seminal vesicles in the infertile male. It may also be used as an adjunct to treatment in these patients. MRI may become a useful adjunct to TRUS in defining male genital ductal anatomy prior to surgical exploration. Vasal exploration including subjective assessment of vasal injection pressure, vasal fluid examination and vasography are important diagnostic tools in the diagnosis and treatment of male genital pathology.

Ultrasound, MRI, contrast studies and new operative diagnostic maneuvers will continue to define the anatomy, physiology and pathology of the male reproductive system.

References

1. Honig, S. C., Lipshultz, L. I. and Jarow, J. (1994). Significant medical pathology uncovered by a comprehensive male infertility evaluation. *Fertil. Steril.*, **62**, 1028–34
2. Schultz-Lampel, D., Bogaert, G., Thuroff, J. W., Schlegel, E. and Cramer, B. (1991). MRI for evaluation of scrotal pathology. *Urol. Res.*, **19**, 282–92
3. Fritzsche, P. J. (1988). MRI of the scrotum. *Urol. Radiol.*, **10**, 52–7
4. Mattrey, R. F. (1991). Magnetic resonance imaging of the scrotum. *Semin. Ultrasound Comput. Tomogr. Magn. Reson.*, **12**, 95–108
5. Baker, L. L., Hajek, P. C., Burkhard, T. K. *et al.* (1987). MR imaging of the scrotum: pathologic conditions. *Radiology*, **163**, 93–8

6. Rholl, K. S., Lee, J. K. T., Ling, D., Heiken, J. P. and Glazer, H. S. (1987). MR imaging of the scrotum with a high resolution surface coil. *Radiology*, **163**, 99–103

7. Thurner, S., Hricak, H., Carroll, P. R., Filly, R. A. and Pobiel, R. (1988). Imaging the testis: comparison between MR imaging and ultrasound. *Radiology*, **167**, 631–6

8. Hricak, H. (1991). The testis/the seminal vesicles. In Hricak, H. and Carrington, B. M. (eds.) *MRI of the pelvis: A Text Atlas*, pp. 313–53. (Appleton and Lange)

9. Horstman, W. G., Middleton, W. D., Melson, G. L. and Siegel, B. A. (1991). Color Doppler US of the scrotum. *Radiographics*, **11**, 941–57

10. Jafri, S. Z., Madrazo, B. L. and Miller, J. H. (1992). Color Doppler ultrasound of the genitourinary tract. *Curr. Opin. Radiol.*, **4**, 16–23

11. Witherington, R. and Harper, W. M. (1982). The surgical management of acute bacterial epididymitis with emphasis on epididymotomy. *J. Urol.*, **128**, 722–6

12. Vordermark, J. S. and Favila, M. Q. (1982). Testicular necrosis: a preventable complication of epididymitis. *J. Urol.*, **128**, 1322–4

13. Kass, E. J. (1990). Evaluation and management of the adolescent with a varicocele. *AUA Update Series*, vol. 9, lesson 12

14. O'Mara, E. M. and Rifkin, M. D. (1991). In Resnick, M. and Rifkin, M. D. (eds.) *Ultrasonography of the Urinary Tract*, 3rd edn, pp. 386–431. (Baltimore: Williams and Wilkins)

15. World Health Organization (1985). Comparison among different methods for the diagnosis of varicocele. *Fertil. Steril.*, **43**, 575–7

16. Rodrigues-Netto, N. Jr, Lerner, J. S., Paolini, R. M. *et al.* (1980). Varicocele: the value of reflux in the spermatic vein. *Int. J. Fertil.*, **25**, 71

17. White, R. I. Jr. (1994). Radiologic management of varicoceles using embolotherapy. In Whitehead, D. and Nagler, E. D. (eds.) *Management of Impotence and Infertility*, pp. 228–40. (Philadelphia: J. B. Lippincott)

18. McClure, D., Khoo, D., Jarvi, K. and Hricak, H. (1991). Subclinical varicocele: the effectiveness of varicocelectomy. *J. Urol.*, **145**, 789–91

19. Geatti, O., Gasparini, D. and Shapiro, B. (1991). A comparison of scintigraphy, thermography, ultrasound and phlebography in grading of clinical varicocele. *J. Nucl. Med.*, **32**, 2092–7

20. Gonda, R., Karo, J., Forte, R. and O'Donnell, K. (1987). Diagnosis of subclinical varicocele in infertility. *Am. J. Roentgenol.*, **148**, 71–5

21. Petros, J., Andriole, G., Middleton, W. and Picus, D. (1990). Correlation of testicular color Doppler ultrasonography, physical examination and venography in the detection of left varicoceles in men with infertility. *J. Urol.*, **145**, 785–8

22. Eskew, A., Watson, N., Wolfman, N., Bechtold, R., Scharling, E. and Jarow, J. (1993). The accuracy of ultrasonographic diagnosis of varicoceles. *J. Urol.*, **149**, 438A

23. Meacham, R. B., Townsend, R. R., Rademacher, D. and Drose, J. A. (1994). The incidence of varicoceles in the general population when evaluated by physical examination, gray scale sonography and color Doppler sonography. *J. Urol.*, **151**, 1535–8

24. Dubin, L. and Amelar, R. (1970). Varicocele size and results of varicocelectomy in selected subfertile men with a varicocele. *Fertil. Steril.*, **21**, 606–9

25. Marsman, J. (1985). Clinical versus subclinical varicocele: venographic findings and improvement of fertility after embolization. *Radiology*, **155**, 635–8

26. Yarborough, M., Burns, J. and Keller, F. (1989). Incidence and clinical significance of subclinical scrotal varicoceles. *J. Urol.*, **141**, 1372–4

27. Bsat, F. and Masabni, R. (1988). Effectiveness of varicocelectomy in varicoceles diagnosed by physical examination versus Doppler studies. *Fertil. Steril.*, **50**, 321–4

28. Dhabuwala, C., Hamid, S. and Moghissi, K. (1992). Clinical versus subclinical varicocele: improvement in fertility after varicocelectomy. *Fertil. Steril.*, **57**, 854–7

29. Nashan, D., Behre, H. M., Grunert, J. H. and Nieschlag, E. (1990). Diagnostic value of scrotal sonography in infertile men: report on 658 cases. *Andrologia*, **22**, 387–95

30. Carter, S. S. C., Shinohara, K. and Lipshultz, L. I. (1989). Transrectal ultrasonography in disorders of the seminal vesicles and ejaculatory ducts. *Urol. Clin. North Am.*, **16**, 787–99

31. Asch, M. R. and Toi, A. (1991). Seminal vesicles: imaging and intervention using transrectal ultrasound. *J. Ultrasound Med.*, **10**, 19–23

32. Secaf, E., Nuruddin, R. N., Hricak, H., McClure, R. D. and Demas, B. (1991). MR imaging of the seminal vesicles. *Am. J. Roentgenol.*, **156**, 989–94

33. Gevenois, P. A., Van Sinoy, M. L., Sintzoff, S. A., Stallenberg, B., Salmon, I., Van Regemorter, G. V. and Struyven, J. (1990). Cysts of the prostate and seminal vesicles: MR imaging findings in 11 cases. *Am. J. Roentgenol.*, **155**, 1021–4

34. Shabsigh, R., Lerner, S. and Fishman, I. J. (1989). The role of transrectal ultrasonography in the diagnosis and management of prostatic and seminal vesicle cysts. *J. Urol.*, **141**, 1206–9

35. Schnall, M. D., Pollack, H. M., Van Arsdalen, K. and Kressel, H. Y. (1992). The seminal tract in patients with ejaculatory dysfunction: MR imaging with an endorectal surface coil. *Am. J. Roentgenol.*, **159**, 337–41

36. Weintraub, M. P., Dermouy, E. and Hellstrom, W. J. (1993). Newer modalities in the diagnosis and treatment of ejaculatory duct obstruction. *J. Urol.*, **150**, 1150–4

37. Honig, S. C., Lamont, J. and Oates, R. D. (1991). Ultrasonographic renal and seminal vesicle anomalies in patients with bilateral congenital absence of the vas deferens. *J. Urol.*, **145**, 326a

38. Thompson, S., Shirvani, A., Honig, S. C. and Lipshultz, L. I. (1993). Transurethral resection of ejaculatory duct cysts: comparison of results in high and low volume azoospermia/severe oligospermia. *J. Urol.*, **149**, 436A

39. Meacham, R. B., Hellerstein, D. K. and Lipshultz, L. I. (1993). Evaluation and treatment of ejaculatory duct obstruction in the infertile male. *Fertil. Steril.*, **59**, 393–7

40. Pryor, J. P. and Hendry, W. F. (1991). Ejaculatory duct obstruction in subfertile males: analysis of 87 patients. *Fertil. Steril.*, **56**, 725–30

41. Sharlip, I. D. (1984). Obstructive azoospermia or oligozoospermia due to Mullerian duct cyst. *Fertil. Steril.*, **41**, 298–303

42. Honig, S. C. (1994). New diagnostic techniques in the evaluation of anatomic abnormalities of the infertile male. *Urol. Clin. North Am.*, **21**, 417–32

43. Jarow, J. P. (1994). Seminal vesicle aspiration in the management of patients with ejaculatory duct obstruction. *J. Urol.*, **152**, 899–901

44. Wessels, E. C., Ohori, M., Grantmyre, J. E., Aihara, M., Gillespie, R. I., Garrett, R. W., Kassabian, V. S., Scardino, P. T. and Lipshultz, L. I. (1992). The prevalence of cystic dilatation of the ejaculatory ducts detected by transrectal ultrasound (TRUS) in a self referral screening group of men. *J. Urol.*, **147**, 456A

45. Anguino, A., Oates, R. D., Amos, J. A., Dean, M., Gerrard, B., Stewart, C., Maher, T. A., White, M. B. and Milunsky, A. (1992). Congenital bilateral absence of the vas deferens. A primary genital form of cystic fibrosis. *J. Am. Med. Assoc.*, **267**, 1794–7

46. Shaban, S. F. (1991). Treatment of abnormalities of ejaculation. In Lipshultz, L. I. and Howards, S. S. (eds.) *Infertility in the Male*, 2nd edn, pp. 409–26. (St Louis: Mosby Year Book)

47. King, B. F., Lewis, R. W., McKusick, M. A. (1994). Radiologic evaluation of impotence. In Bennett, A. H. (ed.). *Impotence*, pp. 52–93. (Philadelphia: W. B. Saunders)

48. Honig, S. C., Thompson, S. T. and Lipschultz, L. I. (1993). Reassessment of male factor infertility, including the varicocele, sperm penetration assay, semen analysis, and *in vitro* fertilization. *Curr. Opin. Obstet. Gynecol.*, **5**, 245–51

49. Honig, S. C. (1993). Use of ultrasonography in the evaluation of the infertile male. *World J. Urol.*, **11**, 102–7

50. Honig, S. C. (1994). Ultrasonography in the care of the infertile man. *Contemp. Urol.*, **6**, 42–64

Imaging of the pituitary gland and relevant parasellar abnormalities

10

D. R. Swearengin and A. W. Litt

INTRODUCTION

The workup of patients with symptoms referable to the pituitary gland or parasellar regions not only requires clinical and laboratory evaluation but often demands correlation with cross-sectional imaging. As in all radiological evaluations, proper communication between the clinician and radiologist ensures that optimal diagnostic information is obtained. State-of-the-art imaging of the sella and parasellar region is performed with magnetic resonance imaging (MRI), which has replaced computed tomography (CT) as the imaging modality of choice. Advantages include the absence of ionizing radiation, the freedom from dental and bone-related artifacts, the avoidance of iodinated contrast and the ability to obtain images in any plane. Disadvantages are few, generally limited to the occasional claustrophobic patient as well as to prolonged imaging times compared with CT. New techniques promise to eliminate much of this time penalty.

The following discussion reviews MRI technique and anatomy, both normal and pathological, relevant to the workup of a patient with a suspected pituitary or parasellar abnormality. Emphasis is placed on representative magnetic resonance images of the normal and abnormal pituitary gland and parasellar structures, and the differential diagnosis is reviewed. The decision for radiological workup of this patient population is, ultimately, a clinical one. In general, patients who require radiographic evaluation include those with pituitary–hypothalamic axis disorders or those in whom neurological or neuro-ophthalmological symptoms are potentially referable to the sella or parasellar region. When the presenting symptom is reproductive failure, pituitary gland imaging is usually performed for the workup of the amenorrheic patient; after pregnancy has been excluded, this should begin with a measurement of the levels of thyroid stimulating hormone and prolactin, and the response to a progestational challenge. Likewise, in male-factor infertility, such as male hyperprolactinemia, pituitary gland imaging may be indicated. Adequate communication of the relevant clinical information to the radiologist is always essential for the performance of an appropriate diagnostic examination.

TECHNIQUE

When it is available, MRI is considered the modality of choice for imaging the sella and parasellar region, although the relative merits of MRI and CT depend, of course, on the specific pathology being imaged. A distinction must be made between microadenomas (those adenomas measuring < 10 mm) and macroadenomas. For pituitary microadenomas, the sensitivity and specificity of these imaging modalities depend on the presence or absence of contrast. Without contrast, MRI and CT produce similar results[1-3]; with contrast administration, the sensitivity and specificity of MRI are greater (in the 85–90% range) than those of contrast-enhanced CT (80–85%)[4].

For pituitary imaging, a basic examination includes pre-contrast sagittal and coronal T_1-weighted sequences (short TR, short TE). If a mass is obvious, as it may be with a macroadenoma, these routine images with non-thin sections (5 mm) will usually suffice. However, in many circumstances, thin-section (≤ 3 mm) imaging, often with magnification views, will also be required, as will intravenous gadolinium contrast. Gadolinium is a rare earth metal, chelated to diethylenetriamine pentaacetic acid (DTPA), and is paramagnetic. This paramagnetic effect results in T_1 shortening, with affected (enhancing) regions thus appearing bright or hyperintense on T_1-weighted images. For example, the normal gland will rapidly enhance, becoming 'bright' or hyperintense on T_1-weighted images, while most adenomas will appear relatively 'dark' by comparison. Studies have shown an approx-imately 20% increase in the detection of micro-adenomas when gadolinium is employed[5–9].

In addition, gadolinium-DTPA has an extremely low level of associated side-effects, such as allergic reactions, especially compared with the incidence with iodinated (CT) contrast. The most frequently associated reactions with gadolinium-DTPA are headache (8.7%) and nausea (3.2%)[10]; anaphylaxis is exceedingly rare (approximately 1/1 000 000). With iodinated contrast injection, however, severe and life-threatening anaphylaxis or cardiovascular complications can be seen, with death occurring in approximately 1/40 000 cases.

Because differences in the amount and rapidity of enhancement between micro-adenomas and the normal pituitary gland may be minimal, an additional increase in sensitivity can often be realized with dynamic imaging. With this technique, a series of rapidly acquired coronal T_1-weighted images is obtained during and immediately following bolus contrast injection, resulting in several sets of identical coronal sections through the pituitary gland, obtained within the first few minutes of active contrast enhancement. Dynamic imaging may show microadenomas not detectable on either pre-contrast or post-contrast static imaging (see example, Figure 7, page 173).

Timing is critical with this technique: imaging must be performed as quickly as possible following bolus contrast injection, to take full advantage of the relatively less rapid and less intense enhancement of adenomas compared with the normal gland[11–13]. Over time, adenomas can enhance to the level of the normal gland and become radiologically 'invisible'. Peak enhancement of the normal anterior pituitary gland occurs within 30–60 s after administration of contrast bolus[5,6], compared with 60–200 s for adenomas.

Fat suppression techniques, which eliminate the T_1 hyperintensity from fat-containing tissues, are occasionally used to differentiate fat from hemorrhage as a source of bright T_1 signal. T_2-weighted images are not always routinely employed, although they may be useful to confirm cystic changes within a lesion[10].

When MRI is not available, contrast-enhanced CT may still provide useful diagnostic information. Axial and coronal thin-section (1.5 mm) images are obtained. Detection rates for microadenomas are stated to be as high as 80–85%[4]. As in MRI, dynamic scanning during contrast administration is most helpful.

If neither of these tests prove diagnostic and localization of the tumor is required preoperatively, bilateral inferior petrosal sinus sampling is occasionally employed[14], most often for the detection of occult adrenocorticotropic hormone (ACTH) micro-adenomas. This technique relies on the relatively constant venous drainage of each half of the anterior pituitary gland into the ipsilateral petrosal sinus. This is an invasive procedure, with a catheter inserted (typically via a femoral vein approach) into the respective petrosal sinuses, and blood samples are obtained. After the procedure, hormonal assays are performed on the venous samples, with higher assay levels indicating the side of the occult microadenoma.

Positon emission tomography (PET) has also occasionally been useful also. Utilizing either F-18 deoxyglucose or C-11 methionine, PET can demonstrate adenomas preoperatively and differentiate residual viable tissue postoperatively from fibrous tissue and/or necrosis[15–17].

The lack of widespread availability of PET and its high cost limit its use.

Finally, even in these days of advanced diagnostic imaging, plain films are occasionally useful. Most often noted as an incidental finding, alterations of the sella turcica can sometimes be revealed in the lateral skull film (or a coned-down view of the sella itself). Processes that slowly enlarge the sella contents can produce an enlarged sella, which may show a thinning of the dorsum. More aggressive processes can occasionally produce destructive changes of the bony sella that are also visible on plain radiographs.

ANATOMY

The pituitary gland is located within the bony sella turcica, which is covered by a dural reflection known as the diaphragm sella (Figure 1). The pituitary infundibulum, connecting the hypothalamus to the pituitary gland, pierces this dural covering. The gland is formed from different embryological structures. The anterior lobe, known as the adenohypophysis, is an epithelial derivative of the pharynx, Rathke's pouch, and comprises approximately 75% of the weight of the adult pituitary gland. The posterior lobe or neurohypophysis is a downward extension of the hypothalamus[4]. The overall weight of the gland is approximately 0.5 g in adult males and has a flat to concave upper margin. The gland may be slightly larger in women, especially in menstruating or postpartum women, and in these patients its superior margin may be mildly convex, especially centrally (additional discussion in the following section). At autopsy the gland averages 5.4–5.7 mm in height, with a range of 3–9 mm[18].

The anterior pituitary gland is composed of three distinct portions. The pars tuberalis is a thin rim of tissue lying along the median eminence and the anterior infundibulum. It is not imaged as a separate structure. The pars intermedius is vestigial in humans[19]. The pars distalis forms the mass of the intrasellar anterior pituitary gland[20], and it appears isointense to white matter in adults on MRI[21].

The pars distalis classically, although not universally, displays a functional anatomical organization that is relevant to imaging. Laterally, cells responsible for the production of growth hormone and prolactin are located. Medially, thyrotrophs, somatotrophs and corticotrophs are located. This functional anatomy often correlates well with the location of adenomas arising from these different cell lines as visualized on imaging studies as well as on pathological section[4].

The posterior pituitary gland is composed of the posterior hypophyseal lobe, the infundibular stem and the median eminence, which is not imaged as a distinct structure separate from the remainder of the hypothalamus. The neurohypophysis releases two major hormones, vasopressin and oxytocin, which are synthesized in the hypothalamus and transmitted via the axons down the infundibulum for storage in the posterior lobe[4]. These neurosecretory substances may account for the markedly different signal of the posterior pituitary compared with the anterior gland. Specifically, in up to 90% of patients, the posterior pituitary gland is imaged as a thin rim of T_1 hyperintensity (compared with the white matter isointensity of the anterior gland). Although the etiology of this 'bright signal' has been variously reported in the radiological literature, and was initially mistakenly identified as a 'fat pad', it is now known to be secondary to the neurohypophysis itself, perhaps secondary to stored neurosecretory hormones or their phospholipid membrane coverings, although the exact source of this T_1 hyperintensity remains unclear[18].

DEVELOPMENTAL AND PHYSIOLOGICAL CHANGES IN GLAND ANATOMY

In order to interpret imaging studies properly, radiological findings must be correlated with normal changes in the size, shape and signal characteristics of the gland throughout life.

In the neonate, the anterior pituitary lobe demonstrates higher T_1 intensity than in the adult, being hyperintense compared with the nearby brainstem. It may also have a convex upper border[22,23]. After 2 months of age, the size and shape assume the characteristics of the pituitary gland in the older child, with a flat superior border and a signal paralleling that of the pons. These changes correlate with the high endocrine activity normally present in the gland in the neonatal period.

During childhood, the pituitary gland displays linear growth and maintains a flat or concave superior border, with the overall gland measuring 2–6 mm in height[24–27]. At this stage of development, there are no significant differences in the gland between the sexes. The stalk should remain smaller in diameter than the basilar artery[28].

During puberty, the pituitary gland undergoes a significant increase in size, obtaining its largest dimensions in life outside the postpartum period (see below)[25,26,29]. In males, it measures up to 7–8 mm in height. In females, however, it obtains greater height, measuring up to 10 mm. It may also project above the superior rim of the sella and have a convex upper border[25].

From young adulthood to middle age, the gland is stable in size and shape[26]. It should not exceed pubertal dimensions, and its superior border should maintain a flat or concave contour. In women, some studies have shown a minimal (< 7 mm) increase in gland size during menses[4].

After 50 years of age, the gland gradually becomes smaller; this may reflect the decrease in pituitary activity seen with menopause and andropause[30,31].

In addition to the above changes, note should be made of significant changes in the pituitary gland during pregnancy. In response to physiological hypertrophy, the gland may increase in weight by 30–100%[32]. During the third trimester, the gland measures up to 10 mm and may display a convex superior border as well as possible increased T_1 signal intensity. The stalk may also increase in size, but should remain ≤ 4 mm in its greatest dimension. The pituitary gland reaches its maximum size in the immediate postpartum period[33], and may normally measure up to 12 mm during this time. After the first postpartum week, the gland quickly returns to normal size, configuration and signal intensity. These changes occur irrespective of the presence or absence of breast feeding[4].

VASCULAR ANATOMY

The vascular supply of the pituitary gland is fairly unusual, and this is important for understanding the gland clinically and radiographically. The gland and hypothalamus are supplied via the superior and inferior hypophyseal arteries and branches of the internal carotid artery[30]. The anterior pituitary gland, however, has no direct arterial feeders; instead, there is a hypophyseal–portal system that provides both the anterior gland's blood supply as well as the route of transport of hypothalamic releasing hormones[4]. This unusual arrangement may explain some clinical and radiological observations. Firstly, the anterior pituitary gland is potentially vulnerable to ischemia, as reflected in Sheehan's syndrome[4] as well as in the tendency for microadenomas to develop areas of infarction and/or hemorrhage[34]. Secondly, there is a slightly delayed enhancement of the adenohypophysis after contrast injection, compared with the more immediate enhancement of the posterior pituitary gland and infundibulum, with their direct arterial supply[11–13].

The gland's venous drainage is via the cavernous sinuses, which in turn flow into the ipsilateral aspects of the petrosal venous system. Each half of the anterior pituitary gland tends to drain into its ipsilateral cavernous and petrosal sinuses. There is, in addition, a rich venous anastomotic network in the parasellar region, and the adjacent cavernous sinuses provide drainage pathways for carotid cavernous fistulas as well as carotid dural fistulas in this region[4]. As expected, MRI demonstrates these changes, which are discussed in detail in a following section.

PARASELLAR ANATOMY

Pituitary pathology can extend past the confines of the sellar turcica to involve adjacent structures. Conversely, parasellar, non-pituitary pathology can involve the sella and/or pituitary gland secondarily. A brief review of parasellar anatomy is, therefore, warranted (Figure 1).

As stated, dura forms the sellar roof. In 80% of people, the optic chiasm is directly above the pituitary fossa and is frequently involved when adenomas present with mass effect. The infundibulum is always posterior to the optic chiasm. Posterior to the stalk is a bulge in the hypothalamus, the tuber cinereum. Further posteriorly one finds the mammillary bodies[18].

Laterally, the sella turcica is bounded by the cavernous sinuses, which are typically iso-intense to the pituitary gland on T_1-weighted images. Laterally located within the sinuses, from superior to inferior, are cranial nerves III, IV, V1 and V2. These may be seen as low-signal foci within the lateral aspects of the cavernous sinuses on high-resolution post-contrast T_1-weighted studies. Additionally, cranial nerve VI travels extradurally along the cavernous sinus. The sinus also contains the siphon loop of the internal carotid artery, which appears as a signal void. Posteriorly and inferiorly within each cavernous sinus are Meckel's caves, which house the trigeminal (Gasserian) ganglia. These appear as cerebro-spinal fluid (CSF) intensity spaces. Finally, the sellar turcica forms the roof the sphenoid sinus, which is immediately inferior to it[18].

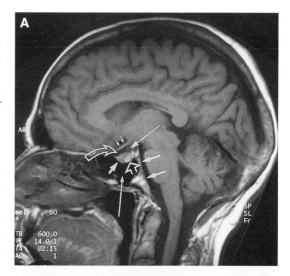

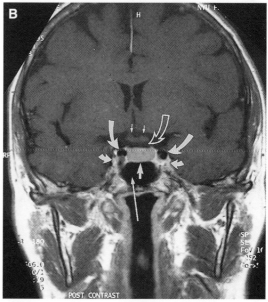

Figures 1 A *and* B *For the legend, please refer to page 166*

PATHOLOGY

Congenital and developmental anomalies

Congenital anomalies of the pituitary gland are rare. Hypoplasia or aplasia of the gland can be seen in some patients with panhypo-pituitarism. The infundibulum is variably present in these patients.

Additionally, 'ectopic' posterior tissue is occasionally seen located within the infundibulum or hypothalamus (Figure 2). This appears as a nodular tissue focus which is isointense to the normally 'bright' T_1 signal of posterior pituitary tissue. These patients are usually asymptomatic, but endocrine dysfunction can occur[18] (for additional discussions of disorders of the infundibulum, please see that section at the end of this chapter).

Encephaloceles

Encephaloceles are most frequently noted in

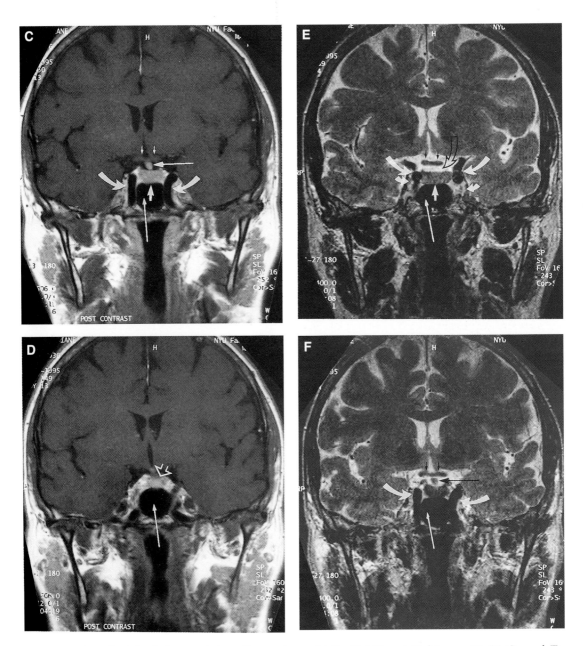

Figure 1 *Normal adult pituitary and parasellar anatomy. (A) Sagittal T_1-weighted image. (B–D) Coronal T_1-weighted images from anterior to posterior, at levels through the anterior pituitary gland, infundibulum and posterior pituitary gland, respectively. (E–F) Coronal T_2-weighted images through the anterior pituitary gland and infundibulum. Indicated are the anterior pituitary gland (medium straight arrows), posterior pituitary gland (straight open arrows), infundibulum (large long arrows), optic nerves/chiasm (small arrows), suprasellar cistern (curved open arrows), sphenoid sinus (small long arrows), clivus (large straight arrows), cavernous sinuses (small curved arrows) and cavernous carotid arteries (large curved arrows)*

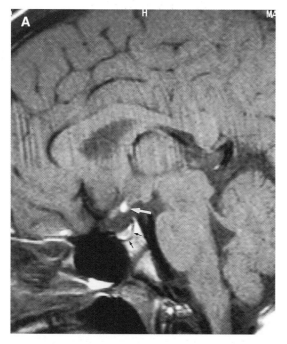

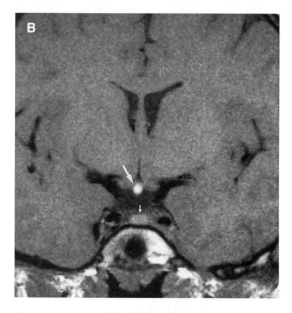

Figure 2 *A 13-year-old boy with delayed growth. (A) Sagittal and (B) coronal non-contrast T_1-weighted images show absence of a normal infundibulum and posterior pituitary, with a T_1 hyperintense 'bright spot' (large arrows) at the expected origin of the stalk. This appearance is consistent with arrested transport of the neurohypophysis, resulting in an ectopic posterior pituitary gland, which the 'bright spot' represents. The anterior pituitary gland is located in its normal position (small arrows)*

the occipital region, but rarely (1/700 000 births) occur through the sphenoid sinus and involve the sella[35]. They are often associated with other midline craniofacial anomalies. The neonates usually present with CSF rhinorrhea or meningitis secondary to accompanying violation of the dura. Adults may display symptoms secondary to herniation of normal pituitary gland and/or optic tissue into the encephaloceles, with resulting hypothalamic or pituitary derangements or visual disturbances[14]. Multiplanar MRI is indispensable in demonstrating the affected anatomy for the purposes of preoperative planning. The encephaloceles may be composed of brain tissue or a CSF space, and would be, therefore, isointense to normal brain matter or CSF in these circumstances.

Pituitary dwarfism

This disease, characterized by short stature with growth hormone deficiency, with or without additional anterior pituitary hormonal derangements, is not truly congenital. It is of uncertain etiology, although a history of birth trauma or other birth difficulty is noted in approximately 50% of cases[36]; consequently this disorder may represent a developmental anomaly. Males are more frequently affected than females in an approximately 2 : 1 ratio. The anatomical and radiological findings include a small sella turcica and small adenohypophysis (Figures 2 and 3). There is hypoplasia or trans-section of the infundibulum, with accompanying loss of the normal posterior pituitary 'bright spot' and corresponding T_1 hyperintensity within the tuber cinereum[14]. This hyperintense focus has been referred to as an 'ectopic' posterior pituitary lobe (further discussion under Disorders of the pituitary infundibulum).

This constellation of findings has been observed in only 40% of cases of idiopathic growth hormone deficiency[37]. The patients with these findings also have a higher incidence of multiple hormone derangements and generally lower growth hormone assays. They are also more likely to have had a

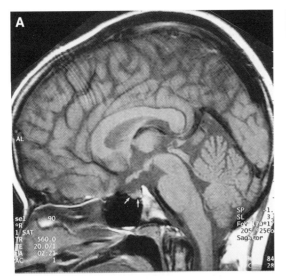

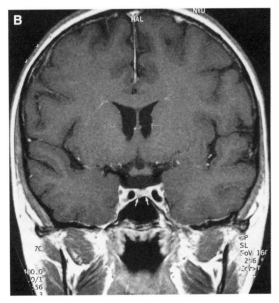

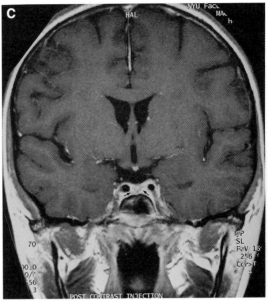

Figure 3 *A 22-year-old woman with pituitary insufficiency. (A) Pre-contrast sagittal and (B) coronal T_1-weighted images. (C) Post-contrast coronal T_1-weighted image. All fail to demonstrate an infundibulum, and the gland (arrows) appears to be hypoplastic, consistent with congenital pituitary hypoplasia*

history of birth trauma[37–41]. The lack of the same MRI findings in other patients with identical forms of pituitary dwarfism has not been explained.

Empty sella

As previously noted, the sella turcica is covered by a thin dura reflection, the diaphragm sella. However, the diaphragm sella is frequently incomplete, and appears to be completely absent in approximately 5% of normal patients[18], with females affected more

often than males in an approximately 5 : 1 ratio[4]. Because of the lack of a competent diaphragm sella, CSF pulsations slowly cause herniation of the arachnoid into the sella turcica, explaining the increasing incidence of this observation with increasing age[14].

Most consider that this finding should be included within the normal range unless the sella is grossly expanded or there are definite referable symptoms[4]. Most patients have normal pituitary function even if the gland appears to be significantly compressed. This is not surprising, as the anterior pituitary has a functional reserve of approximately 90%[42]. In unusual cases, patients may present with non-specific symptoms of endocrine dysfunction, dizziness or headache. In these patients, the empty sella may be the only sign of increased intracranial pressure (pseudotumor cerebri) or altered CSF dynamics[4].

On T_1-weighted studies, the pituitary gland appears to be compressed against the floor of the sella, which is filled with CSF intensity material (Figure 4). The stalk remains in its normal position, differentiating this condition from changes secondary to a space-occupying cyst, which would be expected to show accompanying infundibular displacement[43].

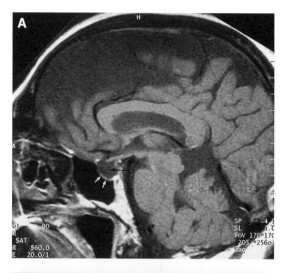

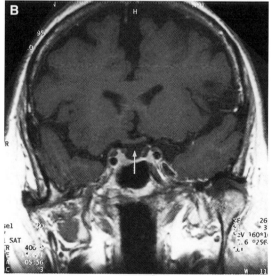

Figure 4 *A 66-year-old woman with increased thyroid stimulating hormone levels. (A) Sagittal and (B) coronal non-contrast T_1-weighted images demonstrate an expanded sella filled with cerebrospinal fluid (long arrows). The pituitary gland (small arrows) appears small and is applied to the sella floor. These findings are consistent with a (partially) empty sella*

Adenomas

Pituitary adenomas are benign tumors of the adenohypophysis and compromise 10–15% of all intracranial tumors[44]. These neoplasms are arbitrarily divided into microadenomas and macroadenomas, depending on whether they are less than or greater than 10 mm, respectively. Endocrinologically active tumors, which account for approximately three-fourths of the total count, tend to be micro-adenomas, simply because they are detected at an earlier stage owing to clinical signs of endocrinopathy. Non-functioning tumors, since they must present secondary to mass effect to become clinically evident, are typically macroadenomas. Occasionally, large non-functioning tumors can present with endocrine derangement, such as secondary hypopituitarism, because of compression of the anterior pituitary gland, infundibulum or hypothalamus[18]. Pituitary adenomas are a common incidental finding at autopsy, seen in approximately 3–27% of the population[14].

Microadenomas

Functioning pituitary adenomas are diag-nosed clinically from recognizable syndromes of pituitary hormonal excess. Their different sizes at discovery reflect the fact that some hormonal derangements are more obvious clinically to both the patient and the physician. Laboratory testing, using stimulation/suppression provocation as well as hormonal assays, can confirm the diagnosis before imaging is pursued. Consequently, the decision to image a particular patient often depends on the individual approach of the referring physician. Additionally, the need for imaging may be determined by its possible effects on treatment, depending on whether treatment is medical (e.g. bromocryptine therapy for an amenorrheic infertile patient with galactorrhea and hyperprolactinemia) or surgical (e.g. an amenorrheic infertile cushingoid patient). When medical therapy is contemplated, imaging serves to exclude an unsuspected source, such as a macroadenoma, as the etiology of the patient's hormonal imbalance before initiating treatment. Additionally, if the diagnosis has been confirmed by laboratory testing, a negative or equivocal MRI scan should not dissuade the physician from treatment, as adenomas can be radiographically occult, even to MRI.

On the other hand, if surgery is being considered, imaging is essential in confirming the location of the microadenoma for preoperative planning. In this case, a negative MRI scan, especially with cortisol-secreting tumors, may prompt more rigorous radiographic workup, such as bilateral petrosal venous sampling. Furthermore, regardless of the treatment option, imaging is often helpful in the evaluation of patients with 'borderline' hormonal elevation, when the diagnosis is not a clinical certainty.

The various pituitary microadenomas are radiographically indistinguishable, although frequently their different locations within the gland may provide a clue to the particular type of adenoma present (for example, prolactin-secreting cells are found laterally within the gland, as are their corresponding microadenomas). With MRI, adenomas are hypointense to the normal gland on non-contrast T_1-weighted images in 80–90% of cases. Less commonly noted is T_2 hyperintensity, seen in one-half to one-third of cases[45]. These tumors are typically hypodense to normal pituitary tissue on CT images. After intravenous contrast, the tumors typically enhance less intensely and less rapidly than normal pituitary tissue on both MRI and CT (Figures 5 and 6). They may occasionally be seen only on the dynamically acquired images (Figure 7). Ancillary findings may be noted. Although these are not diagnostic by themselves, they are valuable as adjuncts, especially if more than one is present. These ancillary findings include focal asymmetry in the upper gland contour as well as asymmetric increase in gland height[10]. Although previously reported as a sign of microadenomas, infundibular shift to the contralateral side is no longer considered a valuable diagnostic

aid, as the stalk displays such a widespread range of normal variation in position. Downward sloping of the sella floor similarly lacks specificity.

The most frequently encountered functioning microadenomas are prolactin-secreting[43], usually presenting with typical symptoms of amenorrhea, galactorrhea and/or infertility in women or with loss of libido and/or impotence in men. If serum prolactin levels are > 200 ng/ml, the clinical diagnosis is essentially confirmed[4]. However, the diagnosis is less certain in the 'low abnormal' range of 25–200 ng/ml, as a number of additional and disparate etiologies are possible, including metabolic disturbances (renal and liver failure), pregnancy or postpartum status, breast stimulation, thoracic wall processes (lesions and trauma), extrapituitary intracranial abnormalities (especially basal processes such as sarcoidosis or tuberculosis) and multiple drugs (including estrogens, phenothiazones, opiates, anti-depressants and antipsychotics, amphetamines, some antihypertensives and cime-tidine)[14]. A negative or equivocal MRI scan in the setting of 'low abnormal' assay values may prompt the clinician to consider such etiologies.

Less frequently encountered are patients with microadenomas resulting in Cushing's disease. Because of the prominent clinical symptoms, these tumors tend to be smaller at presentation, often measuring 1–2 mm in size[43]. As a consequence, ACTH-producing microadenomas are the most difficult to detect, with a decreased sensitivity (approximately 71%)[46] on MRI compared with prolactin and growth hormone secreting tumors (75–100% in multiple small series)[2,45,47,48]. These patients may progress to petrosal venous sampling in order for the tumor to be localized preoperatively. Exclusion of ectopic sources of ACTH is also important, as adrenal tumors (ACTH-independent adenomas or carcinomas) and paraneoplastic syndromes (multiple endocrine neoplasia (MEN) I–II can also produce hypercortisolism.

In contrast to ACTH-producing adenomas, those which secrete growth hormone tend to

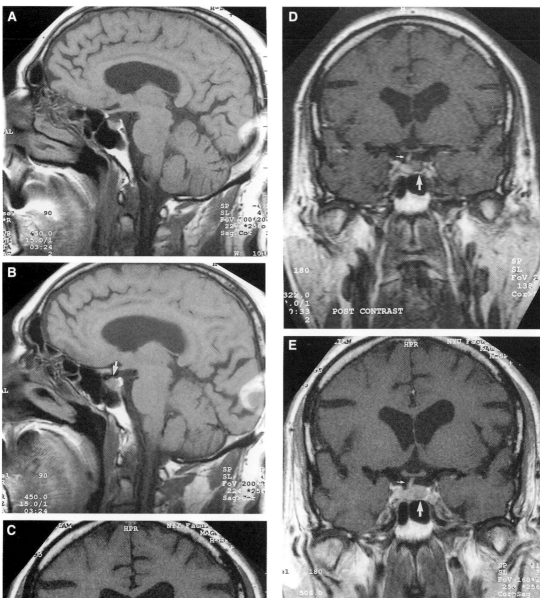

Figure 5 *A 68-year-old man with gynecomastia. (A) Right paramedian and (B) left paramedian sagittal pre-contrast T_1-weighted images. (C) Coronal pre-contrast, (D) dynamic and (E) post-contrast T_1-weighted images. The sagittal views show gland asymmetry on the left, confirmed on the coronal images, all of which show a left microadenoma (large arrows). There is accompanying shift of the infundibulum towards the right (small arrows)*

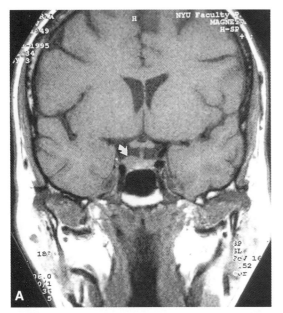

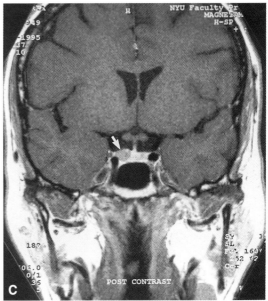

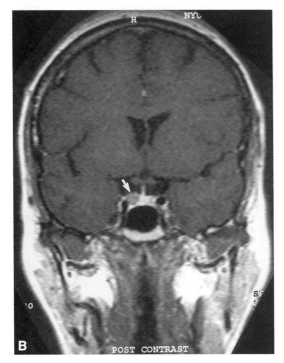

Figure 6 *A 45-year-old woman with galactorrhea. (A) Pre-contrast, (B) dynamic and (C) post-contrast T_1-weighted images all show a right pituitary microadenoma*

adenoma[49,50], with a combination of prolactin and growth hormone secretion seen most often. Thyroid stimulating hormone (TSH), follicle stimulating hormone (FSH) and luteinizing hormone (LH)-secreting microadenomas are less frequently encountered[14].

Macroadenomas

Pituitary macroadenomas, by virtue of their larger size (> 10 mm), do not usually present a problem with radiological detection (Figure 8). They do, however, tend to have more varied radiological appearances than microadenomas. First, they are more often isointense to the normal gland, and differentiation between the tumor and the normal gland is often not possible. This may reflect a lack of MRI signal difference between the two as well as compression and the resultant apparent obliteration of the remaining pituitary tissue. Additionally, macroadenomas often display areas of T_1 hypointensity and T_2 hyperintensity, corresponding to regions of cystic degeneration. Finally, because of their

be discovered at a more advanced stage as a result of the less clinically obvious symptoms of early acromegaly. Therefore, many of these lesions are, in fact, macroadenomas at the time of their discovery[14]. It should be further noted that, in approximately 10% of cases, multiple hormones are produced by a single

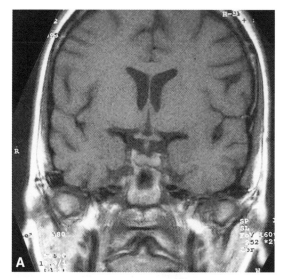

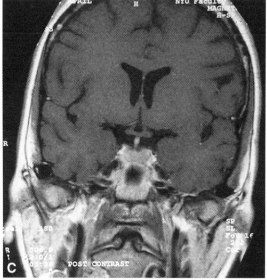

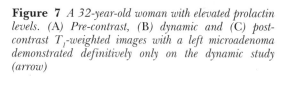

Figure 7 *A 32-year-old woman with elevated prolactin levels. (A) Pre-contrast, (B) dynamic and (C) post-contrast T₁-weighted images with a left microadenoma demonstrated definitively only on the dynamic study (arrow)*

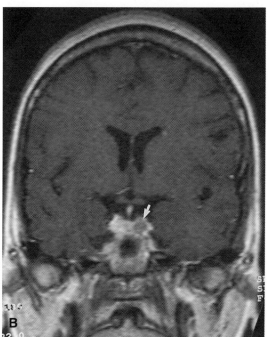

less than robust blood supply, these tumors may display evidence of intratumoral hemorrhage, typically seen as areas of T_1 hyperintensity[34] (Figure 9). Hemorrhage is seen in up to 22% of cases in some surgical series[51]. MRI, because it is very sensitive to the paramagnetic effects of blood products, demonstrates hemorrhage within adenomas more freq-uently than CT.

The presence of associated hemorrhage should not be confused with the clinical syndrome of pituitary apoplexy, which should be used to refer only to the potentially life-threatening syndrome of acute pituitary hemorrhage associated with rapid onset of visual changes as evidenced by chiasmatic field defects, ocular motor palsies and headache or other meningeal signs[4]. Pituitary hemorrhage is most frequently seen without this associated clinical syndrome. For example, in one series over 50% of micro-adenoma patients being treated with bromocryptine displayed evidence of hemor-rhage on follow-up MRI examination, the majority of which were clinically occult[52].

In addition to demonstrating the adenoma itself, imaging also allows for the evaluation of possible complications of tumor growth. Macroadenomas, because of their larger size, are more likely to have associated complica-tions of mass effect and extrasellar extension. Superior extension can result in chiasmatic compression, which is always of clinical concern (Figure 10). Even documented

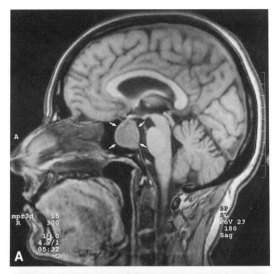

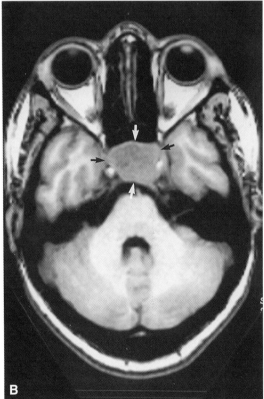

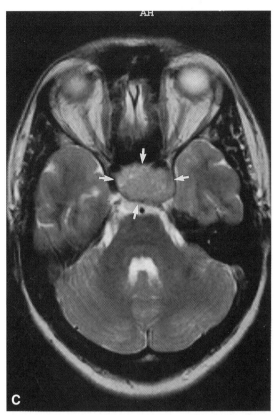

Figure 8 *A 50-year-old woman with double vision for 24 h. (A) Sagittal and (B) axial T_1-weighted images. (C) Axial T_2-weighted image. All demonstrate a low signal mass within an expanded sella. The radiological differential includes atypical adenoma or meningioma. After correlation with pituitary hormonal assays, the patient was given empirical medical therapy for a presumed prolactinoma, which responded with interval decreases in size on follow-up magnetic resonance imaging examinations*

growth to the chiasm without frank compression can warrant surgical intervention.

Lateral extension to involve the cavernous sinus, which is associated with increased morbidity and mortality[53], is often less obvious than suprasellar extension. For example, cavernous sinus invasion may be clinically suspected because of extreme hormonal elevation (e.g. prolactin levels >1000 ng/ml in prolactin-secreting tumors)[54]. On the other hand, sinus invasion may be clinically silent, with only the imaging study suggesting the abnormality (Figure 11). Encasement of the cavernous carotid artery is the most reliable sign of sinus extension[4], and MRI can certainly demonstrate vessel narrowing if it is present. However, the use of indirect signs is most often required as vessel narrowing is infrequently noted. These indirect signs are less specific. For example,

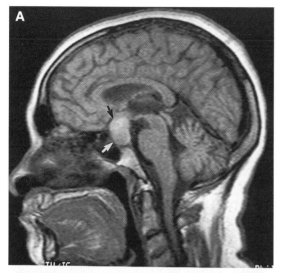

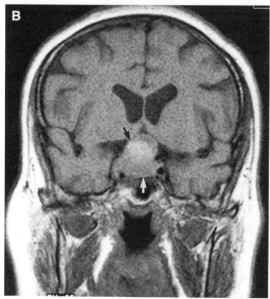

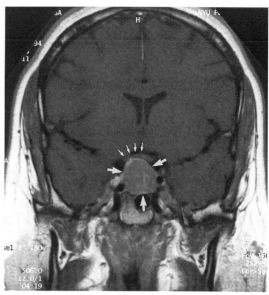

Figure 10 *A 27-year-old woman with 3-month history of amenorrhea. Coronal T_1-weighted image shows a macroadenoma (large arrows) with compression and uplifting of the optic chiasm (small arrows)*

Figure 9 *A 61-year-old woman with known macroadenoma and acute onset of decreased vision. (A) Sagittal and (B) coronal T_1-weighted images with areas of hyperintense hemorrhage (black arrows) on this non-contrast study, confirming the clinical diagnosis of pituitary apoplexy. Note the expanded sella occupied by the macroadenoma (white arrows), with only its superior portion demonstrating acute hemorrhage*

lateral bowing of the intracavernous carotid artery is merely an indication of mass effect, not a definite sign of invasion of the cavernous sinus. Since the adjacent dura separating the sellar contents from the cavernous sinus may be incomplete in normal individuals, and this thin line of signal void is often not visualized in normal patients, its absence cannot be used as supportive evidence for cavernous sinus invasion. Differences in signal characteristics of the two cavernous sinuses compared with each other, however, is suggestive of involvement[10]. Cranial nerve palsies are a late sign of cavernous involvement secondary to their lateral location within this structure[44]. The most reliable sign for absence of cavernous sinus invasion is the visualization of normal pituitary tissue interposed between the adenoma and the ipsilateral cavernous sinus[55].

Inferior extension of tumor past the confines of the bony sella can also be demonstrated. Although coronal images are ideally suited for evaluation of possible inferior extrasella disease, because of the limits of MRI in the demonstration of cortical bone, differentiation between sellar expansion and frank bony destruction may not be possible. In this instance, CT is obviously superior and is the modality of choice if this

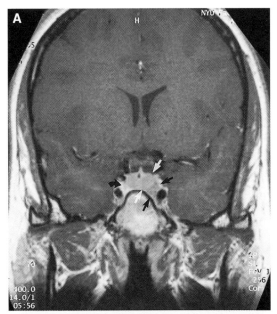

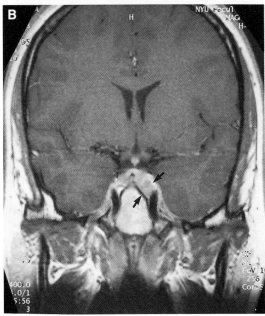

Figure 11 *A 27-year-old woman with gradual onset of amenorrhea. (A, B) Post-contrast coronal T₁-weighted images demonstrate a left macroadenoma (white arrows) with adjacent cavernous sinus invasion (black arrows). Note the normal contralateral cavernous sinus (curved arrow)*

Although adenomas with extrasella spread are more aggressive in terms of local extension, the vast majority are benign[50]. True malignant degeneration of adenomas into adenocarcinomas is rare, but does occur[56]. Metastases from a pituitary carcinoma may involve the central nervous system (CNS) or extraneural sites. The former is most frequently seen with non-functioning macroadenomas that have associated suprasellar extension. The latter is most often noted with hormonally active tumors that have eroded through the sellar floor; corticotropin-secreting adenomas are responsible for nearly 50% of such cases[4].

IMAGING AFTER TREATMENT AND OPERATION

Medical treatment with the use of ergot derivatives (bromocryptine, pergolide) is frequently employed for prolactin-secreting microadenomas and small macroadenomas, and follow-up scanning may reveal an interval decrease in size of tumor bulk after therapy. In one series all macroadenomas decreased in size after treatment with pergolide; 50% decreased in bulk with bromocryptine therapy. With these same agents, micro-adenomas showed size reductions in 33% and 60%, respectively[19]. Additionally, after medical therapy, adenomas frequently show associated intratumoral hemorrhage, occurring in up to 45% of cases (vs. 13% in non-treated patients)[7] (Figure 12).

The follow-up of pituitary adenomas after surgical intervention is, by comparison, both less straightforward and potentially more confusing, because of the resulting anatomical distortion and inevitable post-surgical enhancement (Figure 13). Detailed knowledge of the particulars of surgery, including the approach as well as the use and type of packing materials utilized in the sphenoid sinus, is vital[57,58]. Because of postoperative enhancement, differentiation between post-surgical changes and possible residual tumor can be extremely difficult, if not impossible, in a single postoperative study. For this

possible complication is of clinical concern. Invasion of adjacent marrow-containing structures, such as the clivus, is more readily demonstrated by MRI.

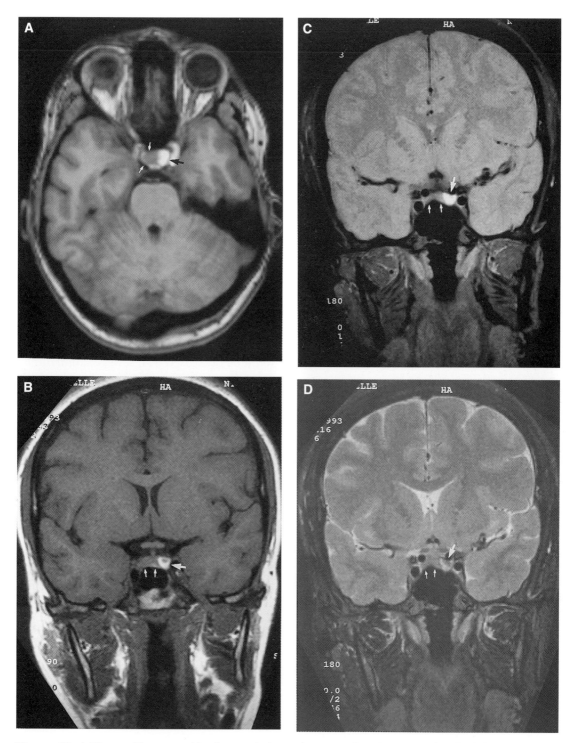

Figure 12 *A 33-year-old woman with a known pituitary adenoma undergoing empirical medical therapy. Previous scans were otherwise unremarkable. Non-contrast, (A) axial and (B) coronal T_1-weighted images as well as coronal, (C) balanced echo (proton density) and (D) T_2-weighted images demonstrate new hemorrhage (large arrows) in the patient's left microadenoma. The blood is hyperintense on most sequences and is most probably subacute in nature. Normal pituitary gland (small arrows) is seen on the right*

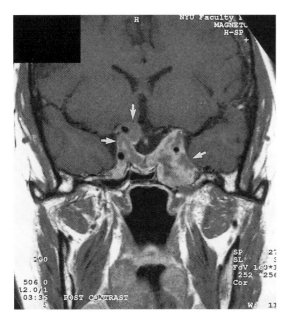

Figure 13 *A 36-year-old woman, status post-transsphenoidal resection for a macroadenoma. Post-contrast coronal T_1-weighted image shows residual tumor with bilateral cavernous sinus invasion*

reason, the initial post-procedure study is performed as a baseline scan for future comparison, with interval changes more important for evaluation of residual tumor than the initial postoperative appearance of the surgical bed.

Recommendations for the timing of initial post-procedure scan vary, but the goal is to wait until adequate time has passed for the expected and temporary postoperative swelling and inflammation to subside. If scans are performed in the initial weeks following surgery, postoperative hemorrhage and other changes may give the false impression that little, if any, tumor has been removed[59]. Additionally, because both acute blood and fat packing in the sphenoid sinus may appear hyperintense on T_1-weighted images, potential confusion may arise. For this reason, in initial postoperative scans, the addition of fat suppression techniques or T_2-weighted sequences to the protocol is recommended. With both techniques, fat will show decreased signal compared with subacute blood, allowing differentiation. However, at this initial stage,

soft tissue in the postoperative bed may represent postoperative change, residual normal pituitary tissue or residual tumor.

Because differentiation among these tissues is not possible, many advocate delaying the initial postoperative scan until 3–4 months after trans-sphenoidal surgery[59]. Compared with this baseline study, enlarging soft tissue within the postoperative bed indicates residual or recurrent tumor. It cannot be overemphasized that serial examinations are necessary in the postoperative patient. Furthermore, in patients with endocrino-logically active tumors, imaging should always be correlated with concurrent serum horm-onal levels[10].

Additional postoperative changes, as well as potential complications, warrant mention. Besides hemorrhage, air within the post-operative bed (seen as signal voids on both T_1- and T_2-weighted sequences), is to be expected in the initial postoperative period. However, it should be decreased with serial examinations; if it is not, a persistent communication between the intracranial compartment and the extracranial space (typically through the surgically violated sphenoid sinus) must be excluded. If displaced and/or compressed preoperatively, the chiasm may also demon-strate postoperative changes in its appear-ance. Frequently, better separation between the chiasm and the postoperative bed is present. Of those patients with visual field compromise preoperatively, many show improvement in their deficits after hypo-physectomy. Finally, after removal of the tumor mass, the chiasm may not only return to its normal position, but may also herniate (or 'fall down') into the sella[4]. This finding is most often an incidental observation with no associated clinical consequence. However, in the rare patient, associated visual field changes may occur, probably secondary to fibrous stretching, and a chiasmopexy may be required[60].

Differential diagnoses

A number of additional sella or extrasella processes can have appearances that mimic adenomas, especially macroadenomas, and can cause diagnostic difficulty from a radiological or even an endocrinological perspective. The latter problem is usually secondary to mass effect upon the hypothalamus, infundibulum or the gland itself, with resulting hormonal derangements.

Craniopharyngiomas

Craniopharyngiomas are benign tumors arising from squamous epithelial remnants of Rathke's cleft within the pars tuberalis[14]. They can occur anywhere along the path of the embryonic Rathke's cleft, from the nasopharynx to the third ventricle, with a suprasellar location most common[10]. Fifty per cent of these display intrasellar extension[61]. Rarely, they can be purely intrasellar. There is a bimodal age distribution, with the largest peak from 5–10 years and a second smaller peak in the 5–7th decades[4,62]. As a consequence, these tumors are not a common cause of reproductive failure. Females are more commonly affected. These neoplasms account for 9% of brain tumors in children and 3% overall[61,63]. In children, the typical presentation is with symptoms of increased intracranial pressure, such as headache or nausea/vomiting. Adults display symptoms of mass effect, most commonly with pituitary insufficiency (secondary to compression of the gland, stalk or hypothalamus) or with visual changes[14]. The overall incidence of endocrine dysfunction in these patients approaches 70%. Some patients may present with symptoms of clinical meningitis secondary to tumor rupture[18].

The radiological appearance of craniopharyngiomas reflects their variable histological composition as well as their extreme variation in size, with tumors ranging from 0.5 to 10.0 cm[4]. Most frequently, they display solid as well as cystic components[14] (Figure 14). The solid components tend to be isointense to brain and display contrast enhancement. The appearance of cystic portions, which occur in approximately 85%, is more varied[63]. Around half will closely parallel CSF in intensity, reflecting a fluid composition with low protein content. However, approximately 50% will display T_1 hyperintensity (these 'motor oil' cysts are so named because of the gross appearance of their contents at surgery[4]). This T_1 hyperintensity may be due to an assortment of substances present, including cholesterol, keratin, necrotic debris, protein or hemorrhage products[14]. Eighty per cent of craniopharyngiomas also have rim-like or nodular foci of calcification, more commonly seen in children than adults[63]. While these areas may be noted as peripheral signal voids on MRI, they are seen to much better advantage with CT. In fact, if the MRI appearance is non-diagnostic, the demonstration of typical calcific foci on CT can establish the diagnosis.

Craniopharyngiomas are histologically benign, but they can be locally aggressive and can recur after surgery. As a consequence, postoperative imaging is routine. Like the follow-up of pituitary adenomas, serial examinations are most helpful, as the initial postoperative MRI scan may be confusing, because of the presence of postoperative hemorrhage and/or other postsurgical changes, such as swelling and inflammation.

Rathke's cleft cysts

Rathke's cleft cysts, as their name implies, also arise from the remnants of this embryonic structure. They tend to be smaller than craniopharyngiomas and are almost always at least partially intrasellar. The fundamental pathological distinction between these two Rathke's cleft derivatives is their wall composition: Rathke's cleft cysts are lined by a single layer of columnar or cuboidal epithelium, whereas craniopharyngiomas have a thicker wall composed of basal cells or squamous epithelium[4]. Rathke's cleft cysts are a relatively common incidental finding at autopsy and are usually asymptomatic, although they occasionally present during life secondary to symptoms of mass effect, such as headache, visual changes or endocrine dysfunction.

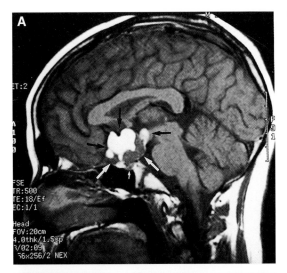

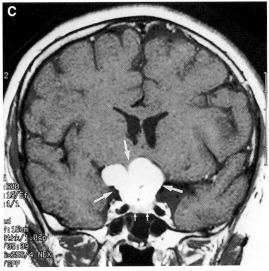

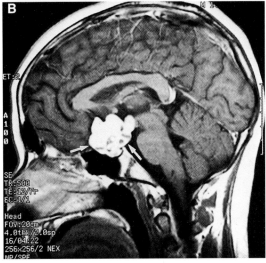

Figure 14 *A 14-year-old boy with visual symptoms. (A) Pre- and (B) post-contrast sagittal and (C) post-contrast coronal T₁-weighted images show a lobulated sellar/suprasellar mass with areas of hyperintensity on the pre-contrast images (large black arrows) consistent with areas of hemorrhage or other material of high protein content. The non-hyperintense portions (large white arrows) heterogeneously enhance after contrast. The pituitary gland (small arrows) is compressed against the floor of the sella by the mass. Pathology was consistent with craniopharyngioma*

These tumors are well-defined and most commonly occur in the midline of the anterior, superior sella[18]. Their MRI appearance varies, depending on the contents of the cyst: if they are purely serous, they may appear isointense to CSF on all pulse sequences[14]; with increasing protein content, the cyst can vary from being isointense to brain to being hyperintense, on T₁-weighted images. Thus, they may be difficult to differentiate from craniopharyngiomas at times. The presence of a solid component excludes the possibility of a Rathke's cleft cyst[10]. They also differ from craniopharyngiomas in their absence of more aggressive local behavior: they are cured without recurrence after surgery or drainage[4].

Other cysts

Not all cystic sellar masses are secondary to pituitary adenomas or Rathke's cleft derivatives. True cysts, arising from rests of mesenchyme, occur here also. These are derived from the developing arachnoid membrane[18] and are benign, well-defined subarachnoid cysts. Although they most frequently arise in the middle cranial fossa, approximately 15% show parasellar extension[64], and some may be purely suprasellar. Occasionally, they may attain significant size and produce symptoms referable to mass effect, such as visual changes or endocrine dysfunction. If the latter is present, precocious puberty is most commonly observed[18].

MRI reflects their purely cystic nature with isointensity to CSF on all pulse sequences (Figure 15). Differentiation from Rathke's cleft cysts, epidermoids, or even parasitic cysts is not always possible[65] (Figure 16).

Occasionally, cysts can be seen within the central portion of the anterior pituitary gland itself. These pars intermedia cysts appear isointense to CSF and are generally small. As expected, they do not enhance (Figure 17).

Meningiomas

Although meningiomas most commonly occur parasagittally at the convexity[18], a suprasellar location is the fifth most frequently encountered[10]. A meningioma arising from the diaphragm sella or posterior clinoids may have secondary sellar extension and can simulate pituitary adenoma[14]. Additionally, meningiomas are rarely purely intrasellar and therefore can be indistinguishable from pituitary adenomas[45].

On MRI, these tumors tend to be hypointense to gray matter on T_1- and T_2-weighted images. Therefore, they may be inconspicuous before the administration of intravenous contrast. The presence of T_2 hypointensity may provide a clue to the diagnosis, as does their typical diffuse, uniform, intense enhancement[18]. Additional factors favoring a meningioma include a normal sella, the presence of accompanying hyperostosis of the planum sphenoidale (a nearly pathognomonic finding seen with some meningiomas), a clear plane of separation between the mass and normal pituitary gland, and demonstrable extension along a dural surface (a dural 'tail')[10] (Figure 18).

Chiasmatic/hypothalamic gliomas

Optic nerve and hypothalamic gliomas are both neoplasms that can affect the sella and suprasellar regions and which can be indistinguishable if they obtain sufficient size.

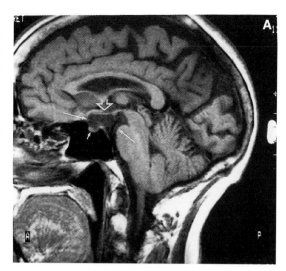

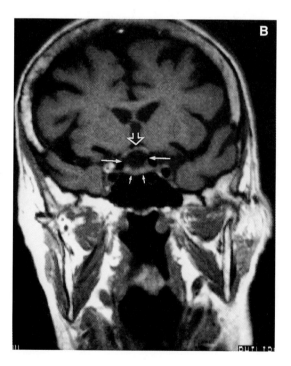

Figure 15 *An 85-year-old woman with pituitary derangements, including increased prolactin and decreased thyroid stimulating hormone levels. Noncontrast (A) sagittal and (B) coronal T_1-weighted images demonstrate a suprasellar 'mass' (long arrows), isointense to cerebrospinal fluid, with sellar extension. The pituitary gland (small arrows) is compressed against the sella floor and the optic nerves and chiasm are displaced superiorly (open arrows). The appearance is consistent with an arachnoid cyst*

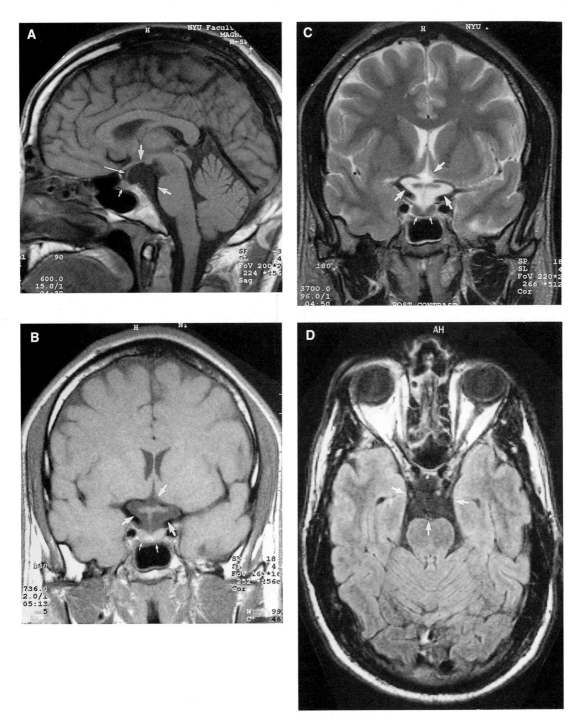

Figure 16 *A 38-year-old man with visual changes and an abnormal ophthalmological examination. (A) Sagittal and (B) coronal T_1-weighted images; (C) coronal T_2-weighted and (D) axial FLAIR images. On all sequences there is a suprasellar 'mass' (large arrows) which is isotense to cerespinal fluid. It is separate from the pituitary gland (small arrows) and displaces the infundibulum anteriorly (long arrow). The findings are most suggestive of an arachnoid cyst; an epidermoid cyst was considered to be less likely*

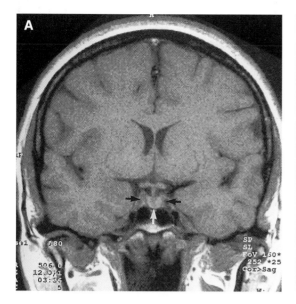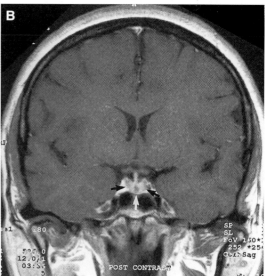

Figure 17 *A 36-year-old woman. (A) Pre-contrast and (B) post-contrast coronal T₁-weighted images demonstrate a non-enhancing central pituitary gland mass (white arrows), slightly hyperintense to cerebrospinal fluid. The normal gland is seen to either side (black arrows). The appearance is consistent with a pars intermedia cyst*

Optic nerve gliomas are more common and most frequently occur in children, with 25% presenting within the first decade[50]. Up to 15% of patients have neurofibromatosis type I, and bilateral gliomas are nearly pathognomonic of the syndrome. These tumors are low-grade malignancies, but vision is usually sacrificed with surgical cure. However, when these malignancies occur in adults, usually middle-aged women, the biological behavior is very different. They are usually glioblastomas and the patient rapidly progresses to blindness and then death[18].

The MRI appearance of these lesions depends on their extent. If they are completely confined to the optic nerve(s), the only abnormality is enlargement of the affected portions of the nerve(s). Before administration of contrast, the tumors are typically isointense to hypointense on T₁-weighted images and hyperintense on T₂-weighted sequences. Enhancement is the rule after contrast and is typically homogeneous. Optic nerve gliomas are low-grade malignancies and typically grow slowly, but they have a tendency to spread along the optic pathways. MRI can document these findings, showing spread, if it is present, along the optic pathways to the lateral geniculate body and optic radiations. Extension to the occipital lobes can also occur. Although larger, locally extensive optic nerve gliomas may be difficult to separate from a possible glioma of hypothalamic origin, extension along the optic pathways is essentially diagnostic of the former[14].

Hypothalamic gliomas are more aggressive and tend to present earlier than their optic nerve counterparts, because of hypothalamic dysfunction. Clinically, patients may have symptoms of diabetes insipidus, syndrome of inappropriate antidiuretic hormone (SIADH), or even problems with temperature regulation. Patients may also present with symptoms secondary to mass effect, such as those of visual disturbances or hydrocephalus, as these tumors have a tendency to obstruct the third ventricle. The occasional patient may have diencephalic syndrome, characterized by cachexia in an otherwise alert child who is euphoric and often displays strong appetite[14].

On MRI, these tumors or portions thereof may be difficult to separate from adjacent

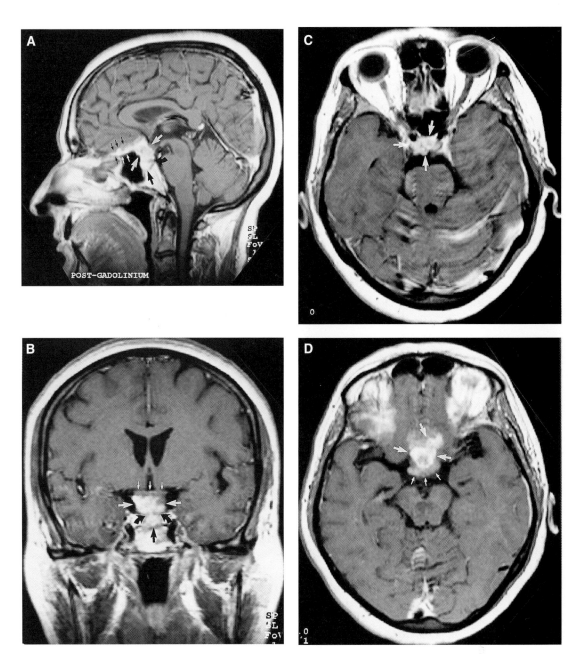

Figure 18 *A 54-year-old woman with decreasing vision. (A) Post-contrast sagittal, (B) coronal and (C–D) axial T_1-weighted images show an enhancing sellar/suprasellar mass (large white arrows). A dural 'tail' (small arrows) seen on the sagittal view indicates a meningioma. On the sagittal and coronal views, note the cleft (curved black arrows) separating the mass from the normal pituitary gland (large black arrows)*

normal brain, as they display variable enhancement. They can be differentiated from a pituitary macroadenoma if normal pituitary tissue is separately identified[10] (Figure 19). Accompanying T_2 signal abnormality may allow differentiation between normal and abnormal tissue, although not between tumor and associated edema.

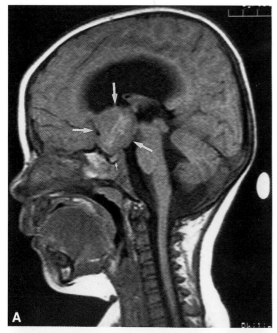

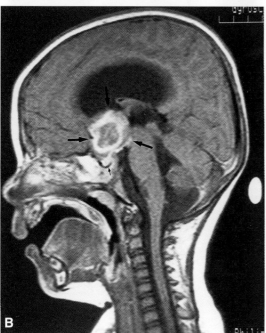

Hamartomas

Hamartomas of the hypothalamus may be incidentally discovered at autopsy or may result in precocious puberty. These benign tumors arise from the tuber cinereum or mammillary bodies and may be either pedunculated or inseparable from the underlying normal tissue. They are usually composed of tissue that is similar to the normal neural tissue of the hypothalamus, although histological variants include lipoma, osteolipoma and tuberous sclerosis[42]. The occasional patient may present with gelastic seizures instead of the more common precocious puberty[66].

MRI reflects the composition of these tumors. As most are composed of neural elements, they tend to be isointense to brain on all sequences and do not enhance[18] (Figure 20). They lack a tendency to invade adjacent structures or grow[14], and do not cause hydrocephalus as a rule, despite their location[18]. MRI merely shows excessive tissue appearing as either a pedunculated or sessile

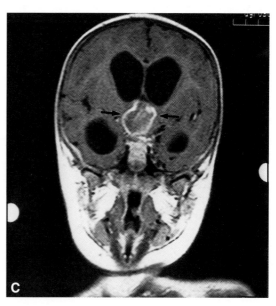

Figure 19 *An 11-month-old boy with symptoms of increased intracranial pressure. (A) Pre- and (B) post-contrast sagittal T_1-weighted images; (C) post-contrast coronal T_1-weighted image. A ring-enhancing suprasellar mass is present (large arrows) which is separate from the normal pituitary gland (small arrows). Pathology revealed a hypothalamic glioma*

mass in the region of the tuber cinereum (Figure 21). The pituitary gland is normal[67].

Germinomas

Although tumors of germ cell origin are more common in the pineal region, they may also occur in the sella or in a suprasellar location. This heterogeneous group of neoplasms of children and young adults is most frequently manifest as a germinoma or teratoma, although less common derivatives, including yolk sac tumors, choriocarcinomas and embryonal cell tumors also occur. Germinomas are the less differentiated tumors of these cell lines and occur in the sella region in approximately 20% of cases. They often present with endocrine dysfunction, most commonly diabetes insipidus secondary to hypothalamic involvement. Patients may alternatively present with other pituitary derangements or with symptoms referable to mass effect, such as hydrocephalus or visual changes. Although males are more commonly affected when these tumors occur in the pineal region, germinomas of the sella region display no sex predilection[14].

MRI demonstrates tumors that are typically isointense to brain before contrast on T_1- and T_2-weighted sequences, although they can be slightly T_2 hyperintense. After contrast they usually markedly enhance (Figure 22). They are frequently large at diagnosis, and are often homogeneous without cystic components. Teratomas, because they are composed of elements from all three germ layers, have a more varied appearance. They may appear as complex, partially cystic, partially solid masses. Areas of signal void may reflect calcification or even teeth, and T_1 hyperintense areas may be caused by fat[14]. The non-fat solid portions typically enhance.

Dermoids/epidermoids

Dermoid and epidermoid tumors are benign, slow-growing neoplasms. Epidermoid tumors arise from congenital inclusion of ectodermal

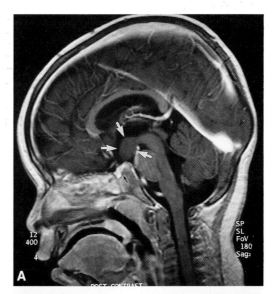

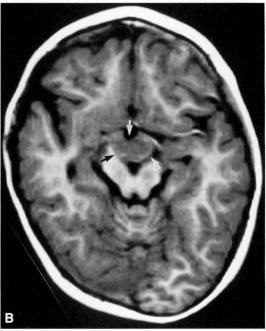

Figure 20 *A 2-year-old boy with a large head, status post-seizure secondary to salt wasting. (A) Sagittal and (B) axial post-contrast T_1-weighted images demonstrate a large mass of the hypothalamic region (large arrows), separate from the sella (small arrow), which does not enhance. Pathology revealed a hypothalamic hamartoma*

elements within the neural tube; with dermoid tumors, both mesodermal and ectodermal derivatives are present. When

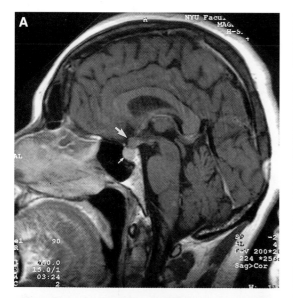

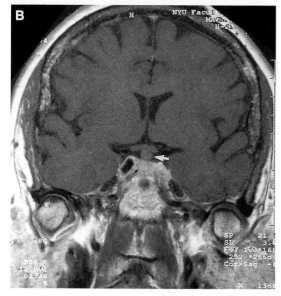

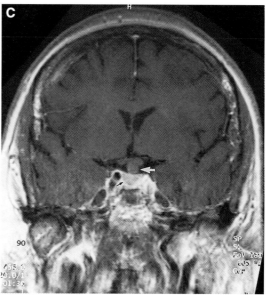

Figure 21 *A 66-year-old woman with facial pain. (A) Pre-contrast sagittal and (B) coronal as well as (C) post-contrast coronal T$_1$-weighted images. A non-enhancing mass (large arrows) is seen superior to and separate from the pituitary gland (small arrows) and infundibulum. The appearance is consistent with a hamartoma of the tuber cinereum*

they occur about the sella, they may cause symptoms referable to mass effect, such as visual changes, endocrine dysfunction (diabetes insipidus or hypopituitarism) or cranial nerve deficits[14].

Dermoid tumors are most frequently noted in the pediatric population. They are typically midline tumors of the posterior fossa, but can occur about the sella. They contain dermal derivatives, such as hair, sebaceous and sweat glands and squamous epithelium[14]. MRI reflects this heterogeneous composition with masses of mixed signal intensity on T$_1$- and T$_2$-weighted sequences. However, some fat is usually present and produces foci of T$_1$ hyperintensity. Fat/fluid levels can be seen. In occasional patients the dermoid tumor may rupture, resulting in a chemical meningitis. In these patients, MRI may demonstrate material, especially fat, scattered within subarachnoid spaces. Calcification may be present, but is seen to best advantage on CT[14]. Unusual dermoid tumors are cystic without fat or calcification[43].

Epidermoid tumors occur in the 4th and 5th decades. These tumors tend to insinuate themselves into adjacent CSF spaces, wrapping themselves around any present neural tissue in the process. The parasellar region is the second most frequently involved area after the cerebellopontine angle[14]. These cysts, lined by stratified squamous epithelium[68], contain variable amounts of desquamated keratin and cholesterol. Not only are they

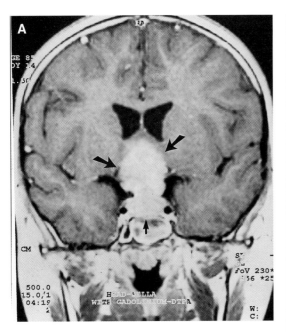

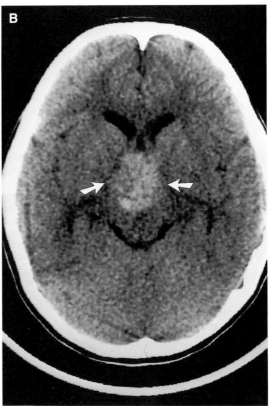

Figure 22 *An 11-year-old girl with decreased vision. (A) Post-contrast coronal T₁-weighted magnetic resonance image demonstrates a large, lobular mass involving the sella as well as the hypothalamus, with accompanying hydrocephalus. (B) Non-contrast computed tomography image shows the mass to be hyperdense. Pathology was consistent with a germinoma*

isointense to slightly hyperintense to CSF on most and sometimes every pulse sequence, they also insinuate into CSF spaces without expanding them, making them notoriously difficult to detect. For this reason, they may be best visualized on balanced echo images. They do not enhance (Figure 16).

Chordomas

Chordomas are tumors of primitive notochord remnants. They are usually sacrococcygeal or clival in location; the latter occasionally involves secondary sellar/ parasellar extension[69]. Although they are benign, these neoplasms are locally aggressive and can produce extensive local destruction. MRI is non-specific, showing a mass with high water content and associated destructive changes[18]. These tumors can be indistinguishable from the rare malignant pituitary

adenocarcinoma or other metastatic disease of the sella or pituitary gland[10] (Figure 23).

Relevant vascular anomalies

As mentioned in the discussion of preoperative workup of pituitary adenomas, careful attention must be paid to the adjacent vascular structures. Such inspection will not only reveal important normal variants but will also occasionally demonstrate true vascular pathology such as cavernous carotid aneurysms. On contrast-enhanced CT, these aneurysms may be indistinguishable from a macroadenoma or meningioma. However, on MRI, characteristic signal flow voids and/or laminated clot formation (with areas of alternating signal intensities creating an 'onion skin' appearance), will be seen on routine T₁- and T₂-weighted sequences and are essentially diagnostic (Figure 24). Angiography confirms the diagnosis. Additional supporting evidence includes the presence of flow-related

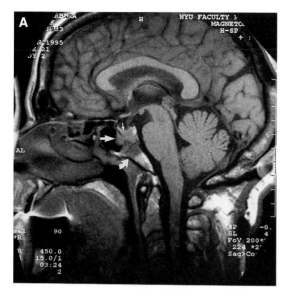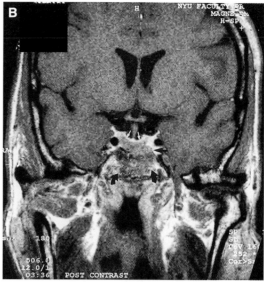

Figure 23 *A 61-year-old woman with acromegaly. (A) Pre-contrast sagittal and (B) post-contrast T_1-weighted images reveal a heterogeneous, partially enhancing mass involving the sella (large straight arrows) and clivus (curved arrows). The superior aspect of the mass is inseparable from the pituitary gland (small straight arrows). The radiographic findings are consistent with metastatic disease of the pituitary gland and/or clivus or a primary clivus chordoma*

registration artifacts as well as visualization of a normal pituitary gland. Patent aneurysms typically do not enhance, because rapid flow still entails a signal void[10] (Figure 25). Other vascular lesions that can occur in this region, such as arterial venous malformations and cavernous carotid fistulas, also have distinctive MRI characteristics (such as enlarged arteries and/or veins with accompanying flow voids, etc.) which allow easy differentiation from primary pituitary processes.

Other pituitary lesions

Although they usually occur as isolated abnormalities, pituitary adenomas infrequently occur as part of a broader syndrome. These rare disorders include MEN I (Wermer syndrome, characterized by tumors of the pituitary gland, parathyroid gland and pancreatic islet cells with a high incidence of peptic ulcers and/or Zollinger–Ellison syndrome), familial amenorrhea–galactorrhea (Forbes–Albright syndrome) and galactorrhea–amenorrhea occurring after pregnancy (Chiari–Frommel syndrome)[70].

Rarely, primary neoplasms other than adenomas may arise within the pituitary gland. In addition to the malignant counterparts (adenocarcinomas) of benign adenomas previously mentioned, primary melanoma may occur. These tumors may produce typical T_1 and T_2 shortening, with resulting lesions appearing 'bright' on T_1-weighted and 'dark' on T_2-weighted sequences[71]. Other rare primary pituitary neoplasms include intrasellar meningiomas[72], germinomas[73], choristomas[74] and gliomas[75].

The pituitary gland may also be involved by metastatic disease, most frequently reflecting metastatic disease to the adjacent sphenoid bone or clivus with secondary extension to involve the sella and/or pituitary gland[14]. The gland can be seeded with direct metastatic deposits, most commonly by primary lung or breast carcinoma or by lymphoma/leukemia[76]. Imaging studies may reveal a focal abnormality indistinguishable from an adenoma[18], frequently involving the stalk or hypothalamus. Rapid growth and/or invasion of adjacent structures, which sometimes occur with these lesions, may make

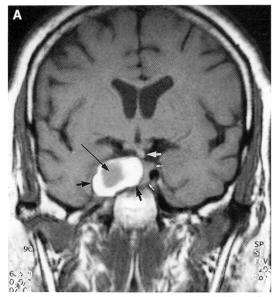

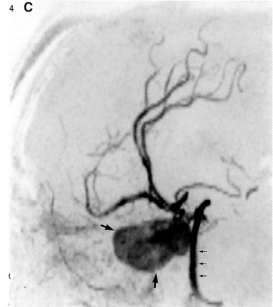

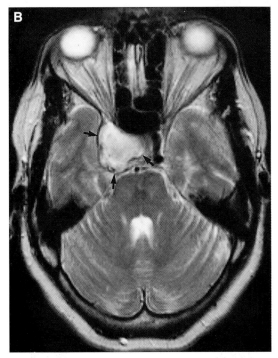

Figure 24 *A 66-year-old woman with a 3-week history of right eye symptoms. (A) Coronal T_1-weighted, (B) axial T_2-weighted and (C) time-of-flight magnetic resonance imaging intracerebral angiogram non-contrast images show a large, thrombosed right supraclinoid carotid artery aneurysm (large black arrows). Differences in signal of its T_1 hyperintense periphery compared with the relatively hypointense center (long black arrow) reflect different stages of clot. The infundibulum is displaced to the left (large white arrow), as is the pituitary gland (small white arrows). The proximal right internal carotid artery (small black arrows) as well as its distal branches appear normal on the magnetic resonance imaging angiogram*

differentiation from benign pituitary adenomas possible, but the typical metastatic deposit is generally indistinguishable from a pituitary adenocarcinoma, a primary sphenoid carcinoma or metastatic disease to the clivus with secondary pituitary/sellar involvement[18]. Patients rarely display symptoms from pituitary metastases, as they tend to die from the primary malignancy before such symptoms become manifest. The gland is, however, more frequently involved at autopsy with metastatic disease than is obvious clinically[14]. If patients do, in fact, have associated symptoms, cranial nerve abnorm-alities are more frequently encountered than endocrine derangement unless there is accompanying hypothalamic involvement[18]. However, diabetes insipidus can herald metastatic disease[77].

Gland enlargement may also be seen secondary to pituitary hyperplasia, which can have a number of causes, some physiological and some pathological. Normal physiological enlargement of the gland occurs in the first 2 months of life, at puberty and during

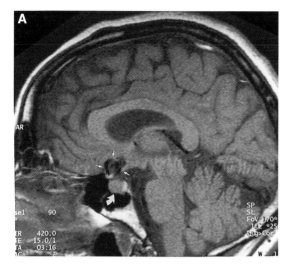

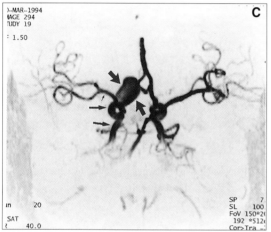

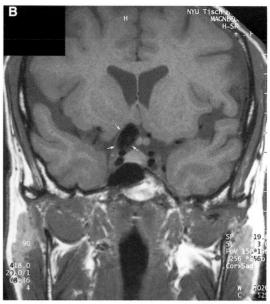

Figure 25 *A 55-year-old woman with increased prolactin. (A) Sagittal and (B) coronal non-contrast T_1-weighted images as well as a (C) time-of-flight magnetic resonance imaging angiogram of the intracerebral circulation reveal a patent right supraclinoid carotid aneurysm (small white arrows and large black arrows), displacing the optic chiasm to the left. A normal pituitary gland is noted separately (curved arrow). The proximal right internal carotid artery (medium black arrows) and distal right middle cerebral artery (small black arrow) are normal*

pregnancy. Pathological causes of gland enlargement include primary pituitary hyperplasia[78–82], precocious puberty (central)[25,83], exogenous estrogen, primary hypothyroidism (secondary to lack of negative feedback from circulating thyroxine with resulting thyrotroph hyperplasia)[84,85], hypothalamic neoplasms[86] and ectopic hormone production in some extrapituitary neoplasms[78]. The resulting enlarged gland associated with any of these conditions typically lacks evidence of a focal abnormality.

Infectious processes

Infection can infrequently involve the pituitary gland. Both tuberculosis and syphilitic infections have been reported in the past, but are rarely seen today. Direct viral infection has not been documented[87]. Bacterial infections occur, but are uncommon, and become apparent only when abscess formation occurs. This rare complication is typically associated with a previously existing pituitary abnormality such as an adenoma[88–90]. The affecting organism is most commonly a Gram-negative coccus, and infection may occur because of hematogenous seeding or direct extension from adjacent sphenoid or cavernous sinus disease. Because of the use of prophylactic antibiotics, infection status after trans-sphenoidal hypophysectomy is an uncommon occurrence. Patients with pituitary abscesses most often present with signs referable to mass effect instead of symptoms of inflammation or infection. Abscesses produce foci of T_1 hypointensity on pre-contrast scans and cannot be differentiated from adenomas. Post-contrast ring enhancement of the inflammatory capsule may allow the two to be distinguished[14].

Cysticercosis can affect the basal cisterns with involvement of the sella[75]. In its racemous form, multiple cystic lesions may be identified. Fungal infections can also affect the gland[91].

Inflammatory disorders

Inflammatory diseases can also involve the pituitary gland. Although they are uncommon, the most frequently encountered inflammatory processes are probably sarcoidosis and Langerhans cell histiocytosis (formerly histiocytosis X). In the former, granulomatous inflammation can affect the basal meninges with secondary involvement of the adjacent neural tissue, including the pituitary gland and/or hypothalamus. If referable symptoms are present, diabetes insipidus is most commonly noted, occurring in 5–10% of cases. Less commonly, panhypopituitarism occurs[14]. Imaging may variably demonstrate thickening of the stalk, a suprasellar/hypothalamic mass or scattered foci of abnormal enhancement within nearby subarachnoid spaces (reflecting meningeal disease) or adjacent brain parenchyma[92]. Stalk thickening can also be seen with Langerhans cell histiocytosis. This disease is more frequently associated with endocrine dysfunction than with neurosarcoidosis, with the 'classic triad' of diabetes insipidus, exophthalmus and lytic bone lesions seen in 25% of cases[43]. Other symptoms may be present, including alternative endocrine dysfunction (delayed puberty, hypothyroidism, hypoadrenalism and hyperprolactinemia) as well as visual changes[93]. Imaging may reveal thickening of the pituitary infundibulum, and contrast enhancement may also be present[94]. The posterior pituitary bright signal is often lost[14], as it is in other causes of diabetes insipidus (additional discussion of this phenomenon under Disorders of the neurohypophysis, below). The demonstration of bone lesions, usually via plain film, may establish the diagnosis.

Other granulomatous diseases can involve the pituitary gland; these include Wegener's granulomatosis (a systemic granulomatous disease manifested by a necrotizing vasculitis primarily affecting the respiratory tract and kidneys, usually in males) and Tolosa–Hunt syndrome (an inflammatory/granulomatous disease affecting tissue of the orbit and/or cavernous sinus or sellar region)[4]. The presence of typical associated clinical and/or radiographic stigmata lead to the diagnoses.

Lymphocytic (autoimmune) adenohypophysitis is a disease of pregnant or postpartum women characterized by lymphocytic and plasma cell infiltrates of this portion of the pituitary gland. The disease is felt to be secondary to the release of pituitary antigens during the puerperal involution of the adenohypophysis, resulting in the autoimmune response described above[95]. Patients present with galactorrhea, amenorrhea, headache and visual disturbances. MRI demonstrates a diffusely enlarged adenohypophysis, which homogeneously enhances.

Deposition diseases

A number of deposition diseases have been shown to involve the pituitary gland, including amyloidosis, selected mucopolysaccharidoses (e.g. Hurler's syndrome) and hemochromatosis[42]. In Hurler's syndrome, the bony dysplasia results in a 'J-shaped' sella. In hemochromatosis, iron overload results in deposition of hemosiderin and ferritin in multiple tissues, especially the liver, heart and pancreas. The pituitary may also be affected, with the gonadotropic cells particularly susceptible. Decreased secretion of LH and FSH owing to functional failure of the gonadotrophs is thought to produce the clinical symptoms of hypogonadism, and manifestations of male gynecomastia, testicular atrophy, hypogonadism and loss of libido[96]. Because of the paramagnetic effects of the deposited iron products, MRI demonstrates an abnormal decrease in signal of the anterior pituitary gland, especially on T_2-weighted sequences. MRI is in fact the only imaging sequence to be able to demonstrate any abnormality in this region in affected patients[14].

Disorders of the neurohypophysis

As mentioned earlier in the discussion of normal anatomy, the posterior pituitary gland 'bright spot' corresponds to the neurohypophysis, although the specific substance or substances that actually produce this T_1 hyperintensity are still somewhat controversial. Nevertheless, this normal finding can serve as an indicator of changes in the functional state of the posterior pituitary gland[97]. Specifically, when present (in up to 90% of normal patients), it confirms the integrity of the hypothalamic–neurohypophyseal axis[4]. Its absence does not necessarily denote pathology; however, its disappearance on serial imaging does. Various disease states can cause this phenomenon, the most frequently reported being diabetes insipidus. In one series, this loss of posterior pituitary bright signal was noted in almost all cases of central diabetes insipidus, but was a less constant finding in its hereditary form[98]. The appearance of the posterior pituitary bright signal has also been demonstrated to change in response to certain pharmacological agents[99] as well as to alterations in serum osmolality[100].

Disorders of the pituitary infundibulum

As previously noted, some inflammatory diseases, including sarcoidosis and Langerhans cell histiocytosis, may demonstrate changes of the pituitary stalk. Several other entities warrant mentioning, as the resulting anatomical alterations reflect the underlying physiological or anatomical derangements.

Specifically, disruption of the normal flow of neurosecretory molecules from the hypothalamus to the neurohypophysis may result in the buildup of these substances within the infundibulum. Such changes produce focal T_1 hyperintensity proximal to the point of obstruction. Accompanying loss of the posterior pituitary bright signal is typically noted. As expected, these changes are typically noted after the stalk has been violated, as occurs in traumatic trans-section[94] or after surgical hypophysectomy[101]. This finding can also be caused by stalk compression, as can occur with pituitary adenomas or other mass lesions[102].

CONCLUSION

In those patients with signs or symptoms referable to the pituitary gland or parasellar structures, MRI has replaced CT as the imaging modality of choice, because of its lack of ionizing radiation, its inherently better soft tissue contrast and its multiplanar capabilities. The patients routinely imaged include those with pituitary–hypothalamic axis endocrinopathies as well as those with neurological or neuro-ophthalmological symptoms potentially related to the sellar or parasellar regions; both disorders can lead to female or male infertility. For the amenorrheic woman presenting with reproductive failure, pituitary gland imaging is usually the final step in the workup, which involves excluding pregnancy, measuring serum TSH and prolactin levels, and performing a progestational challenge test. A 24 hour urine free cortisol should be performed initially for the Cushingoid patient, and serum insulin growth factor-1 (IGF-1) levels for the acromegalic patient. A normal study can aid in categorizing hypothalamic amenorrhea in association with low or normal gonadotropins and a history of stress, weight loss or heavy exercise. If the study is abnormal, imaging most frequently reveals an adenoma, which is the most common structural pituitary abnormality that can be responsible for these presenting symptoms in combination with various endocrinopathies. Rarer causes of pituitary gland and parasellar abnormalities must be entertained in the differential diagnosis, and have been outlined in this chapter. As always, communication of the pertinent clinical information to the radiologist is essential for guaranteeing that the examination provides the relevant diagnostic information.

References

1. Davis, P. C., Hoffman, J. C. Jr, Spencer, T., Tindall, G. T. and Braun, I. F. (1987). MR imaging of pituitary adenoma: CT, clinical, and surgical correlation. *Am. J. Roentgenol.*, **148**, 797–802

2. Pojunas, K. W., Daniels, D. L., Williams, A. L. *et al.* (1986). Magnetic resonance imaging prolactin secreting microadenomas. *Am. J. Neuroradiol.*, **7**, 209–13

3. Stein, A. L., Levenick, M. N. and Kletzky, O. A. (1989). Computed tomography versus magnetic resonance imaging for the evaluation of suspected pituitary adenomas. *Obstet. Gynecol.*, **73**, 996–9

4. Elster, A. D. (1993). Modern imaging of the pituitary. *Radiology*, **187**, 1–14

5. Doppman, J. L., Frank, J. A., Dwyer, A. J. *et al.* (1988). Gadolinium DTPA enhanced MR imaging of ACTH-secreting microadenomas of the pituitary gland. *J. Comput. Assist. Tomogr.*, **12**, 728–35

6. Dwyer, A. J., Frank, J. A., Doppman, J. L. *et al.* (1987). Pituitary adenomas in patients with Cushing's disease: initial experience with Gd-DTPA-enhanced MR imaging. *Radiology*, **163**, 421

7. Macpherson, P., Hadley, D. M., Teasdale, E. *et al.* (1989). Pituitary microadenomas: does gadolinium enhance their demonstration? *Neuroradiology*, **31**, 293–8

8. Newton, D. R., Dillion, W. P., Norman, D. *et al.* (1900). Gd-DTPA-enhanced MR imaging of pituitary adenomas. *Am. J. Neuroradiol.*, **10**, 949–54

9. Steiner, E., Imhof, H. and Knosp, E. (1989). Gd-DTPA enhanced high resolution MR imaging of pituitary adenomas. *Radiographics*, **9**, 587–98

10. Litt, A. W. and Kricheff, I. I. (1991). Magnetic resonance imaging of pituitary tumors. In *Contemporary Diagnosis and Management of Pituitary Adenomas*, pp. 1–19. (New York: AANS Publications)

11. Miki, Y., Matsuo, M., Nishizawa, S. *et al.* (1990). Pituitary adenomas and normal pituitary tissue: enhancement patterns on gado-pentetate-enhanced MR images. *Radiology*, **177**, 35–8

12. Sakamoto, Y., Takahashi, M., Korogi, Y., Bussaka, H. and Ushio, Y. (1991). Normal and abnormal pituitary glands: gadopentetate dimeglumine-enhanced MR imaging. *Radiology*, **178**, 441–5

13. Tien, R. D. (1992). Sequence of enhancement of various portions of the pituitary gland on gadolinium-enhanced MR images: correlation with regional blood supply. *Am. J. Roentgenol.*, **158**, 651–4

14. Chong, B. W. and Newton, T. H. (1993). Hypothalamic and pituitary pathology. *Radiol. Clin. North Am.*, **31**, 1147–83

15. Bergstrom, M., Muhr, C., Lundberg, P. O. and Langstrom, B. (1991). PET as a tool in the clinical evaluation of pituitary adenomas. *J. Nucl. Med.*, **32**, 610–15

16. De Souza, B., Brunetti, A., Fulham, M. J. *et al.* (1990). Pituitary microadenomas: a PET study. *Radiology*, **177**, 39–44

17. Francavilla, T. L., Miletich, R. S., DeMichele, D. *et al.* (1991). Positron emission tomography of pituitary macroadenomas: hormone production and effects of therapies. *Neurosurgery*, **28**, 826–33

18. Chakeres, D. W., Curtin, A. and Ford, G. (1989). Magnetic resonance imaging of pituitary and parasellar abnormalities. *Radiol. Clin. North Am.*, **27**, 265–81

19. Williams, P. L., Warwick, R., Dyson, M. and Bannister, L. H. (1989). The hypophysis cerebri. In Gray, H., Warwick, R. and Williams, P. L. (eds.) *Anatomy of the Human Body*, 37th edn, pp. 1451–6. (New York: Churchill-Livingstone)

20. Reichlin, S. (1992). Neuroendocrinology. In Wilson, J. D. and Foster, D. W. (eds.) *Williams Textbook of Endocrinology*, 8th edn, pp. 135–219. (Philadelphia: Saunders)

21. Baker, B. L. (1974). Functional cytology of the hypophysial pars distalis and pars intermedia. In Greep, R. O., Astwood, E. B., Knobil, E. *et al.* (eds.) *Handbook of Physiology*. Section 7: *Endocrinology*, vol. IV, part 1: *The Pituitary Gland and its Neuroendocrine Control*, pp. 45–80. (Washington, DC: American Physiological Society)

22. Cox, T. D. and Elster, A. D. (1991). Normal pituitary gland: changes in shape, size, and signal intensity during the 1st year of life at MR imaging. *Radiology*, **179**, 721–4

23. Wolpert, S. M., Osborne, M., Anderson, M. and Runge, V. M. (1988). The bright pituitary gland: a normal MR appearance in infancy. *Am. J. Neuroradiol.*, **9**, 1–3

24. Argyropoulos, M., Perignon, F., Brunelle, F., Brauner, R. and Rappaport, R. (1991). Height of normal pituitary gland as a function of age evaluated by magnetic resonance imaging. *Pediatr. Radiol.*, **21**, 247–9

25. Elster, A. D., Chen, M. Y. M., Williams, D. W. III and Key, L. L. (1990). Pituitary gland: MR imaging of physiologic hypertrophy in adolescence. *Radiology*, **174**, 681–5

26. Hayakawa, K., Konishsi, Y., Matsuda, T. *et al.* (1989). Developmental and ageing of brain midline structures: assessment with MR imaging. *Radiology*, **172**, 171–7

27. Konishi, Y., Kuriyama, M., Sudo, M., Hayakawa, K., Konishi, K. and Nakamura, K. (1985). Growth patterns of the normal pituitary gland and in pituitary adenoma. *Dev. Med. Child. Neurol.*, **32**, 69–73

28. Peyster, R. G., Hoover, E. D. and Adler, L. P. (1984). CT of the normal pituitary stalk. *Am. J. Neuroradiol.*, **5**, 45–7

29. Peyster, R. G., Hoover, E. D., Viscarello, R. R. *et al.* (1983). CT appearance of the adolescent and preadolescent pituitary gland. *Am. J. Neuroradiol.*, **4**, 411–14

30. Lee, B. C. P. and Deck, M. D. F. (1985). Sellar and juxtasellar lesion detection with MR. *Radiology*, **157**, 143–7

31. Suzuki, M., Takashima, T., Kadoya, M. *et al.* (1990) Height of normal pituitary gland on MR imaging: age and sex differentiation. *J. Comput. Assist. Tomogr.*, **14**, 36–9

32. Goluboff, L. G. and Ezrin, C. (1969). Effect of pregnancy on the somatroph and the prolactin cells of the human adenohypophysis. *J. Clin. Endocrinol. Metab.*, **29**, 1533–43

33. Elster, A. D., Sanders, T. G., Vines, F. S. and Chen, M. Y. M. (1991). Size and shape of the pituitary gland during pregnancy and post partum: measurement with MR imaging. *Radiology*, **181**, 531–5

34. Reid, R. L., Quigley, M. E. and Yen, S. S. C. (1985). Pituitary apoplexy: a review. *Arch. Neurol.*, **42**, 712–19

35. Smith, D. E., Murphy, M. J., Hitchon, P. W. *et al.* (1983). Transsphenoidal encephaloceles. *Surg. Neurol.*, **20**, 471

36. Craft, W. H., Underwood, L. E. and Van Wyk, J. J. (1980). High incidence or perinatal insult in children with idiopathic hypopituitarism. *J. Pediatr.*, **98**, 397–402

37. Abrams, J. J., Trefelner, E. and Boulware, S. D. (1991). Idiopathic growth hormone deficiency: MR findings in 35 patients. *Am. J. Neuroradiol.*, **12**, 155–60

38. Cacciari, E., Zucchini, S., Carla, G. *et al.* (1990). Endocrine function and morphological findings in patients with disorders of the hypothalamo–pituitary area: a study with magnetic resonance. *Arch. Dis. Child.*, **65**, 1199–202

39. Kuroiwa, T., Okabe, Y., Hasuo, K., Yasumori, K., Mizushima, A. and Masuda, K. (1991). MR imaging of pituitary dwarfism. *Am. J. Neuroradiol.*, **12**, 161–4

40. Maghnie, M., Triulzi, F., Larizza, D. *et al.* (1990). Hypothalamic–pituitary dwarfism: comparison between MR imaging and CT findings. *Pediatr. Radiol.*, **20**, 229–35

41. Yamanaka, C., Momoi, T., Fujisawa, I. *et al.* (1990). Neurohypophyseal function of an ectopic posterior lobe in patients with growth hormone deficiency. *Acta Endocrinol. (Copenh.)*, **122**, 664–70

42. Treip, C. S. (1992). The hypothalamus and the pituitary gland. In Adams, J. H. and Duchen, L. W. (eds.) *Greenfield's Neuropathology*, 5th edn, pp. 1046–82. (New York: Oxford University Press)

43. Kucharcyzk, W. and Montanera, W. J. (1991). The sella and parasellar region. In Atlas, S. W. (ed.) *Magnetic Resonance Imaging of the Brain and Spine*, pp. 625–67. (New York: Raven Press)

44. Elster, A. D. (1988). *Cranial Magnetic Resonance Imaging*, pp. 281–336. (New York: Churchill Livingstone)

45. Kucharczyk, W., Davis, D. O., Kelly, W. M. *et al.* (1986). Pituitary adenomas: high-resolution MR imaging at 1.5T. *Radiology*, **161**, 761–5

46. Peck, W. W., Dillon, W. P., Norman, D. *et al.* (1989). High-resolution MR imaging of pituitary microadenomas at 1.5T: experience with Cushing's disease. *Am. J. Roentgenol.*, **152**, 145–51

47. Kulkarni, M. V., Lee, K. F., McArdle, C. V. *et al.* (1988). 1.5T MR imaging of pituitary microadenomas: technical considerations and CT correlation. *Am. J. Neuroradiol.*, **9**, 5–11

48. Nichols, D. A., Laws, E. R. Jr, Houser, O. W. *et al.* (1988). Comparison of magnetic resonance imaging and computed tomography in the preoperative evaluation of pituitary adenomas. *Neurosurgery*, **22**, 380–5

49. Kovaks, K., Horvath, E. and Asa, S. L. (1900). Classification and pathology of pituitary tumors. In Wilkins, R. H. and Rengachary, S. S. (eds.) *Neurosurgery*. (New York)

50. Russell, D. S. and Rubinstein, L. J. (1989). *Pathology of Tumors of the Nervous System*, 5th edn, pp. 809–54. (Baltimore: Williams & Wilkins)

51. Lacomis, D., Johnson, L. N. and Mamourian, A. C. (1988). Magnetic resonance imaging in pituitary apoplexy. *Arch. Ophthalmol.*, **106**

52. Yousem, D. M., Arrington, J. A., Zinreich, S. J., Kumar, A. J. and Byran, R. N. (1989). Pituitary adenomas: possible role of bromocriptine in intratumoral hemorrhage. *Radiology*, **170**, 239–43

53. Wilson, C. B. (1979). Neurosurgical management of large and invasive pituitary tumors. In Tindall, G. T. and Collins, W. F. (eds.) *Clinical Management of Pituitary Disorders*, pp. 335–42. (New York: Raven Press)

54. Shucart, W. A. (1980). Implications of very high serum prolactin levels associated with pituitary tumors. *J. Neurosurg.*, **52**, 226–8

55. Scotti, G., Yu, C. Y., Dillon, W. P. *et al.* (1988). Magnetic resonance imaging of the cavernous sinus involvement by pituitary adenomas. *Am. J. Neuroradiol.*, **9**, 657–64

56. Scheithauer, B. W. (1984). Surgical pathology of the pituitary: the adenomas. *Pathol. Ann.*, **19**, 269–81

57. Dolinskas, C. A. and Simeone, F. A. (1985). Transsphenoidal hypophysectomy: postsurgical findings. *Am. J. Roentgenol.*, **144**, 487–92

58. Kaplan, H. C., Baker, H. L. Jr, Houser, O. W., Laws, E. R. Jr, Abboud, C. F. and Scheithauer, B. W. (1985). CT of the sella turcica after transsphenoidal resection of pituitary adenomas. *Am. J. Neuroradiol.*, **6**, 723–32

59. Teng, M. M. H., Huang, C. I. and Chang, T. (1988). The pituitary mass after transsphenoidal hypophysectomy. *Am. J. Neuroradiol.*, **9**, 23–6

60. Kaufman, B., Tomsak, R. L., Kaufman, B. A. *et al.* (1989). Herniation of the suprasellar visual system and third ventricle into empty sellae: morphologic and clinical considerations. *Am. J. Roentgenol.*, **152**, 597–608

61. Pusey, E., Kortman, K. E., Flannigan, B. D. *et al.* (1987). MR of craniopharyngioma: tumor delineation and characterization. *Am. J. Neuroradiol.*, **8**, 439

62. Carmel, P. W., Anrtunes, J. L. and Chang, C. H. (1982). Craniopharyngiomas in children. *Neurosurgery*, **11**, 382

63. Young, S. C., Zimmerman, R. A., Nowell, M. A. *et al.* (1987). Giant cystic craniopharyngiomas. *Neuroradiology*, **29**, 468–73

64. Weiner, S. N., Pearlstein, A. E. and Eiber, A. (1987). MR imaging of intracranial arachnoid cysts. *J. Comput. Assist. Tomogr.*, **11**, 236

65. Onda, K., Tanaka, R., Yamada, N. and Takahashi, H. (1989). Symptomatic Rathke's cleft cyst simulating arachnoid cyst – case report. *Neurol. Med. Chir.*, **29**, 1039

66. Marliani, A. F., Tampieri, D., Melancon, D. *et al.* (1991). Magnetic resonance imaging of hypothalamic hamartomas causing gelastic epilepsy. *Can. Assoc. Radiol. J.*, **42**, 335

67. Asa, S. L., Bilboa, J. M., Kovacs, K. *et al.* (1980). Hypothalamic neuronal hamartoma associated with pituitary growth hormone cell adenoma and acromegaly. *Acta Neuropathol.*, **52**, 231

68. Rubinstein, L. J. (1972). *Atlas of Tumor Pathology*, Second Series, Fascicle 6: *Tumors of the Central Nervous System*. (Washington DC: Armed Forces Institute of Pathology)

69. Larson, T. C., Houser, O. W. and Laws, E. R. (1987). Imaging of cranial chordomas. *Mayo Clin. Prox.*, **62**, 886–93

70. Rimoin, D. L. (1990). Genetic disorders of the pituitary gland. In Emergy, A. E. H. and Rimoin, D. L. (eds.) *Principles and Practice of Medical Genetics*, 2nd edn, pp. 1461–88. (Edinburgh: Churchill Livingstone)

71. Chappell, P. M. and Kelly, W. M. (1990). Pituitary sellar melanoma simulating hemorrhagic pituitary adenoma: MR and pathologic findings. *Am. J. Neuroradiol.*, **11**, 1054

72. Michael, A. S. and Paige, M. L. (1988). MR imaging of intrasellar meningiomas simulating pituitary adenomas. *J. Comput. Assist. Tomogr.*, **12**, 944–6

73. Banna, M., Schatz, S. W., Molot, M. J. and Groves, J. (1976). Primary intrasellar germinoma. *Br. J. Radiol.*, **49**, 971–3

74. Cone, L., Srinivasan, M. and Romanul, F. C. A. (1990). Granular cell tumor (choristoma) of the neurohypophysis: two cases and a review of the literature. *Am. J. Neuroradiol.*, **11**, 403–6

75. Scothorne, C. (1955). A glioma of the posterior lobe of the pituitary gland. *J. Pathol.*, **69**, 109–12

76. Kimmel, D. W. and O'Neill, B. P. P. (1983). Systemic cancer presenting as diabetes insipidus. *Cancer*, **52**, 2355

77. Schubiger, O. and Haller, D. (1992). Metastases to the pituitary–hypothalamic axis. An MR study of 7 symptomatic patients. *Neuroradiology*, **34**, 131

78. Horvath, E. (1988). Pituitary hyperplasia. *Pathol. Res. Pract.*, **183**, 623–5

79. Jay, V., Kovacs, K., Horvath, E., Lloyd, R. V. and Smyth, H. S. (1991). Idiopathic prolactin cell hyperplasia of the pituitary mimicking prolactin cell adenoma: a morphological study including immunocytochemistry, electron microscopy, and *in situ* hybridization. *Acta Neuropathol.*, **82**, 147–51

80. Moran, A., Asa, S. L., Kovacs, K. *et al.* (1990). Gigantism due to pituitary mammosomatotroph hyperplasia. *N. Engl. J. Med.*, **323**, 322–7

81. Peillon, F., Dupuy, M., Li, J. Y. *et al.* (1991). Pituitary enlargement with suprasellar extension in functional hyperprolactinemia

due to lactotrophy hyperplasia: a pseudo-tumoral disease. *J. Clin. Endocrinol. Metab.*, **73**, 1008–15

82. Young, W. F. Jr, Scheithauer, B. W., Gharib, H., Laws, E. R. Jr and Carpenter, P. C. (1988). Cushing's syndrome due to primary multi-nodular corticotrophe hyperplasia. *Mayo Clin. Proc.*, **63**, 256–62

83. Kao, S. C., Cook, J. S., Hansen, J. R. and Simonson, T. M. (1991). MR imaging of the pituitary gland in untreated central precocious puberty (abstr.). *Radiology*, **181(P)**, 103

84. Atchison, J. A., Lee, P. A. and Albright, A. L. (1989). Reversible suprasellar pituitary mass secondary to hypothyroidism. *J. Am. Med. Assoc.*, **262**, 3175–7

85. Hutchins, W. W., Crues, J. V. III, Miya, P. and Pojunas, K. W. (1990). MR demonstration of pituitary hyperplasia and regression after therapy for hypothyroidism. *Am. J. Neuroradiol.*, **11**, 410

86. Cusimano, M. D., Kovacs, K., Bilbai, J. M., Tucker, W. S. and Singer, W. (1988). Suprasellar craniopharyngioma associated with hyperpro-lactinemia, pituitary lactotroph hyperplasia, and microprolactinoma. *J. Neurosurg.*, **69**, 620–3

87. Daughaday, W. H. (1985). The anterior pituitary. In Wilson, J. D. and Foster, D. W. (eds.) *Williams Textbook of Endocrinology*, 7th edn, pp. 568–612. (Philadelphia: W.B. Saunders)

88. Dominque, J. N. and Wilson, C. B. (1977). Pituitary abscesses: report of 7 cases and review of the literature. *J. Neurosurg.*, **46**, 601

89. Gupta, R. K., Jena, A. and Sharma, A. (1989). Sellar abscess associated with tuberculosis osteomyelitis of the skull: MR findings. *Am. J. Neuroradiol.*, **10**, 448

90. Selosse, P., Mahler, C. and Klaes, R. L. (1980). Pituitary abscess: case report. *J. Neurosurg.*, **53**, 851

91. Kelly, P. (1982). Systemic blastomycosis with associated diabetes insipidus. *Ann. Intern. Med.*, **96**, 66–7

92. Sherman, J. L. and Stern, B. J. (1990). Sarcoidosis of the CNS: comparison of unenhanced and enhanced MR images. *Am. J. Neuroradiol.*, **11**, 915

93. Ober, K. P., Alexander, E. Jr, Challa, V. R. *et al.* (1989). Histiocytosis X of the hypothalamus. *Neurosurgery*, **24**, 93

94. Tien, R. and Kucharczyk, W. (1991). MR imaging of the brain in patients with diabetes insipidus. *Am. J. Neuroradiol.*, **12**, 533–42

95. Goudie, R. B. and Pinkerton, P. H. (1962). Anterior hypophysitis and Hashimoto's disease in a young woman. *J. Pathol. Bacteriol.*, **83**, 584

96. Bergeron, C. and Kovacs, K. (1978). Pituitary siderosis. *Am. J. Pathol.*, **93**, 295

97. Brooks, B. S., El Gammal, T., Allison, J. D. and Hoffman, W. H. (1989). Frequency and variation of the posterior pituitary bright signal on MR images. *Am. J. Neuroradiol.*, **10**, 943–8

98. Fujisawa, I., Nishimura, K., Asato, R. *et al.* (1987). Posterior lobe of the pituitary in diabetes insipidus: MR findings. *J. Comput. Assist. Tomogr.*, **11**, 221–5

99. Kucharczyk, J., Kucharczyk, W., Berry, I. *et al.* (1988). Histochemical characterization and functional significance of the hyperintense signal on MR images of the posterior pituitary. *Am. J. Neuroradiol.*, **9**, 1079–83

100. Fujisawa, I., Asato, R., Kawata, M. *et al.* (1989). Hyperintense signal of the posterior pituitary on T_1-weighted MR images: an experimental study. *J. Comput. Assist. Tomogr.*, **13**, 371–7

101. Walker, F. O., McLean, W. T. Jr, Elster, A. and Stanton, C. (1990). Chiasmal sarcoidosis. *Am. J. Neuroradiol.*, **11**, 1205–7

102. El Gammal, T., Brooks, B. S. and Hoffman, W. H. (1989). MR imaging of the ectopic bright signal of posterior pituitary regenera-tion. *Am. J. Neuroradiol.*, **10**, 323–8

Application of imaging for ovulation induction and *in vitro* fertilization–embryo transfer

11

L. B. Schwartz, M. J. Nachtigall and N. Laufer

Assisted reproductive technologies are used for the treatment of many causes of infertility. Ovulation induction with clomiphene citrate (CC) has classically been used to treat infertility due to anovulation. Human menopausal gonadotropins (hMG) have been used to treat anovulation, luteal phase defect, endometriosis and unexplained and male factor infertility. Controlled ovarian hyperstimulation induces the growth of multiple follicles for superovulation as well as their growth in conjunction with *in vitro* fertilization and embryo transfer (IVF-ET).

Transvaginal ultrasound (TVUS) has become extremely valuable, if not essential, for monitoring natural as well as induced cycles. The size and number of developing follicles can be determined with TVUS. This enables cycles to be managed safely by maximizing pregnancy outcome and minimizing complications such as hyperstimulation and multiple pregnancies. TVUS also provides information about endometrial thickness and other detailed information about the endometrial lining which aids in determining the adequacy of treatment and the accurate timing for injection of human chorionic gonadotropin (hCG).

Unlike TVUS, other imaging modalities have not proved useful in managing ovulation induction and IVF-ET cycles. Given the accuracy, ease, non-invasiveness and cost-effectiveness of TVUS when used for this purpose, further evaluation of computed tomography (CT) scan or pelvic magnetic resonance imaging (MRI) in this context is not warranted at this time.

THE USE OF TVUS FOR MONITORING THE NATURAL OVULATORY CYCLE

Ultrasound has been used to characterize the normal menstrual cycle in healthy ovulatory women. Recruitment of a cohort of developing follicles occurs in the late luteal phase of the previous menstrual cycle and the early follicular phase of the present cycle. Most of these primordial follicles regress and are too small to be visualized by ultrasound. Some follicles continue to develop past the pre-antral phase and, under the influence of follicle stimulating hormone (FSH), continue to grow with increasing estradiol production. When the follicles achieve a size of 3–5 mm they can be detected by TVUS. The dominant follicle is chosen around cycle day 8 when it measures 8–10 mm[1] and grows about 2 mm/day[2] until ovulation, while the other follicles undergo atresia[3]. One group[4] found that the dominant follicle progressively increased and reached a mean diameter of 21.5 mm at ovulation. Corresponding mid-cycle estradiol levels of 150–200 pg/ml have been reported[3]. Ovulation occurs 36–38 h following the luteinizing hormone (LH) surge[1] and is usually associated with shrinkage or disappearance of the follicle on ultrasound scanning[4,5]. Fluid is seen in the cul-de-sac in only 50% of women and, when present, it is maximal 4–5 days after ovulation[5]. Ultrasound also enables visualization of the corpus luteum. Color Doppler ultrasound may be a better way to evaluate corpus luteum function.

The resistance index (RI) and pulsatility index (PI) are the most reproducible measurements for the evaluation of the corpus luteum. The RI (defined as the systolic peak minus the diastolic peak, divided by the systolic peak) ranges from 0 to 1.0, with 1.0 representing the highest resistance to forward flow. The PI, another measurement of vascular impedance, is defined as the systolic peak minus the diastolic peak, divided by the mean flow velocity[6]. The ovarian artery PI has been shown to have a cyclical pattern. During the follicular phase, it is usually high (> 2.0), with a gradual decrease as follicular maturation progresses. With vascularization of the corpus luteum, diastolic flow increases, with lower PI values[7]. Taylor and colleagues[7] demonstrated that high diastolic blood flow and low-impedance Doppler waveforms (low RI and PI) are present in the ovary containing the active corpus luteum. The inactive ovary shows low diastolic flow and high impedance (high RI and PI). A decreased PI has also been observed in the uterine arteries with formation of the corpus luteum[6]. Therefore, Doppler TVUS shows promise for evaluation of normal and abnormal luteal phase utero-ovarian blood flow, because a healthy corpus luteum is associated with a high diastolic blood flow and low impedance in the ovarian and uterine arteries.

The endometrial characteristics detected on TVUS can also be helpful in evaluating the luteal as well as the follicular phase[8]. The endometrial echo is usually measured in the largest anteroposterior diameter in a sagittal section at the most fundal region. Following menstruation, the endometrium is at its thinnest and displays a 'pencil-line' ultrasound appearance (Figure 1A). As the proliferative phase progresses and estradiol levels increase, the endometrium thickens and is visualized by a widening triple pattern: a hypoechoic interface within the luminal aspects of echogenic endometrial layers ('triple-line' sign)[8] (Figure 1B). The endometrial thickness has been shown to increase from 6.1 mm 4 days prior to the LH surge to 8.7 mm in diameter 1 day after the surge in the natural cycle[6]. The lining develops a homogeneous echogenic appearance after ovulation in response to progesterone[9,10] (Figure 1C). The homogeneously echogenic thickened endometrial ultrasound pattern is seen in the luteal phase and is predictive of ovulation, but cannot replace the accuracy of the endometrial biopsy for confirmation of ovulation and endometrial dating.

THE USE OF TVUS FOR MONITORING OVULATION INDUCTION CYCLES DURING INFERTILITY TREATMENT

The use of TVUS has become critical for accurate monitoring of folliculogenesis and endometrial growth during ovulation induction cycles in patients treated with both CC and hMG.

Clomiphene citrate

CC is classically used to induce ovulation in anovulatory patients with a functioning hypothalamus and pituitary gland such as those with polycystic ovarian disease (PCOD). CC (Clomid®, Serophene®) is a synthetic weak estrogen that competes with endogenous estrogen for estrogen binding sites in the hypothalamus. This results in increased pulse frequency of gonadotropin releasing hormone (GnRH)[1]. GnRH stimulates FSH, which results in increased ovarian follicular development. CC is usually administered for 5 consecutive days (starting on days 3–5 and ending on days 7–9) of the cycle.

TVUS is useful for monitoring the ovarian response to CC with assessment of the size, number and growth of follicles. Ultrasound shows progressive follicular growth throughout the CC-induced cycle, as in the natural cycle (Figure 2). A greater mean follicular diameter is usually attained with CC administration compared with the natural cycle (27.2 mm, range 16.4–31.9 mm vs. 21.6 mm, range 14.4–31.2 mm, respectively)[5]. TVUS monitoring during ovulation induction allows for the prediction of multiple gestations in a patient with many follicles. CC can be used with an ovulation predictor kit for timed

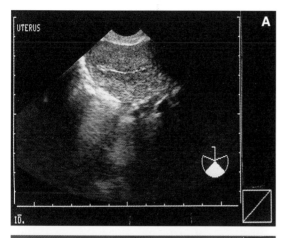

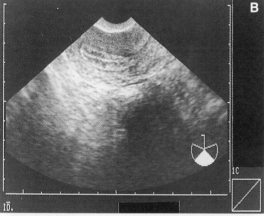

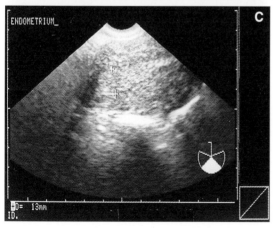

Figure 1 (A) Longitudinal sonographic image of day 3 thin endometrial echo. (B) Longitudinal view of trilaminar endometrial echo immediately prior to ovulation. (C) Longitudinal view of incompletely homogeneous endometrial echo immediately after ovulation. As the luteal phase progresses, the echogenicity will become completely homogeneous

intercourse or intrauterine insemination (IUI). Ultrasound also allows for timely intervention with hCG to trigger ovulation. When the size of the follicle reaches at least 20 mm, hCG can be administered (usually 10 000 IU intramuscularly) and ovulation should occur approximately 36 h later. This can improve accurate timing for intercourse or IUI. One group[11] studied patients treated with CC and IUI for male factor and unexplained infertility and found a significant improvement in pregnancy rates with CC and ultrasound using hCG and timed IUI vs. the natural cycle with LH detection kits and IUI (55% per cycle versus 26.1% per cycle, respectively).

Ultrasound monitoring confirms that the endometrium thickens throughout the follicular phase of CC-induced cycles, as it does in the natural cycle[5]. Endometrial thickness has been shown to increase from 5 mm to 9.6 mm during CC cycles (measured from 4 days prior to the LH surge to 1 day after the surge)[5]. The endometrium in the CC-stimulated group was thinner than the unstimulated endometrium until the day of the LH surge, following which it became thicker[5].

In summary, ultrasound can be helpful in monitoring CC-induced cycles by detecting the number and size of dominant follicles as well as in predicting endometrial receptivity. The follicles should grow 2–3 mm/day and therefore the day for hCG administration can be predicted by a single rather than repetitive ultrasound examinations. This allows for more cost-effectively monitored cycles.

Human menopausal gonadotropins

Ovulation induction with hMG and/or purified FSH has been used to induce the development of multiple follicles in women with many causes of infertility including anovulation, idiopathic etiology, endometriosis and hypothalamic/pituitary dysfunction. The use of hMG does not require the patient to have an intact hypothalamus, since its actions are directed at the ovary.

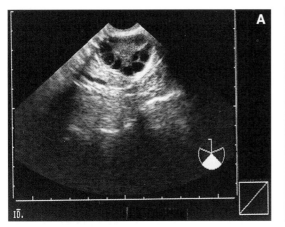 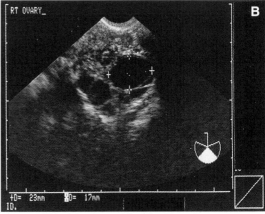

Figure 2 *Transvaginal ultrasound images of an ovary in a patient with a history of polycystic ovary disease (PCOD). (A) Multiple small peripheral follicles characteristic of PCOD, before initiation of clomiphene citrate (CC) treatment. (B) Day 12 in a cycle treated with CC (50 mg/day, days 5–9), showing the development of the dominant follicle*

TVUS has a vital role in monitoring the follicular response to ovulation-inducing agents[11]. For patients in whom luteal phase down-regulation with GnRH agonists (GnRH-a) is first achieved before ovulation induction is initiated, TVUS can be used in combination with low serum estradiol levels to confirm the appearance of 'quiet ovaries' without follicular or cystic activity as well as a thin (< 5 mm) endometrial echo. The incorporation of GnRH-a into various combinations of exogenous gonadotropins provides many advantages, including the prevention of premature luteinization, reduction of cycle cancellation rates and generation of an increased number of follicles and oocytes[12]. Occasionally, such use of GnRH-a can initially inadvertently cause ovarian stimulation before achieving suppression (a 'flare' effect). Resultant ovarian follicular cysts can be detected by TVUS, and this finding could direct the continued sole use of GnRH-a (usually for 2 more weeks) until suppression is achieved, before ovulation-inducing agents are added.

Follicular development in patients undergoing ovulation induction with either GnRH-a and gonadotropins or gonadotropins alone is usually monitored with serial TVUS and serum estradiol levels approximately every 2–3 days, usually beginning on cycle days 7–9[13]. As with CC cycles, follicular growth of 2 mm/day is expected, with simultaneously rising serum estradiol levels. The gonadotropins are usually started on cycle day 3, or once suppression is achieved with GnRH-a down-regulation, and are continued daily until ovulation is induced[13]. TVUS measurement of follicular number and size is critical (Figure 3), since hCG is administered to induce ovulation once the follicles reach 15–19 mm in diameter, corresponding to a serum estradiol level of 200–300 pg/ml per mature follicle[14]. Ovulation should occur approximately 36 h after hCG administration, and intercourse or an IUI is then scheduled 24–48 h later.

Endometrial assessment has been added to the armamentarium of TVUS monitoring of ovulation induction cycles. As with natural and CC-induced cycles, the TVUS endometrial echo in gonadotropin-induced cycles also varies throughout the cycle. During the 'follicular phase' of the induced cycle, the endometrial echo usually appears trilaminar and continuously increases in diameter to a maximum of 8–15 mm at mid-cycle. After the administration of hCG, ovarian progesterone production is initiated and corresponds to a homogeneous endometrial echo, which maintains its thickness until sloughing occurs at menses. In abnormal conditions, such as

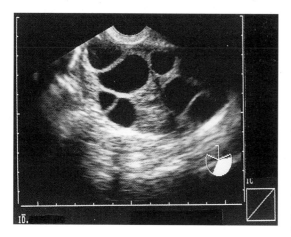

Figure 3 *Transvaginal ultrasound scan of an ovary in an infertile woman treated with GnRH-agonist down-regulation followed by ovulation induction with hMG, showing multiple developing follicles*

premature luteinization experienced by some PCOD patients, incomplete endometrial TVUS patterns can be detected during the follicular phase. Other abnormal TVUS endometrial appearances include thin (< 8.0 mm) or irregular central uterine echoes.

THE APPLICATION OF TVUS TO IVF-ET

IVT-ET has been successfully used for the treatment of many types of infertility for over 10 years. Ovulation induction is used more aggressively for IVF-ET than when performed without the addition of this procedure, in order to stimulate the growth of more follicles and increase the number of aspirated oocytes for optimal chances at fertilization and subsequent embryo transfer, thereby increasing the chance of pregnancy. Similar to its use in non-IVF ovulation-induction cycles, TVUS, in combination with measurement of estradiol levels, is used for serial monitoring of folliculogenesis and endometrial growth during IVF treatment. Also, similar to non-IVF ovulation induction cycles, follicular growth of 2–3 mm/day is expected, with simultaneously rising serum estradiol values. For optimal oocyte quality, hCG is typically administered when at least

2–3 follicles reach 15–19 mm in average diameter, corresponding to estradiol values of approximately 300 pg/ml per mature follicle, and the follicles are then aspirated 34–36 h later[15]. Aberrant folliculogenesis sonographic patterns include slow growth, no growth or decreasing size over time, and are associated with non-fertilizable oocytes[16].

In addition to obtaining fertilizable oocytes, optimal endometrial development is also necessary for adequate endometrial receptivity and successful conception[17], but the literature has not shown a consistent role of endometrial ultrasound monitoring for predicting pregnancy outcome in IVF cycles. An association has been shown between the endometrial TVUS texture and serum estradiol levels[17]. Triple (trilaminar) echogenic patterns seem to be more likely to sustain pregnancy than homogeneous patterns[18–22]. A preovulatory multilayered appearance of the endometrial echo has been associated with a positive pregnancy in contradistinction to incomplete or homogeneous patterns in IVF-ET cycles[23–25].

Some studies report no difference in endometrial thickness between pregnant and non-pregnant IVF cycles[18,26], whereas others find a thicker endometrium in subsequently pregnant patients[27,28]. Cut-off levels of endometrial thickness necessary for successful implantation have been proposed: ≥ 6 mm[18,29], ≥ 10 mm[19,28] or ≥ 13 mm[17,27]. One group[30] studied ultrasound monitoring of IVF cycles and showed a more positive correlation between serum estradiol levels and endometrial thickness than with the number of developing follicles, and a significant inverse correlation between endometrial thickness and plasma progesterone levels. Such data suggest that TVUS-measured endometrial thickness may be useful when combined with follicular measurements and serum estradiol levels for improving decision making about the timing of hCG administration. Moreover, another group[31] found that there were no significant differences in the amount of hMG used, number of oocytes and embryos obtained, pregnancy rates, or rate and severity of ovarian hyperstimulation syndrome (OHSS) in a group of IVF-ET patients whose ovulation induction was monitored by ultrasound only, vs. those followed with both ultrasound and hormonal measurements, suggesting that ultrasound-only monitoring of IVF-ET cycles may be adequate.

The literature regarding the usefulness of color Doppler TVUS for monitoring and predicting pregnancy outcome of IVF-ET cycles has been inconclusive. A PI of < 3[32] or < 3.3[33] was reported to be most favorable for a positive pregnancy outcome. RI was determined to be significantly lower at the time of oocyte aspiration in subsequently pregnant[34] than in non-pregnant outcomes. Another study[35] found a significant difference in RI between pregnant and non-pregnant cycles, but concluded that uterine artery blood flow had less of a predictive value than other endometrial TVUS parameters. One group[36] reported that 35% of women who failed to become pregnant following IVF-ET had a PI of > 3.0 on the day of embryo transfer, and therefore suggested that this measurement may be helpful for clinical decision making about IVF-ET. This could include (1) deciding whether embryos should be cryopreserved until the uterus is more receptive; and (2) reducing the multiple pregnancy rate by indicating that fewer embryos be transferred when this parameter shows the uterus to be most receptive[36]. Others similarly showed that measuring uterine artery PI allows for an accurate prediction of a positive pregnancy outcome in fresh embryo transfer cycles[34]. Steer and co-workers[37] studied women receiving GnRH-a and hormone replacement therapy for frozen embryo transfer cycles. They found that the uterine artery PI was significantly lower in those with successful vs. unsuccessful pregnancy outcomes. They also found significant correlations between the uterine artery PI and endometrial 24-kDa protein, estradiol receptors and histology, but not with endometrial thickness, and they concluded that this measurement was useful for assessing uterine receptivity[37]. In contrast, another group[38] did not find significant differences in uterine or ovarian artery PI between pregnant and non-pregnant women, but reported an insignificant increase in uterine receptivity when the uterine artery PI was in the range of 2.0–2.99 on the day of embryo transfer[38]. In summary, although the technique seems promising, an appraisal of the prognostic outcome of IVF-ET cannot currently be reliably made with Doppler. Therefore, at this time, it does not seem warranted to alter clinical decisions based on Doppler flow values.

Initially, follicular aspiration required an operative laparoscopy. This exposed patients to the inherent risks of general anesthesia and surgery as well as significant time lost from work during recuperation. Advances in ultrasound technology, primarily the development of the transvaginal probe, allowed for more accurate follicular measurements and eliminated patient discomfort from a full, distended bladder that was required with transabdominal scanning. With the proximity that the TVUS probe provides to the posterior cul-de-sac and thus the ovarian structures, it is now widely used for oocyte retrieval procedures, thus eliminating the need for laparoscopy and its inherent risks, costs and longer recovery time. Unlike the laparoscopic approach, TVUS-guided follicular aspiration can be performed in an office setting with minimal sedation. The success rate is comparable to the laparoscopic technique[39], and patient satisfaction is high[40]. The transvaginal approach is preferable for patients with pelvic adhesions, since laparoscopic or transabdominal access may be limited[41].

Needle guides that attach to the vaginal probe have become available for transvaginal follicular aspiration. The probe is covered with a sterile condom and the aspiration needle is passed through the attached needle guide. A long (30 cm) 16–18-gauge needle is used, and the tip can be visualized sonographically. A needle path is generated on the ultrasound screen for the operator to follow when guiding the needle through the cul-de-sac and into the ovary (Figure 4). The desired follicle is brought into the needle path and supported in place with pressure from the vaginal probe. Direct and continuous visualization of the needle is possible as it is advanced into the ovarian follicles. Once the needle is correctly placed inside the follicle, suction is applied and the follicular fluid is aspirated. Simultaneously, the collapsing follicle is visualized on the ultrasound screen. The embryologist concurrently microscopically searches the follicular fluid to identify the oocytes. The number and quality of the oocytes is recorded.

To summarize, technological advances in TVUS have allowed IVF-ET to be performed in a less invasive, more accurate and less costly manner.

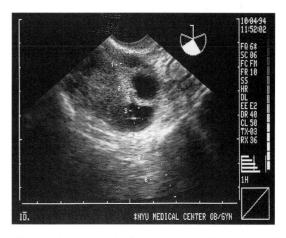

Figure 4 *Transvaginal ultrasonography performed during oocyte retrieval procedure, showing the needle path on the ultrasound screen, with the needle tip inside the follicle*

THE APPLICATION OF TVUS TO COMPLICATIONS ASSOCIATED WITH ASSISTED REPRODUCTIVE TECHNOLOGIES

Not only has the use of TVUS become essential for monitoring induced cycles, the IVF process and the technique of oocyte retrieval, its application is also a cornerstone for the prevention, diagnosis and treatment of several potential complications that can arise from the assisted reproductive technologies. Ovarian hyperstimulation syndrome (OHSS) and multiple pregnancies are two such examples, and, less commonly, difficult oocyte retrievals and ovarian cysts, abscesses and hematomas.

The proximity of the normally situated ovaries to the needle attached to the TVUS probe via the needle guide as it is inserted through the cul-de-sac into the peritoneal cavity and advanced into the ovarian follicles makes the transvaginal approach possible. However, in certain cases, the ovaries may not be located in their normal anatomical position and instead may be located elsewhere, such as anterior to the uterus, perhaps fixed in place by pelvic adhesions. In unusual cases, such as a patient whose ovaries were previously surgically transposed, laparoscopy may provide the only access to the ovaries for aspiration. Transabdominal ultrasound for guidance of transvesical or transurethral aspiration may be the preferred route in some of these cases, since a transvaginal approach may require traversing the uterus and perhaps even the endometrium first before entering the ovary. Such a situation increases the risk of uterine hemorrhage or infection, and may have an adverse effect on implantation following embryo transfer[42]. It has recently been reported that the combined use of TVUS after applying a tenaculum to the cervix in order to manipulate the uterus out of the needle's path to the ovary may enable the transvaginal approach to be used without the uterus first having to be entered[43]. In addition, the use of this combination of TVUS with uterine manipulation by the cervical tenaculum can be extended to stabilize the unstable ovary that moves out of the needle's path as attempts are made to enter the ovary with the transvaginally applied needle[43].

The use of GnRH-a for luteal phase downregulation can be associated with the inadvertent development of ovarian follicular cysts that are sometimes large enough to impair folliculogenesis by either interfering with the production of hormones or causing physical compression on the remainder of the ovarian parenchyma. In such instances, TVUS-guided cyst aspiration can be performed prior to ovulation induction without adversely affecting the pregnancy outcome[44].

Potential complications of the transvaginal oocyte retrieval procedure include infections[45] or bleeding by any pelvic structure that may have been traversed by the needle, either purposefully (e.g. the ovary) or accidentally (e.g. extraovarian structures). Such events are rare, but may involve the ovaries, uterus, iliac vessels or the bowel. TVUS is an important tool for the diagnosis of pelvic abscesses, enabling timely diagnosis and appropriate treatment. Pelvic hematomas are infrequent complications. Accidental introduction of the needle into a pelvic vessel (usually the internal iliac vein) has been reported[46]. The application of TVUS can help to prevent this problem if the operator carefully visualizes all round structures in both the long and short axis to distinguish a vessel from a follicle before introducing the needle. Pelvic hematomas can also result from ovarian or uterine bleeding. TVUS visualization of accumulating free fluid in the pelvis during the procedure enables a timely diagnosis to be made.

Ultrasound guidance also allows for visualization of peristaltic bowel, differentiating it from follicular structures. In this way, its use can aid in preventing bowel injury from needle perforation. Such a complication, therefore, is also extremely rare. However, there is a case report in the literature of appendicitis following transvaginal oocyte retrieval[47]. At subsequent surgery, puncture holes were found in the appendix, which were interpreted to be indicative of a causal relationship between the two events[47].

Following an unsuccessful cycle of ovulation induction, the stimulated follicles usually regress, but sometimes they may persist and even enlarge. The presence of these physiological ovarian cysts, which are detectable by ultrasound, may interfere with induction of ovulation during the immediately following cycle. The response of the remaining ovarian tissue to ovulation induction may be dampened, and the risk of ovarian torsion or rupture and hemorrhage may be increased in these cases. For this reason, it is sometimes recommended to alternate ovulation induction cycles rather than performing them consecutively.

The risk of OHSS is increased in patients with PCOD[48] and in cycles resulting in pregnancy. This syndrome is caused by massive ovarian enlargement resulting from luteinization of multiple follicles and stromal edema. Resulting symptoms include fluid retention, ascites and weight gain, and can progress to include oliguria, electrolyte imbalances, thromboembolism, pleural effusions and hydrothorax. Severe OHSS is rarely associated with the use of CC[49], but is more commonly seen with gonadotropins[48]. Down-regulation with GnRH-a before inducing ovulation may decrease the incidence of OHSS[49], and the aspiration of follicular fluid from all follicles (including the smaller ones) at the time of TVUS-guided oocyte retrieval during IVF-ET is also thought to be protective. Prevention remains the most successful therapy for OHSS, since management is mostly palliative once the symptoms are progressing and may require hospitalization for the most severe cases. A correlation has been shown between OHSS and the presence of multiple intermediate-sized pre-ovulatory follicles on TVUS[50]. An increased risk for OHSS has been associated with serum estradiol levels of > 4000 pg/ml on the day of hCG administration[51]. A combination of serial follicular TVUS monitoring and serum estradiol levels during ovulation induction remains the mainstay for prevention of this disease. Multiple intermediate-sized follicles and high serum estradiol levels serve as predictive tools. When this ultrasound pattern is detected, other options should be considered, such as cycle cancellation by withholding hCG or reducing or withholding gonadotropins for a period of time before resuming them in an effort to continue the cycle. For IVF-ET cycles, another option is to administer the hCG and proceed with the oocyte retrieval but not the embryo transfer. Instead, the patient would continue down-regulation with GnRH-a and the embryos would be cryopreserved for use in a future, safer hormonally prepared cycle.

TVUS provides minimal information during management of OHSS, since knowledge of ovarian size and follicular number and sizes does not alter therapy. Once the disease is in progress, management requires careful attention to fluid and electrolyte balance and prevention of thromboembolic events, when necessary, with heparin prophylaxis. Carefully advising affected patients to limit their physical activity is essential, since their extremely enlarged ovaries increase their risk for ovarian torsion. If symptoms suggestive of torsion arise, the absence of ovarian blood flow on Doppler TVUS can be diagnostic. Ultrasound can also be helpful for diagnosing the presence of associated ascites. Although paracentesis is rarely needed and is reserved only for those patients with severe respiratory compromise, skilled ultrasound guidance to avoid ovarian trauma is essential[52].

A delicate balance exists between stimulating the development of enough follicles and oocytes and transferring enough embryos into the uterus during IVF-ET, to achieve the optimal chance of pregnancy while minimizing the risk of multiple pregnancy. TVUS is valuable in the prevention of multiple gestations when it is applied to follicular monitoring. However, even when strict parameters for TVUS-measured follicular growth and serum estradiol levels are maintained, there still remains an approximately 20% risk of multiple gestations[53]. Most common are twins, but higher-order multiple gestations also occur.

TVUS is also critical to the post-embryo transfer diagnosis of multiple gestations. One study[54] found that, when multiple gestational sacs were seen on first-trimester ultrasound examination, the 'take-home baby' rate improved with IVF. Early first-trimester TVUS monitoring can clearly demonstrate one vs. two or more intrauterine gestational sacs (Figure 5) and can also provide valuable information about the integrity of the sacs. In

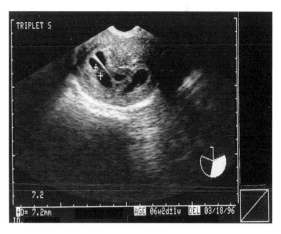

Figure 5 *Triplet pregnancy in an hMG-treated patient. Three intrauterine sacs visualized at a gestational age of 6 weeks 2 days*

this way, TVUS may also have a prognostic role, since irregular sacs that do not contain a yolk sac or fetal pole or fetal heart beat at expected times may indicate an impending pregnancy loss. However, these findings need to be interpreted carefully and in the appropriate clinical context. For example, abnormal sac contents detectable by early ultrasound examination were found by one group[55] to be frequently present on the initial ultrasound scan of pregnant patients after IVF-ET, with 30% eventually delivering at least one live healthy term infant. TVUS is also useful for diagnosing heterotopic pregnancies that may occur after IVF-ET, especially in patients with tubal disease who receive multiple embryos[56].

The early detection of multiple intra-uterine pregnancies by TVUS is clinically important for patient counselling, since the currently available ultrasound-guided procedure of selective reduction is performed during the first trimester. Ultrasound-guided selective reduction of higher-order gestations is a relatively recent medical advance mostly in response to this complication of assisted reproductive technologies. Initially performed with transabdominal ultrasound, this procedure has now been perfected with the TVUS approach. The procedure can be performed as early as 7–8 weeks' gestation, and is reported to be technically simple and relatively safe, with a low pregnancy loss rate[57,58]. The technique involves the ultrasound-guided injection of a toxic substance into selected sacs.

Conversely, one group[59] has advised that iatrogenic fetal reduction be delayed until 12 gestational weeks in triplet or higher-order multiple gestations, and may not even be indicated in twin and triplet gestations. This is based on their finding of a high incidence of spontaneous fetal reduction in multiple gestations assessed by TVUS. In their population of pregnant patients following ovulation induction, spontaneous reduction from twins to a viable singleton approached 100%.

FUTURE DIRECTIONS

We are currently experiencing the results of vast technological advances in TVUS as related to assisted reproductive technologies. TVUS has facilitated the diagnostic and therapeutic processes involved with ovulation induction and IVF-ET. With the use of TVUS utero-ovarian measurements in combination with estradiol levels for monitoring ovulation induction, IVF-ET has been able to be performed more accurately. By virtual elimination of the need for laparoscopy for performance of the oocyte retrieval procedure and its replacement with a TVUS-guided approach, IVF-ET has more recently been able to be performed in a less invasive and less costly manner.

The addition of color Doppler flow parameters has been disappointing in terms of improving TVUS utero-ovarian monitoring during ovulation induction cycles and predicting pregnancy outcome. Results from various centers have been inconsistent and difficult to reproduce. The potential for uterine blood flow parameters to evaluate endometrial receptivity and ovarian flow values to predict egg quality is currently unknown. Hopefully, future work will be aimed at improving standardization and reproducibility of utero-ovarian Doppler parameters so that the value of this technique can be more objectively evaluated and applied.

Evaluation of blood flow in the smaller vessels of the endometrium is also needed.

TVUS in combination with transcervical instillation of sterile saline (sonohysterography) can provide detailed evaluation of the endometrial contour. When applied to the infertile patient, this technique has the potential to provide information previously obtainable only with hysterosalpingography, but without the need for ionizing radiation exposure. The application of sonohysterography to the infertility workup prior to ovulation induction for evaluation of endometrial integrity or for IVF-ET patients with implantation failure despite good fertilization outcome and embryo quality is a worthy area for future investigation.

A preliminary report[60] suggests that three-dimensional ultrasound may be a potentially valuable clinical tool and adjunct to two-dimensional ultrasound. Some gynecological applications of this new technology, such as the evaluation of leiomyomas, are already under investigation[60]. Two-dimensional ultrasound images can sometimes be confusing and difficult to interpret. Three-dimensional ultrasound can facilitate diagnoses by delineating normal and abnormal structures in previously unobtainable planes. Three-dimensional imaging can facilitate the performance and interpretation of ultrasound by creating a spatially oriented display of image position[60], which can be achieved by two-dimensional imaging only by interpretation of several individual images and integration of these results by the clinician. Future work will be needed in order to evaluate the potential for the application of three-dimensional imaging to monitoring of ovulation induction cycles and IVF-ET procedures. Theoretically, more accurate follicular sizes and locations can be obtained by three-dimensional than by two-dimensional imaging, especially when there are multiple follicles superimposed on each other. In addition, perhaps more can be learned about endometrial TVUS parameters with this new technique.

References

1. Mishell, D. R. Jr, Davajan, V. and Lobo, R. (eds.) (1991). *Infertility, Contraception and Reproductive Endocrinology*, 3rd edn, p. 571. (Cambridge, MA: Blackwell Scientific Publications)

2. DeCherney, A. H., Romero, R. and Polan, M. L. (1982). Ultrasound in reproductive endocrinology. *Fertil. Steril.*, **37**, 323

3. Speroff, L., Glass, R. and Kase, N. (1994). *Clinical Gynecological Endocrinology and Infertility*, 5th edn. (Baltimore: Williams and Wilkins)

4. Bakos, O., Lundkvist, O., Wide, L. and Bergh, T. (1994). Ultrasonographical and hormonal description of the normal ovulatory menstrual cycle. *Acta Obstet. Gynecol. Scand.*, **73**, 790–6

5. Randall, J. M. and Templeton, A. (1991). Transvaginal sonographic assessment of follicular and endometrial growth in spontaneous and clomiphene citrate cycles. *Fertil. Steril.*, **56**, 208–12

6. Fleischer, A. C. and Kepple, D. M. (1991). Pelvic anatomy and physiology as depicted by conventional and color Doppler transvaginal sonography. *Infertil. Reprod. Clin. North Am.*, **2**, 659–72

7. Taylor, K. J. W., Burns, P. N., Wells, P. N. T. *et al.* (1985). Ultrasound Doppler flow studies of the ovarian and uterine arteries. *Br. J. Obstet. Gynaecol.*, **91**, 240–6

8. Fleischer, A. C., Herbert, C. M. Hill, G. A. *et al.* (1991). Transvaginal sonography of the endometrium during induced cycles. *J. Ultrasound Med.*, **10**, 93–5

9. Randall, J. M., Fisk, N. M., McTavish, A. *et al.* (1989). Transvaginal ultrasonic assessment of endometrial growth in spontaneous and hyperstimulated menstrual cycles. *Br. J. Obstet. Gynaecol.*, **96**, 954–9

10. Arici, A., Byrd, W., Bradshaw, K., Ketteh, W. H., Marshburn, P. and Carr, B. R. (1994). Evaluation of clomiphene citrate and human gonadotropin treatment: a prospective, randomized, crossover study during intrauterine insemination cycles. *Fertil. Steril.*, **61**, 314–18

11. Tarlatzis, B. C., Laufer, N. and DeCherney, A. H. (1984). The use of ovarian ultrasonography in monitoring ovulation induction. *J. In Vitro Fertil. Embryo Transfer*, **1**, 226

12. Gagliardi, C. L. (1993). Utility of gonadotropin-releasing hormone agonists in programs of ovarian hyperstimulation with intrauterine insemination. *Clin. Obstet. Gynecol.*, **36**, 711–18

13. Schwartz, M. and Jewelewicz, R. (1981). The use of gonadotropins for induction of ovulation. *Fertil. Steril.*, **35**, 3–12

14. Marrs, R., Vargyas, J. and March, C. (1983). Correlation of ultrasonic and endocrinologic measurements in human menopausal gonadotropin therapy. *Obstet. Gynecol.*, **145**, 417–21

15. Hull, M., Moghisii, K., Magyar, K., Hayes, M., Zador, I. and Olson, J. (1986). Correlation of serum estradiol levels and ultrasound monitoring to assess follicular maturation. *Fertil. Steril.*, **46**, 42–5

16. Peluso, J. J., Damien, M., Nulsen, J. C. and Luciano, A. A. (1990). Identification of follicles with fertilizable oocytes by sequential ultrasound measurements during follicular development. *J. In Vitro Fertil. Embryo Transfer*, **7**, 304–9

17. Rabinowitz, R., Laufer, N., Lewin, A., Navot, D., Bar, I., Margalioth, E. J. and Schenker, J. J. (1986). The value of ultrasonographic endometrial measurement in the prediction of pregnancy following *in vitro* fertilization. *Fertil. Steril.*, **45**, 824–8

18. Coulam, C. B., Bustillo, M., Soenksen, D. M. and Britten, S. (1994). Ultrasonographic predictors of implantation after assisted reproduction. *Fertil. Steril.*, **62**, 1004–10

19. Check, J. H., Nowroozi, K., Choe, J. and Dietterich, C. (1991). Influence of endometrial thickness and echo patterns on pregnancy rates during *in vitro* fertilization. *Fertil. Steril.*, **56**, 1173–5

20. Ueno, J., Oehninger, S., Brzyski, R. G., Acosta, A. A., Philput, C. B. and Muasher, S. J. (1991). Ultrasonographic appearance of the endometrium in natural and stimulated *in-vitro* fertilization cycles and its correlation with outcome. *Hum. Reprod.*, **6**, 901–4

21. Sher, G., Dodge, S., Maassarani, G., Knutzen, V., Zouves, C. and Feinman, M. (1993). Management of suboptimal sonographic endometrial patterns in patients undergoing *in-vitro* fertilization and embryo transfer. *Hum. Reprod.*, **8**, 347–9

22. Serafini, P., Batzofin, J., Nelson, J. and Olive, D. (1994). Sonographic uterine predictors of pregnancy in women undergoing ovulation induction for assisted reproductive treatments. *Fertil. Steril.*, **62**, 815–22

23. Glissant, A., de Mouzon, J. and Frydman, R. (1985). Ultrasound study of the endometrium during *in vitro* fertilization cycles. *Fertil. Steril.*, **44**, 786

24. Welker, B. G., Gembruch, U., Diedrich, K., al Hasani, S. and Krebs, D. (1989). Transvaginal sonography of the endometrium during ovum pickup in stimulated cycles for *in vitro* fertilization. *J. Ultrasound Med.*, **8**, 549–53

25. Gonen, Y. and Casper, R. F. (1990). Prediction of implantation by the sonographic appearance of the endometrium during controlled ovarian stimulation for *in vitro* fertilization (IVF). *J. In Vitro Fertil. Embryo Transfer*, **7**, 146–52

26. Fleischer, A. C., Herbert, C. M., Sacks, G. A., Wentz, A. C., Entman, S. S. and James, A. E. Jr (1986). Sonography of the endometrium during conception and nonconception cycles on *in vitro* fertilization and embryo transfer. *Fertil. Steril.*, **46**, 442–7

27. Gonen, Y., Casper, R. F., Jacobson, W. and Blankier, J. (1989). Endometrial thickness and growth during ovarian stimulation: a possible predictor of implantation in *in vitro* fertilization. *Fertil. Steril.*, **52**, 446–50

28. Check, J. H., Nowroozi, K., Choe, J., Lurie, D. and Dietterich, C. (1993). The effect of endometrial thickness and echo pattern on *in vitro* fertilization outcome in donor oocyte –embryo transfer cycle. *Fertil. Steril.*, **59**, 72–5

29. Shapiro, H., Cowell, C. and Casper, R. F. (1993). The use of vaginal ultrasound for monitoring endometrial preparation in a donor oocyte program. *Fertil. Steril.*, **59**, 1055–8

30. Okonofua, F. E., Onwudiegwu, U., Smith, W., Thomas, N., Craft, I. and Dandona, F. (1993). Correlation of ultrasound assessment of endometrial growth and plasma steroid concentrations during superovulation for *in vitro* fertilization. *Afr. J. Med. Sci.*, **22**, 89–93

31. Golan, A., Herman, A., Soffer, Y., Bukovsky, I. and Ron-El, R. (1994). Ultrasonic control without hormone determination for ovulation induction in *in-vitro* fertilization/embryo transfer with gonadotrophin-releasing hormone analogue and human menopausal gonadotropin. *Hum. Reprod.*, **9**, 1631–3

32. Steer, C. V., Campbell, S., Tan, S. L., Crayford, T., Mills, C., Mason, B. A. and Collins, W. P. (1992). The use of transvaginal color flow imaging after *in vitro* fertilization to identify optimum uterine conditions before embryo transfer. *Fertil. Steril.*, **57**, 372–6

33. Coulam, C. B., Bustillo, M., Soenksen, D. M. and Britten, S. (1994). Ultrasonographic predictors of implantation after assisted reproduction. *Fertil. Steril.*, **62**, 1004–10

34. Sterzik, K., Grab, D., Sasse, V., Hutter, W., Rosenbusch, B. and Terinde, R. (1989). Doppler sonographic findings and their correlation with implantation in an *in vitro* fertilization program. *Fertil. Steril.*, **52**, 825–8

35. Serafini, P., Batzofin, J., Nelson, J. and Olive, D. (1994). Sonographic uterine predictors of pregnancy in women undergoing ovulation induction for assisted reproductive treatments. *Fertil. Steril.*, **62**, 815–22

36. Steer, C. V., Campbell, S., Tan, S. L., Crayford, T., Mills, C., Mason, B. A. and Collins, W. P. (1992). The use of transvaginal color flow imaging after *in vitro* fertilization to identify optimum uterine conditions before embryo transfer. *Fertil. Steril.*, **57**, 372–6

37. Steer, C. V., Tan, S. L., Dillon, D., Mason, B. A. and Campbell, S. (1995). Vaginal color Doppler assessment of uterine artery impedance correlates with immunohisto-chemical markers of endometrial receptivity required for the implantation of an embryo. *Fertil. Steril.*, **63**, 101–8

38. Tekay, A., Martikainen, H. and Jouppila, P. (1995). Blood flow changes in uterine and ovarian vasculature, and predictive value of transvaginal pulsed color Doppler ultrasonography in an *in-vitro* fertilization programme. *Hum. Reprod.*, **10**, 688–93

39. Feldberg, D., Goldman, J. A., Ashkenazi, J. *et al.* (1988). Transvaginal oocyte retrieval controlled by vaginal probe for *in vitro* fertilization: a comparative study. *J. Ultrasound Med.*, **7**, 339

40. Taylor, P. J., Wiseman, D., Mahadevan, M. *et al.* (1986). 'Ultrasound rescue': a successful alternative form of oocyte recovery in patients with periovarian adhesions. *Am. J. Obstet. Gynecol.*, **154**, 240

41. Hammerberg, K., Enk, L., Nilsson, L. *et al.* Oocyte retrieval under the guidance of a vaginal transducer: evaluation of patient acceptance. *Hum. Reprod.*, **2**, 487

42. Ashkenazi, J., Farhi, J., Dicker, D., Feldberg, D., Shalev, J. and Ben Rafael, Z. (1994). Acute pelvic inflammatory disease after oocyte retrieval: adverse effects on the results of implantation. *Fertil. Steril.*, **61**, 526–8

43. Licciardi, F. L., Schwartz, L. B. and Schmidt-Sarosi, C. (1995). A tenaculum improves ovarian accessibility during difficult transvaginal follicular aspiration: a novel but simple technique. *Fertil. Steril.*, **63**, 677–9

44. Silverberg, K. M., Olive, D. L. and Schenken, R. S. (1990). Ovarian cyst aspiration prior to initiating ovarian hyperstimulation for *in vitro* fertilization. *J. In Vitro Fertil. Embryo Transfer*, **7**, 153–6

45. Howe, R. S., Wheller, C., Mastroianni, L. *et al.* (1984). Pelvic infections after transvaginal ultrasound-guided ovum retrieval. *Fertil. Steril.*, **49**, 726

46. Feldberg, D., Goldman, J. A., Ashkenazi, J. *et al.* (1988). Transvaginal oocyte retrieval controlled by vaginal probe for *in vitro* fertilization: a comparative study. *J. Ultrasound Med.*, **7**, 339

47. Van Hoorde, G. J., Verhoeff, A. and Zeilmaker, G. H. (1992). Perforated appendicitis following transvaginal oocyte retrieval for *in-vitro* fertilization and embryo transfer. *Hum. Reprod.*, **7**, 850–1

48. Raj, S., Berger, M., Grimes, E. and Taymor, M. (1977). The use of gonadotropins for the induction of ovulation in women with polycystic ovarian disease. *Fertil. Steril.*, **28**, 1280–4

49. Polishuk, W. and Schenker, J. (1969). Ovarian overstimulation syndrome. *Fertil. Steril.*, **20**, 443–50

50. Blankstein, J., Shalev, J., Saadon, T. *et al.* (1987). Ovarian hyperstimulation syndrome: prediction by numbers and size of preovulatory ovarian follicles. *Fertil. Steril.*, **47**, 597–602

51. Haning, R., Austin, C., Carlson, I., Kuzma, D., Shapiro, S. and Zweibel, W. (1983). Plasma estradiol is superior to ultrasound and urinary estriol glucuronide as a predictor of ovarian hyperstimulation during induction of ovulation with menotropins. *Fertil. Steril.*, **40**, 31–6

52. Padilla, S., Zamaria, S., Baramki, T. and Garcia, J. (1990). Abdominal paracentesis for the ovarian hyperstimulation syndrome with severe respiratory compromise. *Fertil. Steril.*, **53**, 365–7

53. Medical Research International, Society for Assisted Reproductive Technology, American Fertility Society (1991). *In vitro* fertilization–embryo transfer (IVF-ET) in the United States: 1989 results from the IVF-ET registry. *Fertil. Steril.*, **55**, 14–23

54. Botchan, A., Yaron, Y., Lessing, J. B., Barak, Y., Yovel, I., David, M. P., Peyser, M. R. and Amit, A. (1993). When multiple gestational sacs are seen on ultrasound, 'take-home baby' rate improves with *in-vitro* fertilization. *Hum. Reprod.*, **8**, 710–13

55. Wax, M. R., Frates, M., Benson, C. B., Yeh, J. and Doubilet, P. M. (1992). First trimester findings in pregnancies after *in vitro* fertilization. *J. Ultrasound Med.*, **11**, 321–5

56. Rizk, B., Tan, S. L., Morcos, S., Riddle, A., Brinsden, P., Mason, B. A. and Edwards, R. G. (1991). Heterotopic pregnancies after *in vitro* fertilization and embryo transfer. *Am. J. Obstet. Gynecol.*, **164**, 161–4

57. Itskovitz-Eldor, J., Drugan, A., Levron, J., Thaler, I. and Brandes, J. M. (1992). Transvaginal embryo aspiration – a safe method for selective reduction in multiple pregnancies. *Fertil. Steril.*, **58**, 351–5

58. Porreco, R. P., Burke, M. S. and Hendrix, M. L. (1991). Multifetal reduction of triplets and pregnancy outcome. *Obstet. Gynecol.*, **78**, 335–9

59. Blumenfeld, Z., Dirnfeld, M., Abramovici, H., Amit, A., Bronshtein, M. and Brandes, J. M. (1992). Spontaneous fetal reduction in multiple gestations assessed by transvaginal ultrasound. *Br. J. Obstet. Gynaecol.*, **99**, 333–7

60. Hamper, U. M., Trapanotto, V., Sheth, S., DeJong, R. and Caskey, C. I. (1994). Three-dimensional US: preliminary clinical experience. *Radiology*, **191**, 397–401

Evaluating efficacy

12

D. L. Olive

INTRODUCTION

A large number of imaging modalities have been made available to the physician for the diagnosis and treatment of reproductive failure. Yet amid this dizzying array of technological wonders, the physician is left to deal with several basic issues. The comparative benefits must be sorted out for alternative diagnostic tests or algorithms. Once their relative values are determined, the applicability of the published data to one's own center must then be determined. Finally, the value of accessory data available to the physician but not heretofore assessed in the published algorithms must be estimated. Generally, these tasks appear so overwhelming that no attempt is made to answer these questions in a rigorous or quantitative manner; that is, no real attempt is made to assess efficacy.

Interestingly, the issue of test value is nowhere more critical than with imaging techniques. Not only must the relative merits of each test be weighed, but also the interpretation of the image must be considered. Finally, the production quality of the image – both day to day and with technological enhancement – must be tossed into the equation. With such a large number of variables at work, it is imperative that those factors that can be assessed accurately are so evaluated. To aid in dealing with these issues, this chapter discusses the principles inherent in defining and evaluating diagnostic tests, along with common pitfalls encountered in attempting to apply these results to clinical practice.

DEFINING THE TEST

With any diagnostic test, a number of characteristics of the test must be ascertained. These

characteristics will vary depending on the group to be tested, the nature of the test itself, other tests available and biases inherent in the study approach. This section deals with these issues.

What is normal?

In selecting a meaning for normal in a given test, several choices are available. For the majority of clinical imaging studies, however, normal can assume two categories of definition: correlated normality and isolated normality[1].

Correlated normality

Correlated normality is a concept in which the designation of normal is associated with a desired state of health. Similarly, it is claimed that abnormal has an association with disease. Determination of threshold demarcations between normal and abnormal are not arbitrary, but rather are dependent upon results in diseased and disease-free individuals. For example, in an attempt to diagnose a cause of reproductive failure, the desired healthy state is one of being able to achieve pregnancy, whereas the diseased state would be an inability to conceive. If a test is designed to estimate fertility potential, a normal test would be one in which the patient could indeed demonstrate fertility; an abnormal test result should correlate with an inability to become pregnant.

A different clinical approach to correlation depends on linking the test results not to disease status, but rather to outcome. The outcome generally involves a treatment or treatments that can somehow be evaluated. For example, the upper limit of normal for a screening test may be chosen as the point below which treatment does more harm than good; in this case the outcome measure is treatment efficacy vs. side-effects[2]. Similarly, an abnormal test might be declared if a treatment could be shown to be cost-effective for the apparent pathology.

Clearly, correlated normality is the ideal, as we are assured that the test results in question indicate exactly what we think they should. However, correlated normality is difficult to achieve for a variety of reasons.

First, the same test may be applicable to a variety of different diagnoses. In this situation, test results must be correlated with each diagnosis separately and a normal range determined that may be unique for each particular disorder. For example, a narrow internal cervical os may represent little risk for incompetent cervix, yet may prove highly correlated with endometriosis. Therefore, the 'normal' cervical diameter for each malady must be separately assessed.

A second problem with correlated normality is that test results must be linked to an outcome rather than a concomitant state. This generally involves long-term studies that may be expensive, difficult to perform and obsolete by their conclusion. For example, if the outcome is fertility, then follow-up of couples attempting conception must generally be completed and may require months or years.

The greatest problem with correlated normality, however, is the fact that multiple variables generally contribute to the outcome in question. It may be difficult to determine the precise importance of a test result in the face of many other confounding variables affecting the outcome. The potential for a 3-cm intramural leiomyoma found on magnetic resonance imaging (MRI) scan to produce infertility may become difficult to assess when the ovulatory status, semen parameters, frequency of intercourse and numerous other variables must be considered simultaneously. Although multivariate statistical methods are designed for just such situations, sufficient data (or information regarding which data to accumulate) may not be available.

Isolated normality

Isolated normality is the more common method of defining normal. This is strictly a univariate concept, with boundaries being placed on the values of a single variable. This range does not correlate with any particular state of health; it is simply derived from the most common values obtained from presumed healthy individuals. In this situation, the range of normal is descriptive, not diagnostic: it describes disease-free individuals; it does not diagnose disease[3].

When isolated normality is utilized, the range of normal becomes a purely statistical grouping based on the mathematical principle chosen to delineate it. Thus, the size of the abnormal group is pre-determined. It must be kept in mind that, in this situation, abnormal and diseased are not synonymous. Furthermore, a value within the normal range does not assure that an individual is disease-free. As stated by Riegelman: 'The range of normal in and of itself tells us nothing about the diagnostic utility of a test. Every test has a range of normal that may or may not help in distinguishing individuals with disease from those without disease'[3].

Examples of isolated normality are the measurement of uterine artery blood flow by Doppler ultrasonography or endometrial thickness by transvaginal ultrasound. Fortunately, in imaging studies most abnormalities are not merely quantitative variations of 'normal' but rather unusual and distinctly different images. Interestingly, in this situation a quantitative threshold is replaced by a univariate threshold for pattern recognition. At what point does a darkened spot in the myometrium on an MRI scan represent a myoma? This is determined by sensitivity of the equipment, skill of the reader and variability within the population. These topics will be discussed shortly.

What is a gold standard?

The gold standard is an accepted reference test or criterion used to identify a disease unequivocally. Examples include confirmation of an ultrasonographically diagnosed ectopic pregnancy by surgical removal and histological specimen, or the visualization of endometriosis confirmed by biopsy. In most cases, true confirmation is attained only with histological specimens. A new test is compared to a gold standard to determine how well it performs in correctly identifying the disease categories in individuals subjected to the test. The use of a gold standard for definitive identification of those with the disease is mandatory in order to evaluate the diagnostic utility of a test, assuming such a standard exists.

Defining the normal zone

The method of establishing limits of normal is clearly different, depending on whether correlated or isolated normality is utilized. In the case of correlated normality, it is presumed that a gold standard exists to define who is diseased and who is disease-free. Given this information, the relationship of the distributions of test results for these populations define both the limits of normal and the value of the test itself. Three possible relationships are illustrated in Figure 1. If the diseased and disease-free populations do not overlap in their test values, the defining demarcation is some value between these two curves; in this case, the test is perfect in providing diagnostic accuracy. At the other extreme is the situation in which the two populations of test results overlap completely. In this case no demarcation is possible and the test is of no value.

The usual situation is one in which there is some overlap of distributions. Clearly, whatever cut-off level is made to distinguish normal from abnormal, some individuals with disease will have normal values and/or some that are disease-free will be called abnormal. The placement of the limit of normal then

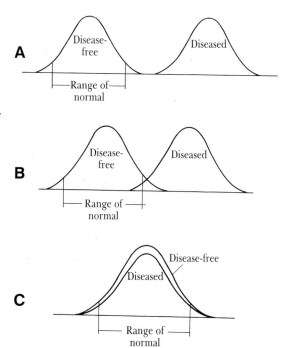

Figure 1 *Possible relationships between test values of normal and abnormal subjects. (A) No overlap between distributions. (B) Partial overlap between distributions. (C) Complete overlap between distributions. From reference 3*

depends to a great extent on how the test is to be used.

Diagnostic tests are used for one of three purposes: discovery (screening), exclusion and confirmation[1]. A discovery test is used to screen a population not clearly exhibiting a disease for latent expression. In this situation, the clinician generally desires to include virtually all diseased individuals in the abnormal test group. The consequence of this is the placement of many disease-free individuals into the abnormal zone; such tests have a high sensitivity and a low specificity. In Figure 2, this would be accomplished by placing the demarcation towards the left of the overlapping values. How far to the left frequently depends on social, psychological, economic and political considerations.

Tests of exclusion are performed to rule out the presence of a disease when one is suspected. Generally, this is used after an abnormal screening test or in the presence of

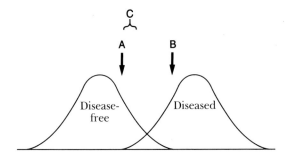

Figure 2 *Demarcations for discovery, exclusion and confirmation tests. A indicates the cut-off for an exclusion test; B indicates the cut-off for a confirmation test; C indicates the range of the cut-off for a discovery test*

symptoms/signs suggestive of the disease. Here, the goal of the test is to be confident that a negative test (normal) truly excludes the disease. This requirement for a very low rate of false-negative (diseased but normal) results again would place the demarcation at the left of the overlap area, but this time probably further to the left. However, the overlap must be small or the test is of limited value.

Finally, a confirmation test is used to confirm the presence of disease when it has been suggested or suspected. This requires a low false-positive test rate; that is, placing a disease-free individual into the abnormal category. The threshold in this instance is to the right of the overlapping regions. However, if too much of the diseased population is termed normal, the utility of the test should be called into question. A good confirmation test thus requires little overlap in the distributions, and placement of the test demarcation at the right edge of the small overlap.

The normal zone using isolated normality is selected by an entirely different process. Decisions must be made (in the absence of disease correlation) about the size of the normal zone, its location within the distribution of values and the symmetry of the zone. The size of the normal zone is determined by answering the question: how uncommon must something be to be called

abnormal? For instance, if the consequence of being called abnormal is having to undergo a more expensive test, then one might more readily term an unusual result abnormal than if the consequence is radical surgery or chemotherapy. The most common size of a normal zone is one that encompasses 95% of the values. However, it is worth noting that the designation of 5% as abnormal has no support from statistical theory and is purely arbitrary[4].

Once the size of the normal zone is determined, the investigator must next choose a location. If the zone encompasses 95%, do the 5% abnormal test results lie on one end of the spectrum or on both ends? If both ends of the spectrum are designated as abnormal, the investigator must decide whether the percentage of abnormal values should be equal at each end or weighted unequally. Generally, if abnormal results are at both ends of the test distribution, each end encompasses 2.5% of the total sample.

A Gaussian (or normal) distribution of test results in a reference population makes such boundaries easy to choose. In this setting, the central 95% is defined by the mean ± 2 (actually 1.96) standard deviations. When the data do not distribute in a Gaussian manner, however, other methods are required. One option is somehow to transform the data into a Gaussian distribution; this can be done in a number of ways, depending on the shape of the original data curve[5]. A second and simpler method is simply to choose the central 95% of values in the reference population as normal, regardless of how they distribute[1].

Defining the reference group

At least as important as demarcation of the normal zone is careful definition of the reference group whose results define normal. Frequently, results of a test will differ considerably, owing to a variety of confounding factors; examples include age, gender and associated clinical conditions. When comparing an individual's test results to a normal reference range, it is imperative that what is termed normal is indeed normal, given that individual's confounders. For instance, one must be cognizant of the stage of the ovarian cycle when attempting to assess the normality of ovarian blood flow, as this will vary considerably from follicular to luteal phase. When known confounding variables exist for a given test result, it seems prudent to stratify the reference population so that a normal range may be found that is applicable to the individual in question.

Another important issue in choosing the reference population lies in appropriate representation. If a reference range is being constructed to define disease-free individuals, the values should indeed derive from those without disease. The principle is a simple one: the normal group should be healthy equivalents of the individual being tested.

Defining the test parameters

When a diagnostic test is being proposed, it must be described in complete detail and compared to the methodology of existing studies. Issues that may affect results include the preparation of the patient, the mechanics of performing the test and the quality of equipment utilized[6]. For example, the image that constitutes an abnormal uterine contour on hysterosalpingogram may vary considerably, owing to the level of resolution of the instrumentation.

Variability of a test

A perfect test would produce the same results each time it was performed and would exactly reflect the true value of the tested sample. In other words, it would be completely reproducible (precise) and completely accurate. Unfortunately, this situation is not practical in the real world. Nevertheless, all too often we neglect to consider this when evaluating a test. Numerical assessment of the precision and accuracy of a test can have a major impact on its clinical utility[3].

Test precision can vary owing to test conditions or test interpretation. Test conditions should be identical with each determination; if they are not, variation results. If a test is performed twice on separate days, conditions may not be exactly duplicated for each test: this is intertest variability. When interpretation is involved, variation can also be seen. Differences in conclusions drawn by the same individual from the same image is termed intraobserver variation, whereas different physicians assessing a single test sample exhibit interobserver variability.

Given that tests show varying degrees of precision, some method of quantification is needed to judge whether the amount of variation is tolerable. This measure is termed the coefficient of variation (CV), defined as the standard deviation divided by the mean for a set of measurements. A CV can be determined for each of the aforementioned types of variations; the larger the value, the less precise the test under the specified conditions.

Precision is not to be confused with accuracy: the ability of a test to come close to the 'true' value. Although accuracy is a desirable property of a good test, the assessment of accuracy requires comparing the test to a gold standard. Unfortunately, gold standards may be unattainable for selected imaging studies, requiring one to compare the new test to a 'best test' that has been deemed the standard after lengthy experience with its use. Thus, it may not always be easy to determine the absolute accuracy of a test, only the comparative accuracy vs. other 'best tests' evaluating the same sample.

When a test is performed multiple times on an individual, a certain amount of variability (from all of the above-mentioned sources) may result. The danger of these sources of variation lie in attempts to assess serial changes in individuals without proper controls or adjustments. An interesting problem is created in deciding what the customary serial change should be. Frequently, alterations in longitudinal testing seem excessive, yet all values fit into the so-called 'normal range'. Care must be taken in interpreting such longitudinal variation as normal or abnormal, and should be based upon appropriately derived norms for variation in serial testing.

Variability of a population

As alluded to earlier, not all 'normal' individuals produce the same result for a test; this variation is the basis for selecting a normal range. This range of acceptable values is graphically illustrated as a distribution of possible normal results. Frequently the distribution is Gaussian in nature and is referred to as a normal distribution. Non-Gaussian distributions can frequently be transformed into Gaussian (normal) bell-shaped curves by mathematical manipulation. By the same token, the abnormal population has a range of test values. If there is no overlap between the normal and abnormal subjects, interpretation of the test is easy. When overlap occurs, however, certain quantitative measures are needed to help us identify the discriminative capacity of a test in a clinical situation.

Recognizing biases

Most tests performed via imaging studies require observational assessment and interpretation. It is important to avoid 'diagnostic suspicion' bias when evaluating diagnostic tests. Such bias may be introduced in both the application of the test and interpretation of the results. It occurs most commonly when the investigator has a prior expectation of what the results will be. To avoid this type of bias, those carrying out the interpretation of the test should not know the status of the patient (i.e. be 'blind' to the disease status). For example, the evaluation of ultrasonography for the detection of hydrosalpinx might be influenced by prior knowledge of a hysterosalpingogram result. If additional diagnostic information is considered, the test performance is no longer being evaluated in isolation; instead, an algorithm including the prior data and test is being assessed in its entirety.

The properties of a diagnostic test will also be distorted if its results influence whether patients undergo confirmatory testing with a reference standard. Such 'verification' or 'work-up' bias is seen frequently, particularly when confirmatory tests are risky, expensive or painful. When evaluating a test, it is important that a consistent evaluation be used, and that it be the same regardless of test results.

EVALUATING THE TEST

Diagnostic tests have several properties, generally termed sensitivity, specificity and predictive value (Figure 3). The first two are stable despite wide variations in prevalence of disease, whereas predictive value is dependent upon the prevalence in the population tested.

Sensitivity

Sensitivity is defined as the proportion of patients with the target disorder who have a positive test result. It is a measure of how many with the disease can be correctly identified as such by the diagnostic test. Sensitivity identifies the proportion of those with disease who are correctly categorized. It does not predict the actual number of individuals who will have the disease if they test positively; this latter measure is known as the positive predictive value (see below).

Specificity

Specificity is defined as the proportion of those without disease who have a negative test result. This term identifies those without the disease who are correctly categorized, but it does not predict the actual number so categorized.

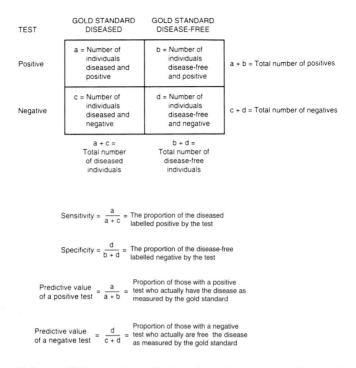

Figure 3 *Calculation of sensitivity, specificity, positive predictive value and negative predictive value*

Predictive values

Although sensitivity and specificity are useful indicators of the properties of a diagnostic test, they are unable to identify how likely it is that the individual with a positive test has the disease, or is disease-free if the test is negative.

The positive predictive value is the proportion of individuals with a positive test who have the disease. The negative predictive value is the proportion of individuals with a negative test who do not have the disease. Before predictive values of a test can be determined, one must know the prevalence of disease prior to the test being applied. Once this is known, the predictive values are calculable. Calculations of these terms are illustrated in Figure 3.

As stated above, predictive values are affected by variation in prevalence of a disease. As the prevalence increases, the positive predictive value increases and the negative predictive value decreases. Thus, the ability of a positive test to predict disease changes dramatically when the test is applied to individuals with different probabilities of having the disease. This situation is particularly evident when the test used is a screening test in a group in whom the probability of disease is very low. For example, with a prevalence of 1%, a sensitivity of 95%, and a specificity of 95%, the positive predictive value is only 16.9%. Thus, even an excellent test with high sensitivity and specificity can have a low positive predictive value when prevalence is low.

Likelihood ratio

A single index frequently used to indicate the utility of a diagnostic test is the likelihood ratio[6]. This measure contrasts the proportion of patients with and without disease at a given level of diagnostic test result, and is defined as the ratio of the probability of obtaining a defined result given the presence of disease compared to the probability in the absence of disease. The likelihood ratio does not change with the prevalence of disease, as do predictive values.

An example of how likelihood ratios are calculated and applied can be seen in a hypothetical study of MRI results for endometriosis of the ovary. If abnormal MRI results are noted in 42/50 individuals (or 0.84) with endometriosis, while an abnormal test is seen in 17/200 (or 0.085) without the disease, the likelihood ratio of the two findings is $0.84/0.085 \cong 10$. In other words, an abnormal MRI scan of the ovary is ten times as likely in women with endometriosis as in women without the disorder.

Likelihood ratios indicate how much a given diagnostic test result will raise or lower the pretest probability of disease. Ratios greater than one increase the probability of the disease being present, while ratios less than one decrease this probability.

A very important property of the likelihood ratio is its ability to help determine the post-test probability of disease.

(A)   Pretest odds for disease × likelihood ratio for test = post-test odds for disease

Note that before this calculation can be performed, it is necessary to convert the pretest probability to odds as follows:

(B)   Pretest odds = pretest probability/1 – pretest probability

Thus, a pretest probability of 0.5 yields pretest odds of 1 to 1, and a probability of 0.8 results in odds of 4 to 1. The post-test odds obtained from equation (A) can then be converted back into probability by the formula:

(C)   Post-test probability = post-test odds/ post-test odds + 1

Using the data from the above example, the post-test probability for ovarian endometriosis with an abnormal MRI result can be calculated as follows:

(1)   Pretest probability of
      endometriosis = 50/250 = 0.2

(2)   Pretest odds = $\dfrac{0.2}{1 - 0.2}$ = 0.25

(3)   Post-test odds = 0.25 × 10 = 2.5

(4)   Post-test probability = $\dfrac{2.5}{2.5 + 1}$ = 71%

Thus, with an abnormal MRI scan, the probability of ovarian endometriosis is increased from 20% to 71%. The point to be emphasized is the role of likelihood ratios in revising the pretest probability of disease to a new, post-test probability.

Comparing tests: the receiver-operating-characteristic curve

Numerous diagnostic tests may be developed for a single diagnosis, and it is our responsibility to be able to determine which test is the best of the lot. It is for this purpose that receiver-operating-characteristic (ROC) curves have been used in the medical literature[7-9]. These curves offer comparisons when use of the dichotomous indices of sensitivity and specificity proves difficult.

An ROC curve is calculated by first choosing a set of potential thresholds that might distinguish a positive test result from a negative result. The sensitivity and specificity can then be calculated for each of the threshold values. The results are plotted, with the ordinate being sensitivity and the abscissa being 1 – specificity. Tests may be compared by calculating the area under the ROC curve: the greater the value, the better the test. One such curve is illustrated in Figure 4.

HANDLING UNCERTAINTY IN CLINICAL DECISION MAKING

Try as we might, absolute diagnostic certainty is usually unattainable. Our task is not to attain certainty but to reduce the level of diagnostic uncertainty enough to be able to make optimal therapeutic decisions. As the cost of infertility care spirals upwards, we as clinicians are frequently confronted with the dilemma of containing patient expenditures while still making the 'correct' diagnosis.

How should we handle this uncertainty? To a large degree, the level of diagnostic certainty needed in a clinical decision is a

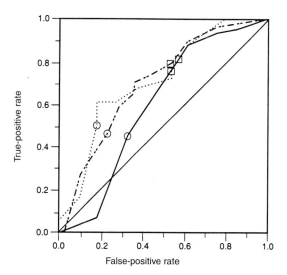

Figure 4 *Receiver-operating-characteristic curves for serum progesterone levels as a predictor of consecutive out-of-phase endometrial biopsies. Lines shown represent curves for a single random progesterone sample (——), a single morning progesterone sample (—— -- ——) and three posted morning samples (···). Circles designate the points on each curve representing a diagnostic threshold of 10 ng/ml. Squares designate the points on each curve representing a diagnostic threshold of 15 ng/ml. From reference 10, with permission*

function of the characteristics of the next step in the process. When a specific therapy for a given diagnosis is high in effectiveness and low in risk, one can handle substantial diagnostic uncertainty. Few tests need to be performed, and their quality need not even be especially good, if the treatment works in those with the disorder yet causes little harm to those who do not have the disease. Any therapy that combines low efficacy with high risk requires substantial diagnostic certainty:

multiple additional tests might be justified in such a situation.

Just as reproductive medicine will never be reduced to a series of flow charts, the employment of diagnostic tests is medicine as an art form. A thorough understanding of each test, its assets and liabilities and its consequences is required for optimal application. Only then can infertility diagnosis rise above the quality of the cookbook as a dynamic, scientific practice.

References

1. Feinstein, A. R. (1985). *Clinical Epidemiology: The Architecture of Clinical Research*. (Philadelphia: W. B. Saunders)
2. Cochrane, A. L. and Elwood, P. C. (1969). Laboratory data and diagnosis. *Lancet*, **1**, 420
3. Riegelman, R. K. (1981). *Studying a Study and Testing a Test: How to Read the Medical Literature*. (Boston: Little, Brown)
4. Murphy, E. A. (1972). The normal, and perils of the sylleptic argument. *Perspect. Biol. Med.*, **15**, 566–82
5. Murphy, E. A. (1982). *Biostatistics in Medicine*. (Baltimore: The Johns Hopkins University Press)
6. Jaeschke, R., Guyatt, G. H. and Sackett, D. L. (1994). User's guide to the medical literature.

III. How to use an article about a diagnostic test. B. What are the results and will they help me in caring for my patients. *J. Am. Med. Assoc.*, **271**, 703–7

7. Metz, C. E., Goodenough, D. J. and Rossman, K. (1973). Evaluation of receiver operating characteristic curve data in terms of information theory, with applications in radiography. *Radiology*, **109**, 297–303

8. Hanley, J. A. and McNeil, B. J. (1982). The meaning and use of the area under a receiver operating characteristic (ROC) curve. *Radiology*, **143**, 29–36

9. McNeil, B. J. and Hanley, J. A. (1984). Statistical approaches to the analysis of receiver operating characteristic (ROC) curves. *Med. Decis. Making*, **4**, 137–50

10. Olive, D. L., Thomford, P. J., Torres, S. E., Lambert, T. S. and Rosen, G. F. (1989). Twenty-four-hour progesterone and luteinizing hormones profiles in the midluteal phase of the infertile patient: correlation with other indicators of luteal phase insufficiency. *Fertil. Steril.*, **51**, 587–92

Economic evaluations of diagnostic interventions

13

J. A. Rizzo and L. B. Schwartz

INTRODUCTION

Concerns over escalating health care costs and the growth of managed care have promoted substantial interest in allocating scarce health care funds more efficiently. Economic evaluations of medical treatment apply the tools of microeconomics to help compare the costs and benefits of alternative treatments, with the ultimate goal of promoting more efficient health care choices.

This volume is particularly concerned with the application of economic evaluations to diagnostic imaging modalities for gynecological care. Before turning to this application, however, it is useful to discuss (1) the basic types of economic evaluations; and (2) the limitations of these approaches.

TYPES OF ECONOMIC EVALUATIONS

There are four main types of economic evaluations: (1) cost analysis; (2) cost-effectiveness analysis; (3) cost-utility analysis; and (4) cost-benefit analysis. We discuss each in turn.

Cost analysis

Cost analysis compares the costs of alternative treatments or therapies, but not the outcomes. This approach is appropriate when the outcomes of two treatments are known to be the same but the costs differ. In such cases, one can choose one treatment or another, on the basis of their relative costs. It is important to understand that cost refers not only to the direct cost of the medical treatment itself, but to other costs (and cost savings) that may

occur as a result of the treatments. For example, if two treatments, A and B, cost the same, but A requires less of the patient's time, then a cost analysis would attempt to value patient time, and include it as part of the analysis. In this example, the cost analysis would indicate that A is preferred to B.

Cost-effectiveness analysis

Cost-effectiveness analysis compares costs as well as outcomes of medical treatments. Cost-effectiveness analysis expresses outcomes in clinically relevant, non-monetary terms, for example, years of lives saved, falls prevented, tumors identified, etc. In conducting a cost-effectiveness evaluation, treatments are compared in terms of their respective costs per unit of outcomes. The intervention with the lowest cost-effectiveness ratio is preferred. For example, if treatment A costs $20 000 per year of life saved, and B costs $30 000, A will be preferred. Note that A may well cost more per patient. Cost-effectiveness analysis in this application is concerned with cost per life saved, however, not cost per patient treated. The reason is that the desired outcome is to save the most lives, not to treat the most patients.

Cost-effectiveness analysis is appropriate when the alternatives being considered involve the same type of outcomes. For example, if one is comparing two interventions to prevent falls in the elderly, cost-effectiveness analysis would be appropriate, since both interventions would have the same objective – to prevent falls. These interventions will generally differ in costs and the extent to which they succeed in preventing falls, however, motivating the application of cost-effectiveness analysis.

Cost-utility analysis

Cost-effectiveness analysis is less useful in situations in which the treatments that are being compared involve different outcomes. In such cases, it may be desirable to measure outcomes in terms of a metric which is comparable across a wide variety of disparate interventions. Cost-utility analysis provides a framework for conducting economic evaluations in these cases. In contrast to cost-effectiveness analysis, cost-utility analysis expresses outcomes in terms of quality-adjusted life years (QALYs). Essentially, QALYs measure morbidity effects, and adjust years of life saved by an intervention to account for quality of life changes. This has the effect of rendering widely disparate interventions comparable, as the following example illustrates. Suppose there are two interventions, one of which is physical therapy for arthritics, the other the availability of neonatal intensive care units (NICUs) for infants of very low birth weight. The first intervention will save very few lives. It may, however, involve substantial improvements in quality of life, particularly if it improves gait, alleviates pain and promotes independence in its target population. Thus, although total life years may not be changed by this intervention, there may be considerable gains in quality-adjusted years of life. On the other hand, NICUs may save substantial numbers of lives. However, if the individuals saved incur major physical and neurological problems, their quality of life may be low, so that the NICU intervention appears far less attractive in terms of quality-adjusted life years.

Like cost-effectiveness analysis, cost-utility analysis compares the ratios of costs to outcomes. Thus, a cost-utility analysis would choose intervention A over B if A cost less per quality-adjusted life year gained. Cost-utility analysis is appealing in that it provides a mechanism for comparing a wide range of alternative interventions, and it captures morbidity effects in addition to mortality. The drawback is that obtaining quality of life estimates may be time-consuming and costly. Moreover, the resulting QALY estimates may be imprecise. Individuals may give widely disparate responses to identical medical conditions, and one cannot be sure whether this variation represents true differences in preferences, or the fact that the QALY instrument is imprecise. A related problem concerns validity. The QALY instrument obtains proxy measures for true quality of life, and it is often difficult to determine how valid these proxies are.

Cost-benefit analysis

Cost-benefit analysis expresses benefits in monetary units. Like cost-utility analysis, cost-benefit analysis makes it possible to compare widely disparate treatments. Benefits may be measured as the monetary value of extended life, reduced morbidity or other outcomes. Sometimes 'benefits' take the form of cost savings. In such cases, it is more appropriate to refer to the study as a net cost analysis, where all costs (costs and cost savings) are tallied.

The drawback to cost-benefit analysis is the difficulty of obtaining reliable and acceptable monetary measures of medical benefits. For example, where the outcome is increased years of life, a cost-benefit analysis must assign a monetary value to this increase in survival. This is not only technically challenging, but politically difficult as well. Early measures of the value of life, such as the present value of future production or consumption, are problematic, in that (1) such measures favor the rich; and (2) there is no guarantee that these crude proxy variables truly measure patient welfare. A more promising approach is to survey subjects to ascertain their willingness to pay for medical interventions. Essentially, this method queries individuals about their willingness to pay for reductions in their risk of death. From this information, one can estimate what is known as the value of a statistical life. For example, suppose individuals in a given population are willing to pay $500 on average for a health care intervention that reduces their individual probability of death by 1 in 100. Then the value of a statistical life is $500 × 100 = $50 000 in this example. Despite much effort and ingenuity on the part of researchers, the willingness to pay approach has substantial methodological problems. It does have the advantage, however, of directly assessing monetary benefits to the potential recipients of the medical intervention.

ECONOMIC EVALUATIONS IN PRACTICE

Economic evaluations and clinical decision making

Economic evaluations provide an important input into clinical decision making, but are not a substitute for it. Even if a carefully conducted cost-utility analysis favors intervention A over B, we cannot say that A should be preferred to B for every patient. Economic evaluations compare medical treatments for the 'typical' patient. In some cases, subgroups of patients are evaluated separately; that is, economic evaluations may be conducted on selected risk groups. But even these types of evaluations are relatively blunt instruments: they cannot dictate what should happen to an individual patient.

Economic evaluations of imaging modalities in the workup and treatment of reproductive failure are particularly important, since they are costly, and in many cases there are various options from which to choose. For example, if a patient is scheduled to undergo a laparoscopy/hysteroscopy during the workup and treatment of infertility, is the added expense of a prior hysterosalpingogram justified? Might the expense of preoperative use of pelvic magnetic resonance imaging (MRI) for suspected endometriomas/endometriosis in patients with otherwise normal infertility workups be justified if it obviates the need for laparoscopy in some cases? Is the initial choice of a hystero-salpingogram for suspected submucosal myoma detection an economically justifiable choice if it can eliminate the need

for a hysteroscopy in patients with normal findings? The application of the types of economic evaluations discussed in this chapter provide a framework for analyzing these difficult issues and arriving at some tentative answers.

Avoidance of unnecessary complications

A second point to bear in mind is that economic evaluations can be very costly, both in terms of money and time. In contemplating such evaluations, the researcher should seek the simplest alternative for the purposes at hand. For instance, there is no need to consider a cost-utility analysis if it is known that the interventions being studied affect survival, but not quality of life. In that case, a cost-effectiveness analysis would be sufficient.

There are a variety of costs and benefits that might be addressed in conducting an economic evaluation. In general, it will be impossible to obtain reliable measures of each. As a rule of thumb, the researcher should strive to list all salient costs and benefits, measuring as many of these as possible. Even if some of these items cannot be measured, they should be discussed in terms of their likely implications for the results. Sometimes, it is clear that including such items would serve to reinforce the conclusions of the analysis.

The importance of perspective

The perspective of the study may be broad – society-wide; or narrow – the perspective of an individual third-party payer. Alternative perspectives affect items to be included or excluded, and indeed whether these items should be tallied as costs or benefits. For example, if a society-wide perspective is adopted, transfer payments should be ignored. Since these are payments from one group of society to another, they cancel out. On the other hand, from the perspective of a recipient of transfer payments, such payments should count as a benefit.

The perspective of the study also cues the audience as to the relevance of the study for their purposes. If the audience is a third-party payer, an economic evaluation conducted from a society-wide perspective will be less relevant than one conducted from the payer's own perspective.

Comparison of relevant alternatives

Ideally, an economic evaluation should compare all relevant treatment alternatives. In practice, however, such a comprehensive evaluation may not be feasible, because of both the inadequacy of data and the prohibitive costs of conducting such a large-scale study. Less comprehensive studies are still valuable, but it is important to note when such studies fail to consider all relevant alternatives.

Economic evaluations that blend art with science

Increasingly, guidelines and checklists for conducting economic evaluations are being published. Such guidelines are valuable, provided they are not misinterpreted to mean that conducting an economic evaluation is like baking a cake. Unlike baking a cake, the recipe for conducting an economic evaluation varies with each study, depending on the data available and the assumptions necessary to deal with situations in which data are missing.

Equity vs. efficiency

A final very important point to understand about economic evaluations is that they address issues of efficiency but not equity. By efficiency, we mean getting the most aggregate benefit (however measured) from a given amount of scarce resources. Economic evaluations generally score well on this dimension. On the other hand, such evaluations say little about how these benefits should be distributed. Society may be willing to trade off some efficiency in the interest of greater equity, but economic evaluations provide little guidance on the nature and extent of these tradeoffs. Thus, the failure to address equity considerations is a further limitation of economic evaluations that must be recognized.

APPLICATION OF ECONOMIC EVALUATIONS TO DIAGNOSTIC IMAGING

To illustrate the usefulness and limitations of economic evaluations, we review and provide a critique of recent work we conducted[1] on the economic impact of MRI on gynecological treatment decisions. We begin our review with a brief overview of the study and its results. The study is then assessed according to a checklist of items used by Udvarhelyi and colleagues[2] in their review of economic evaluations in the medical literature.

Review of reference 1 (Female pelvis: impact of MR imaging on treatment decisions and net cost analysis)

This study included 69 consecutive symptomatic women who were referred for pelvic MRI examinations. Diagnosis and treatment plans were obtained from referring physicians before and immediately after they received verbal reports of MRI results. A majority of women in this study suffered from symptoms associated with endometriosis, leiomyomas and ovarian cysts. Other diagnoses included pelvic adhesive disease, adenomyosis, uterine anomalies and pelvic pain and infertility.

The results indicated that (1) 73% of subjects initially scheduled for surgery either did not undergo surgery or incurred less invasive surgery than planned, following the MRI results; (2) the treatment plan was altered in 84% of patients enrolled in the study because of MRI results; (3) MRI resulted in overall savings of $63 per patient enrolled in the study; and (4) MRI resulted in savings of $1736 per patient originally scheduled for surgery.

On the basis of these findings, the researchers concluded that:

> Use of pelvic MR imaging in diagnosis of some gynecological diseases may alter treatment, decrease the number of invasive surgical procedures performed, and reduce total health care expenditures.
> (Schwartz and co-workers[1], p. 55)

Evaluation of reference 1

In order to be useful, it is important for published economic evaluations to address basic issues of concern to its readership. In their review of the literature on economic evaluations, Udvarhelyi and colleagues[2] used the following six criteria in judging the studies:

(1) Was an explicit statement of the perspective of the analysis provided?

(2) Was an explicit description of the benefits of the program provided?

(3) Were the types of costs included in the study specified?

(4) If costs and benefits accrued during different time periods, was discounting used to adjust for these differences?

(5) Was sensitivity analysis conducted to test important assumptions?

(6) Was a summary measurement of efficiency, such as cost-benefit or cost-effectiveness ratio, calculated?

We evaluate the study by Schwartz and colleagues[1] according to these criteria.

Was an explicit statement of the perspective of the analysis provided?

The study explicitly stated that:

> ... the perspective of the analysis is that of a third-party payer responsible for direct medical costs. Some patient-specific costs, therefore, were not quantified.
> (p. 56)

Was an explicit description of the benefits of the program provided?

This was a net cost analysis. Benefits took the form of cost savings. These costs savings were quantified and discussed qualitatively in the text.

Were the types of costs included in the study specified?

The following costs were listed as part of the analysis: MRI, fees for surgical procedures, hospital room and board, anesthesia services, consultations and medications. Patient time lost from work was not included in the study, as the perspective was that of a hospital or third-party payer. Nonetheless, the researchers argued that including such costs would probably reinforce the study's conclusions, since the use of MRI was likely to lessen time lost from work.

If costs and benefits accrued during different time periods, was discounting used to adjust for these differences?

Patients were followed for an average of 11 months (the researchers contend that this was a sufficient time period for subjects' gynecological problems to resolve). Because of this brief follow-up, the researchers noted that discounting was unnecessary.

Was sensitivity analysis conducted to test important assumptions?

The net cost analysis was conducted using two different methodologies. The first simply costed out projected treatment regimens before and after MRI. The second tracked patients over time to infer actual costs. Thus, the study checked the sensitivity of the results to alternative costing methods. However, ranges of costs for specific items in the cost analysis were not investigated, and a specific section for conducting sensitivity analysis was not included in the paper.

Was a summary measurement of efficiency, such as cost-benefit or cost-effectiveness ratio, calculated?

The study clearly stated that it was a net cost analysis, so that effectiveness measures, QALYs and the like were not included in the study. Net costs (savings) were reported and discussed in the text.

Summary

The study by Schwartz and colleagues[1] addressed most of the items considered by Udvarhelyi and co-workers[2] in their review of economic evaluations in the medical literature. In retrospect, more attention could have been paid to the sensitivity analysis. Nonetheless, five of the six criteria (83%) outlined above were reasonably well addressed in the study. This compares favorably with results reported by Udvarhelyi and co-workers[2]. They found that the median number of principles adhered to was three, or 50%. This figure was lowest in general surgical journals (two), followed by medical subspeciality journals (three) and general medical journals (four).

In addition, Schwartz and co-workers[1] discussed alternative diagnostic approaches besides MRI; specifically, laparoscopy and ultrasound. It is clear from the study that neither of these alternatives are close substitutes for MRI, but have differentiated indications. For example, MRI most accurately depicts small intramural and submucosal leiomyomas and, therefore, its use can guide the surgeon away from performing a laparotomy or laparoscopy for removal of symptomatic leiomyomas that are submucosal and towards less invasive hysteroscopic resection instead. Pelvic MRI can also most accurately differentiate a pedunculated subserosal leiomyoma from an adnexal mass, even when transvaginal ultrasound is inconclusive. Such use can lead to the avoidance of surgery for asymptomatic pedunculated leiomyomas that might otherwise be mistaken for adnexal masses. Whereas pelvic MRI can accurately diagnose ovarian endometriomas, laparoscopy is far superior to MRI for the diagnosis of peritoneal endometriotic implants, with ultrasound even less reliable than MRI for accurate diagnosis of this disease. However, pelvic MRI may be valuable for those cases in which cul-de-sac endometriotic implants are obscured by dense pelvic adhesions at the time of laparoscopy. Clearly, laparoscopy has the advantage over pelvic MRI and ultrasound in diagnostic intervention for pelvic adhesion disease. Pelvic MRI is far superior to ultrasound for the differential diagnosis of Müllerian anomalies when compared with the gold standard of laparoscopy.

CONCLUSION

Economic evaluations are increasingly popular tools for comparing alternative medical treatments and therapies, including appropriate diagnostic imaging interventions. Only recently have these evaluations been applied to diagnostic imaging in gynecology. Such work should be extended, in greater detail, to the imaging techniques commonly used in the evaluation of patients with reproductive failure.

Appropriate diagnostic imaging studies can have important effects on the entire course of patient care, eliminating unnecessary surgery, saving costs and promoting patient welfare. Carefully constructed evaluations can identify such opportunities. Equally important: such studies can identify cases where diagnostic intervention is unnecessary. Helping to distinguish between these two types of case is an important payoff of economic evaluations.

References

1. Schwartz, L. B., Panageas, E., Lange, R., Rizzo, J., Comite, F. and McCarthy, S. (1994). Female pelvis: impact of MR imaging on treatment decisions and net cost analysis. *Radiology*, **192**, 55–60

2. Udvarhelyi, S. E., Colditz, G. A., Rai, A. and Epstein, A. M. (1992). Cost-effectiveness and cost-benefit analysis in the medical literature: are the methods being used correctly? *Ann. Intern. Med.*, **116**, 238–44

Index